THE PRAEGER HANDBOOK OF SOCIAL JUSTICE AND PSYCHOLOGY

THE PRAEGER HANDBOOK OF SOCIAL JUSTICE AND PSYCHOLOGY

Volume 1

Fundamental Issues and Special Populations

Chad V. Johnson and Harris L. Friedman, Set Editors
Jeannette Diaz, Zeno Franco, and Bonnie K. Nastasi, Volume Editors

Foreword by Mary A. Fukuyama

Social Justice and Psychology

PRAEGER

AN IMPRINT OF ABC-CLIO, LLC
Santa Barbara, California • Denver, Colorado • Oxford, England

Library of Congress Cataloging-in-Publication Data

The Praeger handbook of social justice and psychology / Chad V. Johnson [and five others].
volumes cm. — (Social justice and psychology)
Includes index.
Contents: volume 1. Fundamental issues and special populations
ISBN 978-1-4408-0378-9 (hardcopy : alk. paper) — ISBN 978-1-4408-0379-6 (ebook)
1. Social psychiatry. 2. Social justice—Psychological aspects. 3. Psychology, Pathological—Social aspects. I. Johnson, Chad (Chad Vernon) II. Title: Handbook of social justice and psychology.
RC455.P6962 2014
616.89'071—dc23 2014000218

ISBN: 978-1-4408-0378-9
EISBN: 978-1-4408-0379-6

18 17 16 15 14 1 2 3 4 5

This book is also available on the World Wide Web as an eBook.
Visit www.abc-clio.com for details.

Praeger
An Imprint of ABC-CLIO, LLC

ABC-CLIO, LLC
130 Cremona Drive, P.O. Box 1911
Santa Barbara, California 93116-1911

This book is printed on acid-free paper ∞

Manufactured in the United States of America

Dedicated to the Memory of George Albee (1921–2006)

George was a pioneering psychologist whose path was to envision "a world free from exploitation and domination of one group by another, a world in which each person has the freedom and the resources to develop her or his potential to the fullest, a world in which the highest goal would be one person's concern and regard for others" (Kessler, Goldston, & Joffe, 1992, p. 19). And he worked ceaselessly toward these ends. When I first met him in the late 1990s, he and I were keynote speakers at a conference on psychology and juvenile justice. Having my attitudes and values toward professional psychology profoundly shaped by reading many of his contributions, I excitedly blurted out, "you are my hero." Unabashedly George responded, "We all must be heroes."—Harris L. Friedman

Kessler, M., Goldston, S., & Joffe, J. (1992). George Albee: An appreciation. In M. Kessler, S. Goldston, & J. Joffe (Eds.), *The present and future of prevention: In honor of George W. Albee* (pp. 3–32). Newbury Park, CA: Sage.

Contents

Volume 1: Fundamental Issues and Special Populations

Foreword ix
Mary A. Fukuyama

Acknowledgments xiii

Series Introduction: Social Justice and Psychology Series xv
Harris L. Friedman, Chad V. Johnson, and Jeannette Diaz

Set Introduction xvii
Chad V. Johnson and Harris L. Friedman

Introduction to Volume 1 xxi
Jeannette Diaz

Part 1. Fundamental Issues 1

1. The History of Psychology and Social Justice 3
John T. Jost and Aaron C. Kay

2. A Psychological Framework for Social Justice Praxis 33
Jeannette Diaz

3. A Critical Look at Social Justice Ideology in Counseling and Psychotherapy 51
Jonathan D. Raskin

4. Philosophical Reflexivity in Social Justice Work 65
Thomas Teo, Zhipeng Gao, and Raha Sheivari

5. Ideology and the Role of Dialogue in Political Mobilization 79
William R. Earnest and Tod S. Sloan

6. False Consciousness and the Maintenance of Injustice 97
Krystal M. Perkins and William E. Cross Jr.

7. Liberation Psychology, Feminism, and Social Justice Psychology 115
Geraldine Moane

Part 2. Special Populations **133**

8. Healing One Story at a Time: American Indian/ Alaska Native Social Justice 135
Virgil Moorehead and Teresa D. LaFromboise

9. Sexual Orientation and Gender Minorities 155
Linda M. Woolf and Danielle MacCartney

10. Disability Activism and Psychology 177
Daniel Holland, Laura Sturm, Nicolas Culp, and Deidra Holland

11. Vulnerability and Privilege among the Elderly: Social Justice Issues in Gerontology and Psychology 191
Monika Ardelt and Harris L. Friedman

12. Social Justice and Poverty: Perspectives for Psychologists 223
Laura Smith and Riddhi Sandil

13. Criminal Justice and Its Many Injustices: Focus on Prison Psychology within the United States 241
Kathryn M. Whiteley, Tina Bloom, and Harris L. Friedman

Index 269

About the Editors and Contributors 285

Foreword

Mary A. Fukuyama

I am pleased to have been invited to write the foreword for the *Praeger Handbook of Social Justice and Psychology*. Consequently, I offer some observations and reflections on my own experiences with social justice movements, as well as share some recommendations toward the goal of maintaining personal well-being while in the pursuit of well-being for all.

As a psychologist who has followed the development of multiculturalism as a movement within counseling psychology over several decades, I find that social justice advocacy is a natural extension of this movement, both for individual and collective consciousness-raising (Toporek, Lewis, & Crethar, 2009; Vera & Speight, 2003). Psychologists working as researchers, teachers, consultants, therapists, and in a myriad of other roles offer a wealth of resources that can be mobilized for facilitating social change, which are sorely needed to address the multitude of complex social justice issues facing humankind's evolution further into the 21st century and beyond. Read any news headline and there are underlying social justice themes, whether they are related to racism, poverty, environmental and health concerns, human rights, recovery from natural disasters, or more. It is gratifying to see these, and many other, social justice themes addressed from a psychological perspective within the diverse chapters in this handbook. In particular, I see the convergence of many strands within psychology, including multiculturalism, coming together powerfully in its volumes.

As I reflect upon my personal journey, I now understand better how social justice and what has been my main professional focus on multiculturalism (including spirituality) intersect and enrich each other. However, these insights did not come until much later in my life. My first introduction to a social justice movement occurred when I was an undergraduate college student during the Viet Nam War era. I joined my friends in antiwar protests and marched for peace. It was a tumultuous and violent time in U.S. history, and I was stunned when the National Guard shot and killed several student demonstrators at Kent State on May 4, 1970.

The assassinations of Senator Robert Kennedy and Rev. Martin Luther King Jr. also were forever etched in my memory. Feelings of discouragement and disillusionment with the status quo were commonplace, and it was easy for me and many activist members of my generation to get depressed over what seemed such overwhelming odds against creating positive social change.

It was not until I participated in another round of antiwar demonstrations, this time in the 1980s, that I was encouraged to do inner "spiritual practice" to counterbalance the frustration and burn-out that often stems from involvement with social activism. It was recommended that activists do inner work (e.g., centering, meditation, contemplation) as much as extend outwardly (e.g., through demonstrations, letter writing, teach-ins). In the process of engaging in spiritual search, I found inspiring words from important role models for peace, and I was especially comforted by a quote from Rev. Martin Luther King Jr. (1964), "The arc of the moral universe is long, but it bends toward justice."

I also experienced an "aha" moment attending a workshop with cultural anthropologist Angeles Arrien (2013), who offered the following suggestions for being a spiritual warrior: "Show up. Pay attention. Speak your truth. Don't be attached to outcome." I particularly found her advice not to be attached to any outcomes to be liberating. It is quite common to feel helpless when pushing for systemic change. It is also incredibly frustrating to work hard toward a goal and be shut down. With her advice, I could let go of expectations of success, but feel satisfied about having made an effort toward positive change. Working in my own sphere of influence was good enough.

In addition to seeking spiritual wisdom, I have found that affiliating with social movement groups to be essential for social activism. By attending relevant professional conferences and workshops, such as the Teachers College Annual Winter Roundtable on cross-cultural psychology and education in New York City and the American Psychological Association's National Multicultural Conference and Summit, which meets biannually, I found support among like-minded people. It is important not to feel alone in pursuit of social justice. In fact, I believe group energy and effort is not only essential to make desirable social change, but it also nourishes interpersonal connection and reinforces the need to identify with causes larger than one's self. Sometimes the benefits for social justice work operate at the micro-level of personal and interpersonal growth, as well as at the macro-level of larger social issues.

I offer this personal story to suggest that the readers of this book explore the social justice issues that call out to you, approach such challenges with energy and enthusiasm, and carry a bit of wisdom with you whenever possible. For psychologists in particular, but for others who draw upon psychological insights and tools, this handbook offers much of value.

As people look toward the future, it is important to recognize that each person, group, and culture has its own process of reckoning with social justice issues, be that at personal, community, regional, state, national, and even global levels (see

Fouad, 2012). However, as the world becomes smaller through globalization and evolving communications technology, people are more than ever constantly influencing, and sometimes aggravating, one another! We are in an era of extreme polarization. One person's social justice issue may actually be in opposition to another person's social justice issue! Where is the higher ground or common good for all? How can psychologists help mediate conflicts and sort through tough ethical issues? It is through handbooks such as this one that psychology offers a roadmap for negotiating complex, powerful, and humbling social challenges.

It is with this thought that I return to my original premise, that of maintaining personal well-being in pursuit of the common good. As a clinician, I am aware of the need "to care for the care-giver" to prevent burnout. I believe the same applies to social justice activists, as practicing self-care while working toward important change outcomes is essential.

REFERENCES

Arrien, A. (2013). The Four-Fold Path. Retrieved from http://www.angelesarrien.com/

Fouad, N. A. (Ed). (2012). Major section on social justice advocacy. *The Counseling Psychologist, 40,* 326–408.

King, Jr., M. L. (1964). Baccalaureate sermon delivered at the commencement exercises at Wesleyan University in Middletown, CT. Retrieved from http://quoteinvestigator.com/2012/11/15/arc-of-universe/#return-note-4794-9

Toporek, R. L., Lewis, J. A., & Crethar, H. C. (2009). Promoting systemic change through ACA advocacy competencies. *Journal of Counseling and Development, 87,* 260–268.

Vera, E. M., & Speight, S. L. (2003). Multicultural competence, social justice, and counseling psychology: Expanding our roles. *The Counseling Psychologist, 31,* 253–272.

Acknowledgments

We would like to thank the contributing authors for their highly informative chapters, diligence, and responsive to requests for revision. We are deeply indebted to our editorial assistant, Lindsay Plott-Buckner, who worked tirelessly, superbly, and without complaint throughout the editing process. We are also grateful for additional editorial assistance provided by Heather Threadgill and Eamon Slattery. Finally, we acknowledge all those, both within psychology and without, who struggle with oppression and injustice and work toward social justice and peace.

Series Introduction: Social Justice and Psychology Series

Harris L. Friedman, Chad V. Johnson, and Jeannette Diaz

The *Social Justice and Psychology series* provides cutting-edge books emphasizing the social justice implications of various topics within psychology. It is predicated on the notion that psychology is never value neutral, and that all psychological endeavors are embedded in rich implications for social justice—from the questions psychologists choose to explore, the methods they choose to seek answers, and the uses for which they choose to apply their findings. The objective of the series is to bridge theoretical and applied psychology through making explicit many of these social justice implications and, by doing so, facilitate psychology as a science and profession to be more concerned about doing good in the world. It is fitting that we launch this series with *The Praeger Handbook of Social Justice and Psychology*, a three-volume compendium of chapters addressing a wide variety of key topics in the area. This handbook serves as a broad overview of many, but not all, topics relevant to social justice and psychology. As such, it provides an excellent starting place for understanding the diverse interfaces between social justice and psychology, but it is neither exhaustive of all possibly germane areas, nor does it go into great depth in any one area. Consequently, future volumes in the series will address specific topical areas more deeply.

Set Introduction

Chad V. Johnson and Harris L. Friedman

Although there are many scattered writings on social justice and psychology, and many volumes and papers devoted to specific aspects of it, there has been no singular source with which one can gain an overview of this vast and intersecting literature; this is the role we hope *The Praeger Handbook of Social Justice and Psychology* will play. The idea for this handbook originated through a conversation between Harris L. Friedman and our Praeger editor, Debbie Carvalko. Harris had previously published two books through Praeger and, while talking to Debbie about some of his social activism projects, she mentioned that Praeger would probably be interested in a handbook on psychology and social justice, as well as a possible book series thereafter. This seemed an exciting and worthwhile project, so Harris agreed to be the series lead editor, and approached Chad V. Johnson to take the lead role with the editing of the handbook. Together Chad and Harris, realizing the magnitude of this effort, decided to recruit additional co-editors, namely Zeno Franco, Bonnie K. Nastasi, and Jeannette Diaz. As a team, the co-editors wondered how to fairly cover a terrain as large and complicated as needed in such a handbook. From the beginning, the co-editors were planning for the handbook to be a multivolume set, starting with the idea of five volumes—so that each co-editor would take the lead on one. However, due to concerns about the cost of five volumes, the co-editors decided three would suffice.

Next, the co-editors faced the difficult decision about how to select content to include and exclude within the handbook, as well as how to equitably recruit a group of chapter contributors who would reflect the multiple diversities in accord with prevailing ideals among social justice advocates. The editorial team considered various ideas about setting up advisory boards, including one composed of notable professionals familiar with different areas of psychology and social justice and another of nonprofessional stakeholders (e.g., members from the various groups being discussed in terms of social justice, so that those who might be disenfranchised would have voice in how they were portrayed in the handbook). This led to many discussions about how to "walk the talk," insofar as how to include social justice principles into the design and implementation of the handbook. Despite noble aspirations, the pragmatics of deadlines in moving the project forward resulted in limited outside input, but efforts were made to obtain maximum diversity among the chapter authors, and they became the primary informal voice guiding the direction of the handbook. In addition, in our recruitment materials we requested that contributing authors include a global and "community voice" in their chapters, and strongly encouraged the inclusion of nonprofessional, community partner co-authorships. However, two individuals besides the chapter authors and co-editors did, in particular, play an important role in shaping the handbook, namely Marc Pilisuk and Mary A. Fukuyama, whom the co-editors unofficially deemed to be the "senior advisory board." Mary has written the foreword and Marc the afterword, according to the helpful roles they played.

As the handbook took its final form, its three volumes were loosely divided into themes, notwithstanding that there is overlap in some of these and, when that occurred, the co-editors made sometimes arbitrary decisions as to chapter placements within each volume. The first volume contains a section on fundamental issues that undergird the area of social justice and psychology. These include chapters focusing on the history of social justice within psychology, providing a psychological framework for guiding applications, a critical appraisal of ideology, philosophical reflexivity on applications, potential for dialogue on decolonization, consideration of false consciousness, and liberation psychology and feminism. Together these foundational chapters set the stage for what follows. Next in this volume are chapters focusing on several special populations, examining concerns about indigenous people, sexual orientation and gender minorities, the disabled, the elderly, the impoverished, and prisoners.

The second volume focuses on the theme of well-being and also an assortment of professional issues for psychologists related to social justice. The part on well-being includes an overview chapter on this topic, as well as chapters on stress in urban minority girls, sustainability and environmental issues, dignity and mental illness, workplace issues, community-based health promotion and veteran services, disasters, moral and jurisprudential issues, neuroscience implications, and socially engaged spirituality. The last part of this volume includes informative chapters on pedagogical tools, a model for psychology doctoral training, and research methods.

The third volume focuses on two themes, youth concerns and how varying disciplines within psychology deal with social justice issues, as well as contains the afterword and several appendixes that provide relevant resources. Chapters in the first part of this volume addressing youth issues include human rights, social justice within schools, families, and urban communities, as well as empowering youth advocates and dealing with injustices related to educational deprivation. Its second part contains chapters on how specializations within applied psychology handle social justice issues, including counseling and clinical psychology, community psychology, industrial-organizational and consulting psychology, and school psychology.

Together the three volumes constituting the handbook and its chapters provide an overview of many of the most crucial areas at the interface of psychology and social justice. Although much is missing, as there is too much to include—even within three-volumes, readers can gain a good overview of the field by reading the handbook in its entirety, or can simply sample individual chapters as a way to become more familiar with particular issues. Our hope is that subsequent volumes in this series will provide coverage for many of its gaps, as well as opportunities to explore some issues introduced in the handbook in much greater breadth and depth.

Although we strove to provide as comprehensive a survey of what we thought were the most pressing and timely issues facing psychology today, we recognize that we did not cover every important topic. In fact, there are so many areas that could not be covered in this handbook that, although we feel we have given a good overview, we lament how much is not addressed. One area that is of particular interest to us involves social justice for other species on our planet, ranging from animal treatment within scientific and commercial settings to the destruction of ecological systems supporting animals (and our own) existence. Another is the controversial American Psychiatric Association's new diagnostic criteria (*DSM-5*), which have just been released, and this evolving area merits further consideration of its potential use, as well as misuse, in clinical practice. Psychologists' involvement in torture and war also stands out as an important area with many social justice implications to which we did not give adequate coverage. Last, we wish the handbook could have been more globally focused as we recognize social justice is a topic that reaches far beyond the borders of Western countries. Nonetheless, we hope this handbook provides a valuable starting place from which psychology students and scholars might inform their own social justice work, and from which psychologists might be inspired to take up the social justice mantle by utilizing their knowledge and skills to genuinely make the world a more favorable and sustaining place for all beings.

We conclude that social justice is no longer only the purview of politicians and activists. Psychology and its various specialties, with its many approaches to understanding and changing individual and social behavior, have an obligation to use its skills and knowledge to further the common good. To quote parents everywhere, the world is not fair. At times, it is quite unjust, and this injustice has very real and regrettable consequences in terms of human life and well-being. Psychologists who teach, research, practice, and engage in other professional activities have many tools to make a meaningful difference related to social justice.

In addition, we think social justice is not just an "add-on" to psychology, something superfluous to spend a week discussing in a graduate capstone seminar—and then to be forgotten when newly minted psychologists enter the "real" world. Instead we believe social justice should form the very basis of all psychology, as decisions regarding social justice permeate all areas of professional life, ranging from the topics psychologists choose to research to the clients with whom they choose to work. In essence, we believe that psychology is not value-neutral, but involves people in every way, and therefore is unavoidably related to social justice.

Lastly, we acknowledge that social justice issues are often ambiguous and relative. The problem is not that most psychologists, coming from diverse perspectives (e.g., class, ethnic, political, religious), do not agree that the world, at least in part, is in need of repair, but many hold legitimate disagreement over how it is broken and what should be done to fix it. Perhaps the call for social justice is appropriate—as long as it avoids prescribing exactly what kind of justice to enact. That is, if considered from an expanded and more inclusive vantage that recognizes structural and systemic, as well as individualistic, problems in society, psychologists can attempt to address these from their own respective positions. There will be disagreements, of course, but none should argue that others with good intentions from their perspectives are not also attempting to pursue and achieve more social justice. From this framework, there is room for different approaches for addressing the myriad of social justice problems. As a quick take-away, we end with some questions involving the importance to community participation and involvement, voice, empowerment, challenging the status quo, recognizing and addressing oppression and injustice, and more:

- Can psychologists reconcile being both scientists and advocates for social justice (and how can they take a more balanced and reflective, and less ideologically driven, view without being paralyzed toward inaction)?
- Can psychologists escape reductionary biological and brain disease models, and its concurrent overemphasis on the individual, to work toward understanding the importance of the wholeness of persons and their interconnectedness with all aspects of world?
- Can psychologists develop a critical stance that places social justice within its mainstream, rather than cynically marginalizing it as something only for naïve do-gooders to pursue?

Introduction to Volume 1

Jeannette Diaz

The chapters in this first volume provide us with the theoretical and practical challenges of engaging in psychologically informed social justice work, research, and theory development. Jost and Kay begin this volume, and our series, with a description of the historical underpinnings of the current psychological concept of social justice. Their chapter moves readers from the early writing of Aristotle on justice and its relationship to equality, to the writings of Karl Marx who, in spite of eschewing a direct discussion of social justice, nevertheless provided the seeds for subsequent philosophical critiques of capitalist systems of production, and an understanding of the material and structural base of human existence. In reviewing utilitarian and deontological approaches to social justice and accompanying social psychological research, Jost and Kay help us see that individual decision makers are influenced not just by abstract notions of justice, but by personal experience and internalized cultural norms. Jost and Kay also highlight the extent to which individuals holding liberal, socialist, or "left" ideologies differ in their understanding of social justice from those holding conservative or "right" ideologies, with the former more concerned with fairness and the avoidance of harm and the latter more focused on loyalty and respect for authority. The authors then turn to a review of central social psychological theories of justice—equity theory, procedural justice, and interactional justice. Based on their review of the accompanying empirical literature in social psychology, Jost and Kay conclude that social justice holds both subjective and objective elements that lead to conflicting notions of what social justice is, and situations where individuals may tolerate situations that, by objective measures, would be considered unjust (see also Chapter 6 by Perkins and Cross). The divergence in objective and subjective understandings of justice suggests that social justice is a multifaceted concept, thereby precluding a solely normative approach to social justice. In spite of the complexity raised by the subjective aspect of social justice, the authors are optimistic in their assessment of what social psychology can contribute to the development of normative theories of social justice that reflect a psychological understanding of human decision making and behavior.

Diaz further illuminates the subjective underpinning of the enactment of social justice through a critical review of central notions of justice—distributive, procedural, relational/interactional, restorative, and retributive. In each case, she highlights the extent to which the implementation of these norms of justice is highly impacted by perceptions of the relationship between self and other, as well as attributions regarding the characteristics and motives of the other. Using moral exclusion theory as a way of explaining situations of injustice such as racially biased criminal proceedings, Diaz highlights the difficulty of implementing normative and outcome-based social justice approaches, particularly since such approaches are typically developed by individuals and groups in power. Reframing social justice within a globalized world, Diaz points out that globalization requires an expanding understanding of social justice that includes individuals and communities geographically separated but nevertheless united by globalized political and economic structures. Focusing on relational models of morality and justice, her chapter helps the reader see the extent to which social justice is, inherently, a psychological/interpersonal construct and, as such, one that can be effectively realized only within the context of relationship between Self and Other. Drawing upon recent work on the comparative and neurological understandings of empathy, she offers the possibility that social justice can be realized only to the extent that people are able to enhance their capacity for empathy; in this way, social justice is less an idealized outcome state and more the process of continually engaging with the Other in relationships characterized by compassion and understanding.

Raskin's chapter provides an important critical commentary on the social justice endeavor in psychology. We expect some readers will find this chapter provocative, and perhaps uncomfortable, but a project on social justice is not complete without turning a critical and reflexive stance onto the very notion of social justice, particularly since so much of social justice works is founded upon liberal/progressive traditions that call for clear advocacy and system change. In this chapter, Raskin calls for careful and thoughtful clarification of social justice terms, beliefs, and values. For example, what is the "common good" or "self-determination" and according to whom and for whom? Social justice psychologists frequently critique (deconstruct) the underlying assumptions and biases inherent in status quo thinking and practice. Unfortunately, as Raskin points out, it is far too common for social justice advocates and psychologists to fail to sufficiently practice reflexivity and critical self-analysis, thereby resulting in iatrogenic harm and the imposition of the very types of biased processes and values of which they themselves are critical. Raskin challenges us to determine whether or not social justice work in psychology is based on sound theoretical principles or is simply ideologically based advocacy parading as academic/scholarly practice. Can psychologists dispassionately study issues such as capitalism, discrimination, environmentalism without the indignation demanding change that often characterizes the left, or the unwavering support for preserving the status quo that often characterizes the right? Can these issues be seen as worthy of study not because of a preconceived notion of what is a correct approach but rather, because the issues themselves are gravely important as scientific concerns? These are the challenging issues posed by Raskin.

In a similar vein, Teo, Gao, and Sheivari critique a limited application of reflexivity that focuses primarily on self-reflection noting that, while self-reflection is an important element in developing critical and informed approaches to research, it nevertheless runs the risk of conflating structural issues with intrapersonal ones. For these authors, the tools of reflexivity can be of service to social justice work to the extent that reflexivity encompasses a critical awareness of the Other that includes an awareness of one's own subjective and biased beliefs regarding the Other. Similar to Raskin's chapter, Teo et al. critique social justice work that holds the perspective of the Self as more informed or more legitimate than the perspective of the Other. Is the Other oppressed if he or she does not believe he or she is oppressed? Is social justice work viable if the perspective of the Other is not directly addressed or incorporated? Teo et al. challenge social justice work that presumes to know what is best for the Other, without clearly understanding what the Other's believe is best for him or her. These authors call for social justice workers to use the tool of ontological reflexivity in order to clearly delineate: their philosophical positions regarding human nature and activity, the very nature of social justice and social justice work, and the role of violence. They also call for epistemological reflexivity to minimize the risk of social justice workers imposing upon others their own views of health, empowerment, and resistance. Epistemological reflexivity results in an understanding of the typically privileged position of social justice workers, as well as an expansion of Self through the direct incorporation of the experience and views of the Other. Finally, they call for ethical reflexivity, noting that social justice work is, unabashedly, about values and morals.

The two subsequent chapters in Part One of this volume address the troubling phenomenon that oftentimes occurs, namely "why do oppressed individuals and groups allow themselves to be oppressed or, worse, unwittingly participate in their own oppression?" Although addressing the same issue, each chapter provides somewhat divergent response. Earnest and Sloan's chapter (Chapter 5) provides a psychodynamic perspective on the perpetuation of oppression, and Perkins and Cross (Chapter 6), provide a psycho-structural perspective.

Drawing upon traditional Freudian theory regarding family dynamics, the internalization of these dynamics, and the projection of these dynamics onto systems and individuals outside of the family, Earnest and Sloan hypothesize that oppression exists because individuals internalize conditions of oppression and self-worth from the family structure (i.e., the traditional Oedipal complex as discussed by Freud) onto dynamics of the workplace. For example, they posit that a woman who accepts an oppressive work environment does so because she has internalized the power dynamics that existed between herself and her father and, as a result, finds herself unable to confront an abusive or oppressive work environment. At question here, however, is the extent to which traditional psychodynamic concepts are cross-culturally and globally applicable, particularly given recent critiques regarding the uncritical use of Western ideas of the psyche to understand cultures dramatically different from those that the theories were initially patterned after. Also left unaddressed by these authors is the extent to which material conditions oftentimes require that individuals accept conditions of oppressions. For example, it is not difficult to find examples throughout the world of poor women who continue to return to oppressive work environments in order to make money to buy food, medicine, and/or schooling for their children, siblings, and/or aging parents. While poststructuralists have correctly pointed out that human behavior cannot be solely understand by the material conditions of existence, neither can we ignore these conditions. By explaining human acceptance of oppression through a psychodynamic lens, Earnest and Sloan suggest that intrapsychic or intrafamilial dynamics may be as important as sociopolitical and socioeconomic dynamics in understanding the acceptance of oppression, a position certainly worthy of empirical examination.

Perkins and Cross draw upon the work of critical theorists, such as Fanon, Gramsci, Habermas, Marx, and Engels, by invoking the concepts of false consciousness, hegemony, and miseducation to understand why some low-status individuals and groups endure ongoing social and economic inequality and why oppressed individuals sometimes actively participate in their own oppression. While these authors do attend to individual-level psychological dynamics, their analyses encompass ideological, situational, and structural conditions that, together with personal dynamics, help explain the perpetuation of injustice. They refer back to Fanon's (1952, 1986) classic work on the relationship between the colonizer and the colonized who explained how relationships of power becomes psychologically internalized. Expanding beyond these early philosophers and writers, Perkins and Cross review recent social-psychological theories and ideas such as system justification theory and racial colorblindness. Within the broader context of false consciousness, they review research on individual and group identity development, social identity, political ideology, and social comparison. The authors then bring these theories up to date with a conversation regarding intergroup dynamics within a globalized context, pointing out that the globalized nature of our world means that group comparisons are made not just within communities or nations, but across nation-states and geographically dispersed cultural groups. They discuss how hegemonic aspects of globalization extend Fanon's ideas regarding the relationship between the colonized and the colonizer. Similarly, the globalization of education brings new meaning to earlier discussions on the role of miseducation and the perpetuation of oppression.

Moane's chapter on liberation psychology, feminism, and social justice concludes Part One on fundamental issues in social justice and, in many ways, addresses some of the challenges posed in earlier chapters. Through a review of the convergent and divergent elements of these two social justice traditions in psychology, Moane pulls out central concepts to assist in a critical and reflexive approach to social justice work: structural analysis of conditions; practice based on the lived experience of individuals; critical consciousness; problematizing and de-ideologizing situations of oppression; the recovery of historical memory; and attention to the intersectionality of human experience, a concept unique to feminist approaches to social justice. By bringing these two social justice traditions together, Moane creates a cultural and praxis-based bridge joining academic traditions that stem from dramatically different philosophical grounds. A significant methodological outcome that emerges from the theoretical and philosophical traditions of liberation and feminist psychology is participatory approaches to research that help social justice workers circumvent ideologically based approaches to social justice (as critiqued by Raskin in Chapter 3) or interventions that impose narrowly framed ideas of what is just or good for the other (as highlighted by Teo et al., in Chapter 4). Her case studies of social justice workshops held in Ireland help the reader understand how concepts from liberation and feminist psychology are brought to bear in pedagogical encounters, the first with women and the second with lesbian, gay, bisexual, and transgender, queer/questioning, and intersex (LGBTQI) participants,. These workshops, and the voices of the participants themselves, also provide avenues by which to address the pernicious dynamics of false consciousness discussed by Perkins and Cross (Chapter 6).

SPECIAL POPULATIONS

Although a reader of this series is likely familiar with many of the human rights and social justice issues that confront our world today, the chapters in Part Two inform readers of the immediacy and poignancy of oppression, discrimination, and social injustice throughout the world. These chapters illustrate the challenges of populations typically ignored or devalued: sexual orientation and gender minorities; indigenous people, the physically disabled, the elderly, poor. These chapters offer suggestions for uniquely psychological engagement with such individuals and groups and with the larger social political structures within which they reside.

Moorehead and LaFramboise address arguably one of the most poignant examples of social injustice in U.S. history, the lives and experiences of American Indians/Alaska Natives. They center their chapter on significant historical moments (e.g., the boarding school era and tribal relocation) and how these experiences inform advocacy and social change programs. Finally, they emphasize the power of story-telling, a hallmark of American Indian cultures, particularly when focused on stories of healing, resilience, and victory over trauma and suffering. Native peoples have suffered a great deal of historical and present-day oppression. The authors note the influence of historical trauma and its transmission from generation to generation, and the effects of racism and frequent microaggressions. Yet, the authors emphasize, these challenges have served to call forth the strength and resilience of Native people and their healing traditions (e.g., story telling), and innovative applications of these salubrious practices (e.g., digital story telling and remembering historical resistances). Moorehead and LaFramboise close their chapter with the admonition that Native people, and those who support them, focus on their stories of resilience and success, as these will move them forward in healing and empowerment.

Woolf and MacCartney focus the reader's attention on the human rights violations experienced throughout the world by lesbian, gay, bisexual, transgender, queer, intersexed (LGBTQI) individuals. Their nuanced discussion of the definition of terms highlights how the meaning of terms such as *male* or *female* are as much social and political realities as they are biological facts. As such, the rights assigned to individuals who fall outside mainstream notions of heterosexuality are based on morality rather than the material determinism of biology. Woolf and MacCartney describe the human rights violations of LGBTQI individuals throughout the world, including issues of direct and indirect violence, political discrimination, educational discrimination, and discrimination in the workplace. While many countries have come a long way in terms of socially just treatment of LGBTQI individuals, as evidenced by United Nations (UN) Declarations, there is need to go farther; for psychologists, there have also been historical shifts within the American Psychological Association (APA), but also there is a still quite a long way to go. Woolf and MacCartney provide a critical perspective on the role of psychologists, citing the history of APA regarding diagnostic categories and ongoing practices, such as "reparative therapy," regarding sexual orientation, while at the same time reviewing the increasing amount of resources available to psychologists who work with this population. By linking the work of national organizations, such as the APA, to the work of international organizations, such as the UN, Woolf and MacCartney situate the social justice concerns of LGBTQI individuals within a broader global conversation regarding human rights and psychosocial well-being for this population. Their chapter, like many others in Part Two, is a call to informed action.

Holland, Sturm, and Culp in Chapter 10 take us to post-Communist Central and Eastern Europe (CEE) for a description of not only the human rights violations experienced by people with physical disabilities prior to the fall of communism, but also the challenges these individuals continue to face even as the region quickly moves toward a democratic system of governance. As with Woolf et al. they place their discussion within the context of global declarations from the UN, which specifically address human rights issues and issues of social justice for special populations and point out that even as democratic advances characterized CEE countries, the human rights of differently abled individuals have lagged, mirroring the situation in so many other parts of the world. These authors point out that charitable approaches to individual with disability fall short of human rights approaches and, through descriptions of the work of activists and NGOs in CEE countries, outline for us the various steps required to ensure the human rights of people with disabilities, ranging from advocacy, providing social support for individuals and their families, to movement along legislative and policy routes. Their description of the work of disability rights activists highlights the important role of the civil sector. The authors conclude with a discussion of the role of psychologists in the arena of disability of rights, noting that only few psychologists are actively engaged in the disability rights movement. They question the traditional bifurcation of advocacy and clinical care and point to the need to focus on the sociopolitical context of disability as well as individual clinical needs, pointing out the ecological models such as that offered by Bronfenbrenner (1979) allow for the development of a hybrid psychology that merges social advocacy and clinical practice.

Ardelt and Friedman's chapter turns attention to the challenges associated with changing demographics in the United States resulting in an increasingly aged population. The dynamics they write about are certainly not unique to the United States, but mirror changing demographics throughout the world, and the resultant global discussion on how to address the socioeconomic changes that naturally follow from the confluence of lower fertility rates and longer life expectancy. Although their chapter brings up many of the social justice issues associated with an aging population—elder abuse and limitations of the built world, to name a few—the central focus of their chapter is the equitable allocation of resources across the life span. If correctly or incorrectly, economic resources are viewed as a zero-sum game, what are the consequences of allocating greater amounts of social and economic resources to the end of the life span? Does this inequitable distribution of resources result in diminished attention to the resources needed by infants and children at the beginning of their life span? Their analysis of economic resource allocation helps us understand the importance of implementing developmental perspective that emphasizes how intervention at one point in the life span impacts development at other points in the life span. Ardelt and Friedman's chapter challenge the notion that a zero-sum understanding of resource allocation, as manifest in countries such as the United States, can effectively nurture development across the life span?

Issues of poverty and development are explicitly addressed by Smith and Sandil, who call for increased attention to the intersection of class and psychosocial well-being with a specific attention to classism—the systematic oppression of the poor through institutions, attitudes, cultural images, and practices. The authors provide a description of poverty throughout the world and discuss the ramifications of classism. They then turn their attention to the role of psychologists in both the perpetuation (through classism) and the amelioration of the negative psychosocial consequences of poverty. Like Teo et al. in Chapter 4, Smith and Sandil in Chapter 12 invite critical reflection on conscious and unconscious involvement in the perpetuation of classism, noting that, as a relatively privileged group in society, psychologists are oftentimes not aware of the barriers that people in poverty experience, some of which include differential access to basic services such as education and medicine, chronic stress, and economic inequity perpetuated by minimum wage standards that are not living wage standards. Similar to Moane (Chapter 7), the authors then turn to the role of social action within the psychologist's tool box, examining participatory action research (PAR), a well-developed methodology focused on decreasing power disparities in society. In their discussion of PAR, these authors explain that the participatory research process provides a continuum of participation that allows researchers to operate as either informed outsiders or fully engaged insiders. Smith and Sandil close with a discussion of the implications of globalization on poverty, helping us understand the intersectionality of gender and global poverty, and the extent to which globalized systems of production can exacerbate poverty and, in turn, intensify mental health concerns in low- and middle-income countries and communities throughout the world.

Whiteley, Bloom, and Friedman note that the criminal justice system is based on rule of law and is, at its best, supposed to support social justice aims—such as ensuring that retributive justice is fair and not just a reflexive reaction of those injured. But the laws themselves are often based on societal power differentials, often resulting in the opposite of these ideals. The authors point to numerous examples of this, noting for example, that the conviction of a felony disenfranchises many young, Black men, effectively limiting their political influence over a lifetime even if their infractions were minor. Furthermore, inappropriate sentencing of youth as adults disproportionately impacts minorities. Differences in sentencing suggest that the criminal justice system itself is far from being just, especially when white-collar criminals are incarcerated in different facilities or simply go free. The authors present strong scientific evidence showing that community based re-offending treatment efforts are better than prison in rehabilitating people and reducing recidivism, few changes seem possible within the U.S. criminal justice system. Limited prison and community then point out how mental health services perpetuate the pro-longed incarceration of the mentally ill rather than the treatment of underlying mental health issues. The authors point out that although the public often thinks of imprisonment as protecting society, incarceration oftentimes disrupts important social structures, since imprisoned individuals are no longer able to work, ultimately resulting in numerous ripple effects, such as poorer performance of their children in school. Whiteley et al. pointedly hold psychology accountable as a discipline for often being complicit in blaming the individual for antisocial behavior, while ignoring broader social factors and influences. For example, they discuss the ways in which psychological language adds to the view of incorrigibility for some offenders, resulting in unjustly withholding treatment for some prisoners who might benefit. Finally, the authors also hint at a range of complex ethical conundrums that are daily realities for prison psychologists.

Together, the chapters in this volume set the stage for the handbook. They provide a critical conceptual base for social justice work among psychologists and review the role and work of psychology with several important special populations. Taken as a whole, the chapters in this first volume prepare readers for thinking critically about conceptions and applications of social justice and provide poignant examples of social justice work.

REFERENCES

Bronfenbrenner, U. (1979). *The ecology of human development.* Cambridge, MA: Harvard University Press.

Fanon, F. (1952). *Black skin, White mask.* Paris, France: Editions Du Seuil.

Fanon, F. (1986). *The wretched of the earth.* New York, NY: Grove Press.

Part 1

Fundamental Issues

Chapter 1

The History of Psychology and Social Justice[1]

John T. Jost and Aaron C. Kay

Social justice is a term that originates in philosophical discourse but is widely used in both ordinary language and social science, often without being clearly defined. We trust the reader to forgive the temerity that is inherent in our offering up a general definition here, given that the alternative of plodding on in conceptual dusk (if not total darkness) is hardly an attractive option. For the present purposes, *social justice* may be said to represent a state of affairs (whether actual or ideal) in which (1) benefits and burdens in society are dispersed in accordance with some justifiable allocation principle (or set of such principles); (2) procedures, norms, and rules that govern political and other forms of decision-making protect (rather than violate) the basic rights, liberties, and entitlements of individuals and groups; and (3) human beings (and perhaps other species as well) are generally treated with dignity and respect not only by authorities but also by other relevant social actors, including fellow citizens (see also Feinberg, 1973; Frankena, 1962; Miller, 1999).[2] Social justice, defined in this way, is a property of social systems—or perhaps a "predicate of societies" (Frankena, 1962); a just social system is to be contrasted with those systems that foster unnecessary or unjustified suffering, exploitation, abuse, tyranny, oppression, prejudice, and discrimination. Thus, Toynbee (1976) wrote: "The best safeguard against fascism is to establish social justice to the maximum possible extent" (p. 204).

The foremost problem for scholars or practitioners of social justice is that widespread disagreements persist, even after centuries of debate, concerning each of the elements incorporated in our definition (see Boucher & Kelly, 1998; Campbell, 2001; Miller, 1999; Solomon & Murphy, 2000). What is to be considered a truly fair dispersion of benefits and burdens and why? Is it on the basis of equity, equality, need, or some other principle of allocation? Similarly, how does one determine what constitutes an appropriate or reasonable set of rights, liberties, and entitlements? Finally, what does it mean to treat others with dignity and respect? These and related questions have been broached by some of the greatest minds in Western civilization, including Plato, Aristotle, Hobbes, Locke, Hume, Rousseau, Kant, Hegel, Marx, Mill, Rawls, and legions of others, but no consensus has yet emerged. Given this historical context, it may be considered highly ambitious to think that social psychological science can contribute something of value to the study of social justice, but we dare to suggest that in the long run it can.

A TYPOLOGY OF SOCIAL JUSTICE CONCERNS

One of the first empirical research programs explicitly devoted to the study of social justice focused on issues of distributive fairness, especially considerations of equity in the allocation of resources (Adams, 1965; Blau, 1968; Homans, 1961; Walster, Walster, & Berscheid, 1978). Next came work on procedural justice, which addressed not only outcomes but also the decision-making rules used to determine those outcomes (Folger, 1977; Lind & Tyler, 1988; Thibaut & Walker, 1975). Before too long, a third type of justice was investigated—namely, interpersonal or interactional justice—to incorporate concerns about informal as well as formal treatment by others in everyday life (Bies & Moag, 1986; Colquitt, 2001; Greenberg, 1993). In the remainder of this chapter we will focus on distributive, procedural, and interactional justice concerns; interested readers are directed elsewhere for consideration of two additional types of justice concerns, namely retributive and restorative justice concerns (see Braithwaite, 1989; Carlsmith, Darley, & Robinson, 2002; Jost & Kay, 2010; Vidmar, 2002).

DISTRIBUTIVE JUSTICE

Aristotle and the History of the Concept

One of the earliest influential accounts of distributive justice—that is, the issue of how to allocate resources, especially under conditions of scarcity, fairly and appropriately[3]—was Aristotle's. In Book V of the *Nicomachean Ethics*, Aristotle (ca. 322 BC) notes that "we call just the things that create and preserve happiness and its parts for the citizen community" (2002, p. 159) and inquires about different types of justice and ways of being just (or unjust). According to one prominent interpretation, for Aristotle:

> The hallmark of a just apportionment is *equality*. In distribution, this consists in maintaining the same ratio of quantified good or burdens to quantified merit for all recipients. In rectification, it consists in restoring the parties to the relative position (schematized as "equality") they were in before one harmed the other. (Broadie, 2002, p. 36, emphasis in original)

Interpretational ambiguity arises from the fact that in Homeric Greek the same word (*isotes*) is typically used to mean both justice and equality; the word is best translated as "geometrical equality" or "proportionality" (Vlastos, 1962/1997). Thus, Aristotle says that a just distribution is one that is impartial in the sense of "treating equals as equals" (see also Feinberg, 1973; Frankena, 1962; Mansbridge, 2005), but his conception of distributive justice emphasizes what social scientists today would call principles of equity, proportionality, or merit (Deutsch, 1975; Lerner, 1974).

Aristotle (2002, p. 162) anticipated one of the chief difficulties of justice theories based exclusively on equity or proportionality principles—namely, that decision makers disagree about which inputs (or merits) should be utilized in determining proportional outcomes (or rewards):

> The matter of distribution "according to merit" also makes this clear, since everybody agrees that what is just in distributions must accord with some kind of merit, but everybody is not talking about the same kind of merit: for democrats merit lies in being born a free person, for oligarchs in wealth or, for some of them, in noble descent, for aristocrats in excellence. (1131a24–29)

Indeed, the notion that political or ideological factors influence one's conception of social justice is a central theme of this chapter, and we will return to it in our review of the research literature. The fact that ideology can be said to influence (subjective) justice preferences does not mean, however, that disagreements over what is (objectively) just are simply tantamount to ideological conflicts or that they are empirically intractable and ultimately irresolvable.

The Socialist Tradition

The writings of Karl Marx have probably inspired more social justice movements than any other piece of literature, with the possible exceptions of religious texts (regarding the latter, see Adelson, 1995; Solomon & Murphy, 2000). It is ironic, then, that Marx himself was notoriously suspicious about the meaning and use of the term *justice*, which he equated with the concept of *jurisprudence*.[4] Marx saw justice as an inherently bourgeois (perhaps liberal) concern along the lines of *noblesse oblige*, and he expressed disdain for the "vulgar socialists" of his era who, in his view, championed empty slogans such as "a fair day's wages for a fair day's work." He was also skeptical about philosophical attempts to develop abstract or universal conceptions of justice that would transcend specific social and historical circumstances, such as those proffered by Kant or Hegel (Jost & Jost, 2007). Thus, most scholars agree that Marx generally eschewed justice-based arguments in making the case for revolution and the overthrow of the capitalist system (Tucker, 1969; Wood, 1972/1980; but see Husami, 1978/1980). Instead, Marx appealed to collective self-interest, as in the famous line from *The Communist Manifesto*: "Workers of the world unite; you have nothing to lose but your chains!" That is, he saw it as obviously in the objective interests of the working class to overthrow the capitalist system, and he assumed that their material life circumstances would (eventually) shape their subjective perceptions of the system in accordance with objective realities. In so doing, Marx may have underestimated the problem of false consciousness (Jost, 1995; Jost & Banaji, 1994).

Even if Marx saw little revolutionary potential in appeals to social justice, many of his followers have discerned in his writings the seeds of a powerful justice-based critique of capitalism (e.g., Campbell, 2001). For instance, Marx argued that capitalism depends for its very existence on "surplus value" being created through the labor process. The idea is that no worker is ever paid what his or her work is actually worth (to the employer, that is, the value of what is produced); otherwise, there would be no profit (or profit motive). But the worker who wants to survive and provide for his or her family has no real choice in a capitalist society but to produce wealth for those capitalists who control the means of production. Marx clearly denounced this situation as a form of exploitation, and it is one of the reasons that he predicted (and longed for) the transition from capitalism to socialism and communism, which he believed would finally put an end to class-based exploitation. Thus, Marx objected to the stark economic inequality between social classes that inevitably characterizes the capitalist mode of production on grounds that are indistinguishable from considerations of social justice, as we use the term here (see also Campbell, 2001; Husami, 1978/1980; Konow, 2003). At the same time, he worried that certain conceptions of justice would be used to provide ideological cover for the status quo.

There is also Marx's normative claim, in his *Critique of the Gotha Program*, that under socialism the appropriate principle of distribution will be "from each according to their ability, to each according to their needs" (1875/2008, p. 27; see also Miller, 1999, for a discussion). As Lerner (1974) and Deutsch (1975) point out, taking into account the needs of individuals is a principle of distributive justice that is not necessarily included in other theories of social justice, including Aristotle's. Schwinger (1986), among others, has argued that "need considerations are more than a reaction to actual deficiencies of resources" (p. 223) and that they function much like other distributive justice principles, especially in trusting, favorable interpersonal relationships. Similarly, value is often attached to the principle of equality of outcomes (as well as opportunities) across individuals and social classes, and many interpret Marx's demand for a classless society as a call for thoroughgoing egalitarianism with respect to distributive outcomes (e.g., Campbell, 2001).

It is possible that as a practical matter Marx's condemnation of "utopian socialists" led him to underestimate the extent to which perceptions of social injustice based on principles of equality or need contain revolutionary potential. Research throughout the social and behavioral sciences reveals that anger in response to felt injustice—that is, moral outrage—is in fact one of the most robust predictors of participation in collective action and motivation for social change (e.g., Gurr, 1970; Martin, Scully, & Levitt, 1990; Montada & Schneider, 1989; Moore, 1978; Solomon, 1990; Tyler & Smith, 1998; Van Stekelenburg & Klandermans, 2007; Van Zomeren, Postmes, & Spears, 2008; Wakslak, Jost, Tyler, & Chen, 2007). Although Marx was deeply angered by the exploitation of workers in capitalist society, he set out to develop a dispassionate historical analysis and therefore said much less about social justice than he might otherwise have done, for better or for worse.

The Liberal-Progressive Tradition

Due at least in part to Marx's skepticism, the concept of " 'social justice' was more readily embraced by liberals and progressives than by socialists proper," as Miller (1999, p. 3) notes. There are two major Western liberal traditions that are most responsible for scholarly and practical interest in questions of social justice. Sandel (1998, p. 184) sums up these traditions succinctly in posing the following question: "Should justice be founded on utility, as Jeremy Bentham and John Stuart Mill argue, or does respect for individual rights require a basis for justice independent of utilitarian considerations, as Kant and Rawls maintain?" These two possibilities are generally referred to as the utilitarian and deontological perspectives, respectively, and we consider each in turn.

Utilitarianism

Utilitarianism is a consequentialist theory of justice, insofar as it emphasizes the hedonic and moral consequences of various decisions about how to allocate benefits and burdens in society. The central idea is that the most just outcome or procedure is whatever results in the greatest happiness of the greatest number. Utilitarian philosophers disagree, however, about how to gauge happiness (or "well-being" or related terms, such as "public interest" or "general good;" see Bowie & Simon, 2007).[5] Bentham took the concept to mean simply pleasure minus pain (1962), whereas Mill advanced a more robust conception that included related notions such as virtue, rationality, and truth. Even today, support for the welfare state, which redistributes wealth and other valued resources in such a way as to reduce the misery of those who are worst off without extracting an equivalent amount of suffering from those who are better off, is justified or—in the language of Frankena (1962) and Feinberg (1973)—"justicized," that is, shown to be just on largely utilitarian grounds (e.g., Campbell, 2001; Konow, 2003; Sen, 1979).

Although philosophical utilitarianism is quite clearly a normative theory about how people ought to behave, descriptive research in psychology suggests that in many situations people are indeed highly sensitive to the perceived consequences of an action (e.g., the degree of harm that results from it) when evaluating its moral soundness. In a series of ingenious experiments involving the well-known trolley problem, which requires decision makers to make hypothetical but morally troubling life-and-death decisions about appropriate and inappropriate ways of minimizing harm to innocent bystanders, research participants do make cost-benefit calculations and favor utilitarian solutions (e.g., taking action so that one bystander is killed while five others are spared), as long as the emotional salience of the costs is relatively low for either situational or dispositional reasons (e.g., Greene, 2007). Interestingly, cognitive load manipulations interfere with the type of moral reasoning that gives rise to utilitarian solutions to dilemmas of this type (Greene, Morelli, Lowenberg, Nystrom, & Cohen, 2008). When emotional processing predominates, this research suggests that participants look much more like deontological theorists adhering to moral absolutes than utilitarians making complex calculations (see also Baron, 1993).

Deontological Approaches

Deontologists hold that determinations of right and wrong depend not only on the consequences of human action but also on other considerations, including transcendent justice principles, such as the assumption that it is wrong to kill an innocent, healthy person under any circumstances. One of the most famous proponents of a deontological approach to justice, Immanuel Kant, argued that objective, universally applicable principles of justice can be derived on the basis of abstract human reasoning (i.e., rationality). He proposed, for example, that a "categorical imperative" (1785/2005, p. 79) exists for each of us to treat others in a manner that we would ourselves like to be treated.

Rawls (1971) proposed that the most just social system is the one that would be chosen by rational decision makers under a *veil of ignorance*, that is, in the absence of any specific knowledge of their own status or position within the social system that is adopted; he referred to this hypothetical decision-making situation as *the original position*. Drawing in part on psychological theory and research, including the work of Piaget (1932/1965) and Kohlberg (1969), Rawls concluded that under these circumstances rational individuals ought to (and in fact would) choose a social system that, *ceteris paribus*, (1) minimized the degree of inequality in social and economic outcomes (the equality principle) and (2) maximized the social and economic outcomes of those who would occupy the worst position in the new system (the so-called maximin principle). Taken together, these principles imply that some degree of inequality in society is tolerable, but only to the extent that it ultimately benefits those who are relatively disadvantaged, for example, by creating enough wealth that everyone benefits. This conclusion is a hallmark of political liberalism, insofar as it contains a limited commitment to egalitarianism (i.e., one that falls short of socialism; see Nielsen, 1985) and at least some attention to the satisfaction of those basic needs that are required for human welfare (Rawls, 1993; Sandel, 2005). Thus, Rawls' work constitutes, among other things, a normative theory of justice that is meant to be "consistent with the laws of psychology," and, ultimately, a complex philosophical defense of liberalism in the Kantian tradition of developing and enforcing a rational social contract, that is, the consent of the individual to participate in society.[6]

One measure of the profundity of Rawls' (1971) contribution to scholarship and research on social justice is the sheer number and illustriousness of contemporary critics that it has attracted (see, e.g., Blocker & Smith, 1980; Daniels, 1989; Solomon & Murphy, 2000). It would take us astray to delve into the extensive secondary philosophical literature, so we will confine the remainder of our discussion of Rawls's theory to the empirical research literature it has generated. In so doing, we should be very clear that—as most researchers also acknowledge—empirical studies cannot actually determine what Rawls hypothetical decision makers ought to choose under the veil of ignorance or even what they would choose under the constraints he envisioned. This is because it is, as a practical matter, quite impossible to divorce actual decision makers from their own personal characteristics, experiences, beliefs, opinions, and so on. Some philosophers have suggested that this practical impossibility represents a fatal flaw in Rawls' theory (rendering it, if not incoherent, then at least not very useful for determining what justice principles real people would prefer). Without dismissing the force of this criticism, we can appreciate that the purpose of the original position is simply to develop an objective conception of social justice by insuring impartiality with respect to decision making and eliminating all potential sources of bias (i.e., self-serving, group-serving, and system-serving motivations). Findings from experimental and survey research inspired by Rawls' theory do speak to the question of what distributive justice principles people tend to prefer when these sources of bias are at least muted (though not entirely removed).

The empirical literature provides mixed evidence for the notion that actual decision makers tend to favor the equality and maximin principles over viable alternatives, such as sheer wealth maximization. In some studies, research participants who lack information that would enable them to act on the basis of self-interest and related motives do indeed evaluate the fairness of various distributional schemes in ways that are at least somewhat similar to how Rawls theorized they should behave (Bond & Park, 1991; Brickman, 1977; Michelbach, Scott, Matland, &

Bornstein, 2003; Schulz & May, 1989). For instance, Mitchell, Tetlock, Mellers, and Ordóñez (1993) found that a majority of research participants exhibited a preference for maximizing the minimum standard of living in their society. However, there are studies that show clear departures from what Rawls would have expected (Curtis, 1979; Frohlich & Oppenheimer, 1990; Frohlich, Oppenheimer, & Eavey, 1987a, 1987b). A comprehensive research program summarized by Frohlich and Oppenheimer (1992) revealed that most of the participants in their experiments, which were conducted in the United States, Canada, and Poland, opted for a "floor constraint" (some safety net) without any "ceiling" (i.e., limitation on maximum income). Their participants, in other words, preferred a social system that contained more inequality than Rawls' theory would suggest.

Although such evidence does not disconfirm Rawls' (1971) theory of what is (objectively) just, it does suggest that it is very difficult for actual decision makers to leave behind much of their own personal experiences and cultural baggage in order to place themselves in the original position (i.e., behind a veil of ignorance). The fact that social group and ideological differences are frequently observed in experiments involving hypothetical societies (Bond & Park, 1991; Mitchell et al., 1993; Mitchell, Tetlock, Newman, & Lerner, 2003; Scott, Matland, Michelbach, & Bornstein, 2001) suggests that people are anchored to a considerable extent by the economic realities and justice beliefs that seem to operate in their own societies, even when they are explicitly instructed to ignore them. In other words, empirical studies of Rawls' theory cannot help but reveal the presence of ego, group, and system justification motives (e.g., see Jost & Banaji, 1994)—despite the fact that the veil of ignorance was intended as a device to exclude influences such as these—in addition to *bona fide* attempts to engage in justice-based reasoning.

Conservatism and the Critique of the Liberal-Socialist Tradition

It should be clear from the foregoing that most philosophical conceptions of social justice, especially those that emphasize egalitarian and welfare (i.e., need-based) principles, were developed historically by theorists of the liberal or socialist left who were critical of traditional social, economic, or political arrangements. In fact, the concept of social justice is invoked most often by those who seek to challenge a social system that they regard as intrinsically unjust (Barry, 2005). Miller (1999) notes, for example, that "social justice has always been, and must always be, a critical idea, one that challenges us to reform our institutions and practices in the name of greater fairness" (p. x). This explains why the very concept of social justice is sometimes rejected by political conservatives, libertarians, and others on the political right who seek to vindicate existing institutions that they regard as—if not always just—at least efficient, natural, or otherwise defensible.[7]

Intellectual historians usually trace the origins of modern political conservatism to Edmund Burke, an Irish-born Member of Parliament in England who famously opposed the French Revolution and encouraged his fellow citizens to "look backward to [the authority of] their ancestors" rather than turning to revolution (Burke, 1790/1987, p. 30; see also Viereck, 1956; White, 1950). Burke and his followers thus rejected liberal and socialist ideas as well as the broader intellectual context of the Scientific Enlightenment in which those ideas were developed (e.g., Jost, 2009). As noted by Shapiro (2003), Burke expressed "contempt for all forms of egalitarianism, which struck him as a doctrine that is profoundly at odds with all the evidence of nature and history" (p. 152). He also emphasized the importance of tradition and favored gradual, incremental reforms over more radical social change, because he believed that "conserving an imperfect inherited world from the worse imperfections that human beings are capable of contriving is the business of political leadership" (p. 152). To this day, political conservatism is aptly characterized in terms of two major principles, namely traditionalism (or resistance to change) and acceptance of inequality or hierarchy (Jost, 2006, 2009; Jost, Glaser, Kruglanski, & Sulloway, 2003; but see Greenberg & Jonas, 2003; Wildavsky, 1989).

Haidt and Graham (2007) have argued that liberals and conservatives possess different moral intuitions, such that liberals are more likely than conservatives to emphasize the importance of fairness and the avoidance of harm, whereas conservatives are more likely than liberals to prioritize ingroup loyalty, deference to authority, and purity. It can be granted that such value differences do indeed exist and can be traced back to the writings of Edmund Burke, if not earlier. Questions can be raised, however, about whether adherence to tradition, custom, authority, and ingroup norms should really be considered moral virtues (or justice principles) rather than ideological commitments. Indeed, the glorification of ingroup, authority, and purity concerns, in extreme cases, tends to be associated with authoritarianism and even genocide (e.g., Altemeyer, 1996; Kelman & Hamilton, 1989; Rummel, 1997; Sidanius & Pratto, 1999; Staub, 2011). This makes them unlikely candidates to be considered moral or justice principles in any normative philosophical sense (see also Jost, 2012). A stronger case can be made for moderate conservative principles such as desert, merit, prosperity, and personal freedom (e.g., Mitchell et al., 2003; Nozick, 1974; Smith, 1776; Solomon & Murphy, 2000). Ideological disputes arise when these conservative values inevitably come into conflict with liberal-socialist principles such as equality, welfare, and improving the lot of those who are worst off in society. We turn now to a review of the social psychological theories and evidence bearing on the use of these various justice principles in resource allocation and other decision-making contexts.

Social Psychological Theories and Evidence

Equity Theory

Probably no theory has been more broadly influential to the empirical study of social justice than the one that arguably came first: equity theory. Aristotle (384–322 BCE), as we have seen, argued that justice requires proportionality, that is, "equality of ratios" (2002, p. 163; 1131a31). This insight provides the starting point for equity theory, as developed by Homans (1961), Adams (1963, 1965), Blau (1968), Walster, Berscheid, and Walster (1973), and Walster et al. (1978). The theory holds that in rendering judgments about distributive justice, people seek to determine whether there is a proportional relationship between their inputs (e.g., degree of effort, ability, time, training) and the outcomes they receive (e.g., payments and other rewards as well as costs or punishments). To make this determination in practice, people typically draw interpersonal comparisons involving similar or relevant others (e.g., Festinger, 1954) or intrapersonal comparisons, that is, relative judgments based on their own prior experiences and expectations (Adams, 1965).

If an individual concludes that the ratio of inputs to outputs in a given case is disproportionate, psychological distress is theorized to ensue; such distress, in turn, is expected to motivate the individual to restore equity (Walster et al., 1973). An important aspect of equity theory—an aspect that arguably is what makes it a theory of justice rather than simply a theory of attribution, social judgment, or preferences—is that people are hypothesized to dislike being overbenefited (i.e., rewarded in a disproportionately favorable manner) as well as being underbenefited. However, the latter situation is especially aversive because it violates both justice and self-interest (Walster et al., 1978; see also Boll, Ferring, & Filipp, 2005; Loewenstein, Thompson, & Bazerman, 1989; Peters, Van den Bos, & Bobocel, 2004). In terms of emotional responses, those who are underbenefited are assumed to feel angry and resentful, whereas those who are overbenefited are assumed to feel guilty (Chen & Tyler, 2001; Hassebrauck, 1986; Hegtvedt, 1990; Homans, 1961; Jost, Wakslak, & Tyler, 2008; Schmitt, Behner, Montada, Müller, & Müller-Fohrbrodt, 2000).

How do people cope with the aversive reactions engendered by the presence of inequity? According to Hatfield and Sprecher (1984), individuals can choose between two options: (1) they can restore equity in actuality (i.e., objectively), by increasing or decreasing inputs (e.g., by working harder or withholding effort) or outputs (e.g., by giving or taking more or less in terms of benefits or burdens); or (2) they can restore equity psychologically (i.e., subjectively), by rationalizing or otherwise reconstruing the nature or relative evaluation of inputs and outputs so as to make the situation or relationship seem equitable. According to equity theory, the individual engages in these processes whether he or she is directly involved in the inequitable situation or not; in other words, it is psychologically aversive to observe inequity in the relationships of others as well as in one's own relationships.

The evidence has supported the basic tenets of the theory to an impressive degree (Ambrose & Kulik, 1999; Greenberg, 1990; Mowday, 1991). For this reason, equity theory has had tremendous impact on several areas of social science, ranging from the study of close relationships (Utne, Hatfield, Traupmann, & Greenberger, 1984; Van Yperen & Buunk, 1990) to organizational behavior (Ambrose & Kulik, 1999; Bolino & Turnley, 2008). Studies have shown, for example, that inequity produces physiological arousal (Markowski, 1988) and that the desire to establish (or restore) equity is an important factor in children's resource allocations

(Leventhal & Anderson, 1970). Greenberg (1980) found that participants were especially likely to follow the equity norm when distributing rewards between themselves and a competitor in the presence of a mirror, which presumably increases adherence to salient social norms. Perceptions of equity are related to perceptions of stability and contentment in new marriages and other close relationships (Utne et al., 1984; Van Yperen & Buunk, 1990; but see Montada, 2003; Sprecher & Schwartz, 1994), and perceptions of inequity (i.e., feeling overbenefited) may also help to explain negative reactions that are (ironically) caused by increased social support (Gleason, Iida, Bolger, & Shrout, 2003). Similarly, perceptions of inequity explain a wide range of behavior in workplace settings (Greenberg, 1988), including employee theft of property that belongs to an organization that is seen as underrewarding its employees, relative to the latter's efforts and other inputs (Greenberg, 1993).

Principles of Equality and Need

A number of authors have pointed out that equity is by no means the only appropriate principle of distributive justice (e.g., Clark & Mills, 1979; Deutsch, 1975; Feinberg, 1973; Konow, 2003; Leventhal, 1980; Miller, 1999). They take what is sometimes referred to as a multidimensional approach to justice norms (Cohen & Greenberg, 1982; Mikula, 1984; Reis, 1984). Along these lines, Lerner (1974) observed that people's conceptions of justice can take various forms, and that different situations call for different justice principles (see also Törnblom & Foa, 1983). When recipients share a common identity, as in the case of families, the Marxian principle of allocation based on need is much more likely to be adopted than when no such identity exists (see also Deutsch, 1975; Lamm & Schwinger, 1980; Lerner, 1974). For example, the idea of dishing out relative dinner portions to one's children on the basis of their report cards (i.e., merit)—regardless of their ages, sizes, or appetites—strikes one as inherently unjust if not downright absurd. Rather, a need-based allocation seems far more appropriate. Similarly, circumstances exist in which members of close-knit groups prefer norms of parity or equality in dispersing benefits and burdens, presumably because of the value placed upon the maintenance of harmonious social relations among members (Deutsch, 1975; Konow, 2003; Wenzel, 2000).

Of all of the putative justice principles, equality has received far and away the most philosophical attention (e.g., Frankena, 1962; Miller, 1999; Nagel, 1991; Rawls, 1971; Solomon & Murphy, 2000; Vlastos, 1962/1997; Walzer, 1983). Demands for equal rights and equal treatment under the law have been fundamental causes of political revolution and constitution-building in Europe and the Americas since the time of the Enlightenment. As we have seen, equality is central to the liberal-socialist tradition, and leftists today are distinguished largely by their advocacy for greater social, economic, and political equality (or, perhaps more accurately, less inequality in each of these spheres). Although earlier generations of conservatives, such as Burke (1790/1987), objected to egalitarianism in various guises, most conservatives today endorse political equality (e.g., one person, one vote) and equality of opportunity in education and economic domains. But, as Parfit (1998) notes, to subscribe to egalitarianism as a justice principle also requires being "concerned with people's *being equally well off,*" that is, to believe, "It is in itself bad if some people are worse off than others" (p. 3; see also Williams, 1976/2000).[8] By contrast, conservatives, libertarians, and other critics of egalitarianism claim that privileging equality of outcomes as well as opportunities is indefensible (e.g., Wildavsky, 1991).

According to Lerner (1974), equity is deemed the fairest principle in situations in which individuals feel both dependent on and nonequivalent to other social actors, as in marketplace environments (see also Deutsch, 1975). Consistent with this notion, research indicates that the importance of equity considerations (relative to other justice norms) depends upon perceptions of social relations, that is, the ways in which people see themselves as connected to others (or not) when it comes to sharing resources (Clayton & Opotow, 2003; Skitka, 2003; Wenzel, 2001, 2002).[9]

Far and away the most popular equity principle in common circulation is the principle of merit, that is, the rewarding of individuals on the basis of contributions or entitlements such as ability, effort, motivation, and achievement (e.g., Frankena, 1962; Hayek, 1976; Nozick, 1974). Justifications for this principle are frequently utilitarian in nature, insofar as they suggest that a meritocratic system creates incentives for productivity that are beneficial to society as a whole. Miller (1999) has suggested that principles of equality and merit are compatible in certain ways and that social justice may require an integration of the two. For one thing, equality and merit "stand opposed to a distribution of advantages on the basis of luck" (p. 201); this suggests that the extent to which the capitalist system may be considered just by egalitarians and meritarians depends in part upon the extent to which outcomes are not due to chance (or nepotism or simply being in the right place at the right time). Furthermore, Miller argues, on normative grounds, that the principle of merit should never be used to allocate "those goods and services that people regard as necessities, such as health care" (p. 200). On this point, there is at least some agreement between subjective and objective conceptions (Lupfer, Weeks, Doan, & Houston, 2000). Research participants do feel that different types of resources should be allocated on the basis of different justice principles (Fiske & Tetlock, 1997; Törnblom & Foa, 1983), and that burdens and necessities should be distributed with regard to considerations of need and equality rather than merit (e.g., Gamliel & Peer, 2006; Matania & Yaniv, 2007; Norton & Ariely, 2011).

Do Liberals and Conservatives Prefer Different Justice Principles?

Given that one of the core ideological differences between political liberals and conservatives concerns the value that is placed on equality of outcomes (Jost et al., 2003), it is not too surprising that justice preferences and judgments covary with political orientation (Christiansen & Lavine, 1997; Rasinski, 1987; Skitka & Tetlock, 1993). In hypothetical society paradigms, for instance, liberals generally prefer more egalitarian distributions of wealth that also offer protections for those who are in greatest need, whereas conservatives are more likely to prioritize equity, efficiency, and individual merit (Mitchell et al., 1993, 2003). These differences in justice preferences are clearly consistent with the philosophical differences among socialists, liberals, and conservatives that go back several centuries, as noted earlier.

Mitchell et al. (1993) observed that ideological polarization was greatest for judgments of hypothetical societies containing moderate degrees of meritocracy. Presumably, this is because liberals saw the justice glass under such circumstances as half-empty (emphasizing the role of chance), whereas conservatives saw it as half-full (emphasizing ability and effort). Research by Napier and Jost (2008) demonstrates that ideological differences in reactions to economic inequality have consequences for subjective well-being. Specifically, they found that increasing economic inequality in U.S. society from 1974 to 2004 (as measured in terms of the Gini coefficient and other macro-economic indices) negatively impacted the self-reported happiness of liberals (vs. conservatives) to a significantly greater extent, apparently because the conservative assumption that inequality is often legitimate and meritorious provides a kind of ideological buffer against the negative hedonic effects of inequality. Given our quest for objective indicators of social justice, it is worth pointing out that even moderate conservatives experienced a decline in subjective well-being as economic inequality increased.

PROCEDURAL JUSTICE

Although the terms *social justice* and *distributive justice* are often used interchangeably by philosophers and laypersons (e.g., see Miller, 1999), social scientists in recent decades have come to recognize that justice considerations pertain not merely to the allocation of resources but also to the methods or procedures by which decisions are made at work, in political life, in the family, and so on. A major thrust of contemporary social psychological research has demonstrated that justice appraisals are determined at least as much, if not more, by the perceived fairness of procedural than distributive factors (e.g., Tyler & Smith, 1998). The concept of equality is fundamental to conceptions of procedural as well as distributive justice: people want to be treated with fairness and respect; that is, they want to be treated as equals (i.e., not as social inferiors).

The pioneers of this research tradition, Thibaut and Walker (1975), were primarily interested in third-party decision making, such as legal decisions made by judges or juries. Their work showed that the perceived fairness of the specific procedures used to render a verdict or decision influences research participants' evaluations of both the final outcome and the decision maker. Researchers have not looked back since; there has been far more research on aspects of procedural justice than on other types (including distributive justice) over the past quarter of a century. Work in this area focuses on the subjective perceptions of fair (vs. unfair) treatment, but by describing the social-structural (and other) antecedents of such perceptions, researchers are also moving us closer to identifying the objective circumstances that foster social justice in a normative sense (Miller, 1999; Tyler & Jost, 2007).

According to Walker, Lind, and Thibaut (1979), "the belief that the techniques used to resolve a dispute are fair and satisfying in themselves" (p. 1402) follows from two major procedural features, which Brockner and Wiesenfeld (1996) defined as: "(a) process control, referring to how much people are allowed to present evidence on their behalf before the decision is made, and (b) decision control, that is, whether individuals have any say in the actual rendering of the decision" (p. 189). That is, people want to know that they will have input into (and are therefore able to exert at least some influence over) the decision-making process as well as the decision itself. Thibaut and Walker (1975) proposed that when people possess these two types of perceived control, they are able to trust that procedures will be fair and that their short-term and especially long-term outcomes will be favorable in general.

Research has been supportive of the notion that process control is a fundamental determinant of justice appraisals (e.g., Houlden, LaTour, Walker, & Thibaut, 1978; Thibaut & Walker, 1975). Thibaut and Walker's pioneering work has influenced myriad research programs, including research on the voice effect, that is, the demonstration that the opportunity to express one's views or feelings during the course of the decision-making process significantly increases perceptions of procedural fairness (Folger, 1977; Lind & Tyler, 1988; Van den Bos, 2005). Studies show that the presence of voice affects not only justice judgments but is also associated with increased positive affect, decreased negative affect, and greater trust in authorities (inter alia, Brockner et al., 1998; Folger, Rosenfeld, Grove, & Corkran, 1979; Lind & Tyler, 1988; Tyler & Lind, 1992; Van Prooijen, Van den Bos, & Wilke, 2004).

Voice is by no means the only variable that influences perceptions of procedural justice. Leventhal, Karuza, and Fry (1980) identified six different factors that can contribute to justice appraisals. To be considered fair, they argued, decisions must be made (1) consistently across instances and time periods, (2) neutrally, that is, without bias, preconceptions, or self-interest, (3) on the basis of accurate information, (4) with an opportunity to make corrections if necessary, (5) in consideration of the interests of all relevant parties, and (6) ethically. Although these six characteristics were theorized to be the most important criteria for determining whether procedural justice exists in a given situation, Leventhal (1980) pointed out that they should not necessarily be weighted equally. Depending upon the specific circumstances, some rules may be weighted more heavily than others. Consistent with this general notion, situational differences (e.g., variability in the formality of a given decision-making setting) affect the criteria that people use in making judgments of procedural fairness (Barrett-Howard & Tyler, 1986). Nevertheless, aggregating across a wide range of situations, people tend to prioritize three of the criteria—consistency, accuracy, and ethicality—in determining whether procedural justice requirements have been satisfied (Barrett-Howard & Tyler, 1986; Lind & Tyler, 1988).

Interactional (or Informal) Justice

The philosopher Frankena (1962) observed that "society does not consist merely of the law or the state: it has also a more informal aspect, comprised of its cultural institutions, conventions, moral rules, and moral sanctions." Thus, he argued, "In order for society to be fully just, it must be just in its informal as well as in its formal aspect" (p. 2). If this is correct, then it is possible to speak of social injustice as arising not merely as a consequence of unfair treatment proffered by institutionally sanctioned authority figures such as politicians, judges, police officers, bosses, teachers, and so on, but also on the basis of how citizens tend to treat one another. It is in this sense that prejudice, discrimination, and authoritarianism on the part of ordinary citizens can contribute to a social climate that is undemocratic and fundamentally unjust, as Lewin (1939/1948) and Toynbee (1976), among many others, noted with regard to fascist society. Several models of interactional justice have been put forth by social and organizational psychologists over the years; few of them deal explicitly with behavior or circumstances that are as extreme as those associated with fascism, but the models clearly do involve a broader conception of social justice than is suggested by more formal models of distributive or procedural justice.

Tyler and Lind (1992) deserve credit for highlighting a number of ways in which aspects of social interaction affect perceptions of procedural justice (cf. Leventhal, 1980; Thibaut & Walker, 1975). The idea was taken further by Bies and colleagues (Bies & Moag, 1986; Folger & Bies, 1989; Tyler & Bies, 1990), who distinguished between structural and interactional components of decision-making procedures. In stressing the importance of the latter, Bies and Moag (1986) noted that people are sensitive not merely to the structure or content of a given procedure but also to the "quality of interpersonal treatment they receive during the enactment of organizational procedures" (p. 44, see also Colquitt, Greenberg, & Zapata-Phelan, 2005). In other words, people do not just want fair procedures at work and elsewhere; they also want fair treatment in a much broader sense.

Concluding Remarks

Students of social justice—like those who dare to confront questions of rationality or truth—must grapple with the uneasy relationship between the subjective and the objective or, relatedly, descriptive facts about how people actually think, feel, and act with respect to justice considerations and normative standards about how they ought to behave if their actions are to be considered just (see also Baron, 1993; Konow, 2003; Miller, 1999; Payne & Cameron, 2010; Tyler & Jost, 2007). Aristotle (384–322 BCE) captured the dilemma this way: "People think that acting unjustly depends on them; hence they also think that being just is easy. In fact it is not" (2002, p. 173; 1137a4–6). Behaving justly, in other words, involves doing the right thing for the right reasons, and therefore possesses a subjective dimension that can be studied descriptively and an objective dimension that must be approached normatively.[10]

Another difficulty is that reasonable parties can disagree about what justice entails, and many long-standing, seemingly intractable conflicts, such as the Arab-Israeli conflict, involve interpersonal or intergroup disputes over what is considered fair and legitimate (e.g., Deutsch, 2006; Gibson, 2008; Kelman, 1983, 2001; Leung & Stephan, 2000; Mikula & Wenzel, 2000). Conversely, it is unsatisfactory to conclude simply that justice (like truth or beauty) is in the "eye of the beholder," although it may be tempting to leave it at that. As Miller (1999) observed, "Popular beliefs about social justice may turn out to be defective in various ways; for instance, they may prove to conceal deep contradictions, or involve serious factual errors" (p. x).[11] Thus, one cannot merely assume that justice consists in what people *think* is just (e.g., Sampson, 1983), though (as the philosophers know) it may be an extraordinarily difficult—but not, in principle, impossible—task to determine what actually *is* just in any given situation.

One important reason why one cannot simply interpret the subjective acceptance of a given state of affairs as objective evidence of its rightness is that people sometimes tolerate circumstances that seem obviously unjust to outsiders, or in retrospect, or from the point of view of normative standards of just treatment (Crosby, 1984; Deutsch, 1985; Lerner, 1980; Martin, 1986). Some such cases are said to reflect "false consciousness" (Fox, 1999; Jost, 1995; Lind & Tyler, 1988; Tyler & McGraw, 1986).[12] They may even suggest the presence of system justification motivation, that is, the desire to exonerate the existing social system and, in so doing, to minimize or overlook its injustices, whether petty or grand, thereby perpetuating them (see Jost, Banaji, & Nosek, 2004; Jost & Van der Toorn, 2012). It is essential for the scholar of social justice to bear in mind at least the possibility that there are objective standards of justice, even if specific candidates are bound to be controversial (e.g., Feinberg, 1973; Hare, 1981; Miller, 1999; Rawls, 1971). Just as researchers are able to use scientific means to study the objective causes of subjective well-being (or happiness) of individuals (e.g., Kahneman, Diener, & Schwarz, 1999), it should be possible for social scientists to discover which characteristics of social systems are more and less likely to maximize equity, equality, need, liberty, and other putative principles of social justice, and which characteristics lead disproportionately to unjust outcomes such as suffering, exploitation, abuse, prejudice, and oppression. An objective, scientific approach is needed because, as Frankena (1962) pointed out, "even the prevailing moral principles of a society may be unjust or oppressive" (p. 3). Under these circumstances, system justification motivation will obstruct the path to social justice, and researchers cannot afford to rely purely on the subjective perceptions of the citizenry. In reviewing the history of social psychological theory and research on the topic of social justice, we have tried to keep in mind this fundamental truth about our subject matter, which renders it especially challenging from an empirical perspective: subjective and objective conceptions of justice often diverge.

With respect to subjective conceptions, John Stuart Mill (1910) wrote:

> Not only have different nations and individuals different notions of justice, but, in the mind of one and the same individual, justice is not some one rule, principle, or maxim, but many, which do not always coincide in their dictates. (p. 51)

It is possible to grant this important point without abandoning the enterprise of developing objective, normative standards of social justice altogether. Indeed, many topics that fascinate psychologists—such as motivation, self-regulation, social influence, rationality, happiness, culture, political ideology, and so on—have no single determinant or simple solution to the problems they highlight. Each of these phenomena is likewise beset by complex determination, subjective ambivalence, and the tension arising from conflicting forces that are internal and external to the individual. The study of social justice, as with other indispensable topics, requires the search not for one answer but for several (see Walzer, 1983). That is, the most compelling normative conception of social justice may well combine elements of utilitarian and deontological approaches and reconcile multiple, potentially conflicting justice principles—such as equity, equality, need, merit, and liberty—in some hierarchical structure that weights such principles differentially as a function of contextual variables and local contingencies.

In any case, we think that normative questions about social justice themselves are too important to leave entirely to philosophers, legal scholars, and experts in other, nonempirical fields, as if withholding scientific data from the conversation serves society well. For one thing, empirical research has a crucial role to play in clearing away common misconceptions—including erroneous assumptions, stereotypes, and misunderstandings about the causes of human behavior—and thereby updating and elevating public discourse about matters of social justice and morality (Greene, 2003; Payne & Cameron, 2010; Tyler & Jost, 2007). Over time, scientific findings have the capacity to change culturally prevalent representations of free will, responsibility, and so on, and these changes will (eventually) manifest themselves in legal transformations (Blasi & Jost, 2006; Greene & Cohen, 2004). Furthermore, philosophers, including Rawls (1971), often strive to develop normative theories of justice that satisfy the principle of minimal psychological realism, that is, theories that are at least consistent with what is known about the laws of human psychology. Legal authorities, too, have a vested interest in prescribing laws that are psychologically realistic in the sense that most citizens will be able to follow them.

Despite the existence of these legal and philosophical marketplaces for social psychological ideas (and especially data) concerning social justice, researchers frequently suggest that they cannot help to determine what is actually just and that they must confine their efforts to offering purely descriptive or subjectivist accounts of what people think is fair (*inter alia*, Adams, 1965; Mikula & Wenzel, 2000; Skitka & Crosby, 2003; Tyler & Smith, 1998). This approach to the problem, which Sampson (1983) described as "truncated subjectivism" (p. 146), is understandable for its scholarly prudence, but we think that it may be overly modest about what social psychology has to offer. It is useful to bear in mind that cognitive psychologists and other scientists have contributed mightily to refining normative theories of rationality (e.g., Kahneman, Slovic, & Tversky, 1982; Thaler, 1991) as well as formerly philosophical (and even metaphysical) treatments of epistemological questions in general (e.g., Goldman, 1992; Kornblith, 1999). In recent years, philosophers have incorporated evidence from social and personality psychology in evaluating Aristotelian and other normative (as well as descriptive) theories of ethics, virtue, and moral character (Appiah, 2008; Doris, 2002; Flanagan, 1991; Harman, 1999). We see no reason to assume that social psychological research will be any less useful in forging the kinds of normative conceptions of justice and injustice that have traditionally been the bread and butter of moral philosophy and legal scholarship (Greene, 2003; Jasso, 1999; Tyler & Jost, 2007).

The founder of modern social psychology, Kurt Lewin was unapologetic—some might even say heroic (e.g., Ring, 1967)—about the normative use of social science to serve the ends of social justice and, in so doing, to improve society. The evidence suggests that considerable progress toward this most ambitious goal has been achieved (e.g., Jost & Kay, 2010; Konow, 2003; Lerner, 2003; Miller, 2001; Payne & Cameron, 2010; Tyler, 2006; Tyler & Jost, 2007). At the same time, the jury is still out on whether the theories and methods of social psychology can offer unique, indispensable insights that—when combined with those gathered from philosophy, law, history, anthropology, sociology, economics, organizational behavior, political science, and other disciplines—will allow scholars and practitioners to attain the highest degree of social justice and to overcome its most stubborn, pernicious obstacles. We follow Lewin in supposing, however optimistically, that they can.

NOTES

1. Material for this chapter is taken and adapted from selected portions of the following: Jost, J. T., & Kay, A. C. (2010). Social justice: History, theory, and research. In S. T. Fiske, D. Gilbert, & G. Lindzey (Eds.), *Handbook of social psychology* (5th ed., Vol. 2, pp. 1122–1165). Hoboken, NJ: Wiley. We thank Stephanie D. Hawkins, Erin P. Hennes, Kristina Howansky, Benjamin C. Ruisch, and Audrey E. Vera for assistance with manuscript preparation.

2. The three aspects of our definition correspond, roughly, to distributive, procedural, and interactional justice, as we use these terms in this chapter. By offering this definition, we are not suggesting that a theory of social justice must address all three aspects, but we do assume that it will address at least one of them.

3. Frankena (1962, p. 9) writes: "Justice, whether social or not, seems to have at its center the notion of an allotment of something to persons—duties, goods, offices, opportunities, penalties, punishments, privileges, roles, status, and so on. Moreover, at least in the case of distributive justice, it seems centrally to involve the notion of *comparative* allotment."

4. Friedrich Engels, too, believed that justice was merely "the ideologised, glorified expression of the existing economic relations" (see Miller, 1999, pp. x–xi). Although we review evidence in this chapter that ideological perspectives are indeed correlated with preferences for specific justice principles, we do not assume that the study of social justice as a whole is a purely or hopelessly ideological endeavor.

5. It is also customary to distinguish between (1) "act utilitarians," who believe that justice should be calculated on a case-by-case basis for each individual decision, and (2) "rule utilitarians," who believe that justice requires adherence to general principles that, if consistently applied, will be associated with the most favorable consequences for society over time. Disagreement persists over whether Mill should be considered an act or rule utilitarian (e.g., see Hooker, 2011).

6. Dworkin (1972) pointed out that Rawls's (1971) account differs from other well-known philosophical theories of the social contract in that Rawls argues that people *would* agree to a certain set of principles under certain (counterfactual) circumstances, whereas other theories assume that justice results from the honoring of actual (not hypothetical) agreements made by decision makers in advance.

7. One of the most well-known examples is Hayek (1976) in *The Mirage of Social Justice.* Other libertarians, such as Nozick (1974), have developed their own theories of justice, in which principles of equality and need are subordinated to principles of individual liberty and merit. A more extreme example of the right-wing rejection of the very concept of social justice comes from the writings of Pareto, who argued that the concept of justice is "void of all meaning." At the same time, it has been noted that Pareto's "condemnation of state intervention and trade union activities exuded moral outrage; he assumed that every strike, every subsidy, every protective tariff involved a seizure or destruction of rightfully acquired wealth" (Femia, 1998, pp. 76–77).

8. Egalitarians assume, in other words, that the "demand for equality is built into the very concept of justice" (Frankena, 1962, p. 20), but they do not necessarily assume that justice always requires perfect equality or that equality is the only relevant principle of social justice. Frankfurt (1987) has suggested that in many cases what really bothers egalitarians is not that some have less than others but that some simply do not have enough to meet their basic needs; this may explain why principles of equality and need are frequently bundled together in liberal-socialist conceptions of social justice.

9. Equity theorists have argued that often what looks like the application of (or preference for) an equality principle is really the application of an equity principle under circumstances in which "the scrutineer perceived the relevant inputs to be equal" (Reis, 1984, p. 39). This returns us to the Aristotelian injunction to "treat equals as equals."

10. By suggesting, with Aristotle, that "good intentions" matter, we are not denying the adage that "the road to hell is paved with good intentions." This is why it is crucial to

distinguish between subjective and objective conceptions of justice: people can sincerely believe that they are doing what justice requires when in fact they are not. At the same time, intentions are often relevant to justice considerations; this is why the law (appropriately) treats premeditated homicide as a more serious violation of justice than cases of wrongful death with no "malice aforethought."

11. Taking Miller's observation seriously would seem to pose a problem for so-called moral intuitionist theories, which assume that "people have a built-in moral sense that creates pleasurable feelings of approval toward benevolent acts and corresponding feelings of disapproval toward evil and vice" (Haidt, 2001, p. 816). Although this is an intriguing notion, it overlooks the systematic ways in which people can be wrong about justice and morality. For instance, some people experience a disgust reaction when confronted with homosexual behavior and are therefore convinced that such behavior is immoral (Haidt & Graham, 2007; Schnall, Haidt, Clore, & Jordan, 2008). Social history is replete with such examples, including expressions of disgust and outrage at interracial relationships that are now widely and appropriately understood to be beyond moral reproach.

12. It is noteworthy that Aristotle (384–322 BCE) excludes the possibilities that a person could "receive unjust treatment voluntarily" or act unjustly against himself or herself (2002, pp. 169–176; 1135a15–1138b11). His conclusions therefore appear to contradict the notion that people could accept or tolerate injustice (or engage in false consciousness), but this is because Aristotle defines just and unjust actions as requiring the conscious (voluntary) intention to behave in a manner that is either just or unjust, respectively. (He does, however, introduce the concept of "incidental [in]justice," whereby individuals' actions result in just [or unjust] outcomes in the absence of intention.) The discovery of implicit (or nonconscious) motivation in social and cognitive psychology raises certain possibilities that were not addressed by Aristotle. Thus, modern discussions of false consciousness (and system justification) assume that people can be driven by nonconscious cognitive and motivational factors that can contribute to the perpetuation of social injustice (e.g., Blasi & Jost, 2006; Jost & Banaji, 1994; Jost, Rudman, Blair et al., 2009; Payne & Cameron, 2010).

REFERENCES

Adams, J. S. (1963). Toward an understanding of inequity. *Journal of Abnormal Social Psychology, 67,* 422–436.

Adams, J. S. (1965). Inequality in social exchange. In L. Berkowitz (Ed.), *Advances in experimental social psychology* (Vol. 2, pp. 267–299). New York, NY: Academic Press.

Adelson, H. L. (1995). The origins of a concept of social justice. In K. D. Irani & M. Silver (Eds.), *Social justice in the ancient world* (pp. 25–38). Westport, CT: Greenwood Press.

Altemeyer, B. (1996). *The authoritarian specter*. Cambridge, MA: Harvard University Press.

Ambrose, M. L., & Kulik, C. T. (1999). Old friends, new faces: Motivation research in the 1990s. *Journal of Management, 25,* 231–292.

Appiah, A. (2008). *Experiments in ethics.* Cambridge, MA: Harvard University Press

Aristotle (2002). *Nicomachean ethics* (Trans., Eds. S. Broadie & C. Rowe). Oxford, UK: Oxford University Press. (Original work written 384–322 BCE).

Baron, J. (1993). Heuristics and biases in equity judgments: A utilitarian approach. In B. A. Mellers & J. Baron (Eds.), *Psychological perspectives on justice* (pp. 109–137). New York, NY: Cambridge University Press.

Barrett-Howard, E., & Tyler, T. R. (1986). Procedural justice as a criterion in allocation decisions. *Journal of Personality and Social Psychology, 50,* 296–304.

Barry, B. M. (2005). *A treatise on social justice.* Berkeley, CA: University of California Press.

Bentham, J. (1962). Principles of penal law. In J. Bowring (Ed.), *The works of Jeremy Bentham* (pp. 396). Edinburgh, Scotland: W. Tait. (Original work published 1843).

Bies, R. J., & Moag, J. S. (1986). Interactional justice: Communication criteria of fairness. In B. Sheppard (Ed.), *Research on negotiation in organizations* (pp. 43–55). Greenwich, CT: JAI Press.

Blasi, G., & Jost, J. T. (2006). System justification theory and research: Implications for law, legal advocacy, and social justice. *California Law Review, 94,* 1119–1168.

Blau, P. M. (1968). Social exchange. In D. L. Sills (Ed.), *International encyclopedia of the social sciences* (Vol. 7). New York, NY: Macmillan.

Blocker, G. H., & Smith, E. H. (Eds.). (1980). *John Rawls' theory of social justice: An introduction.* Athens: Ohio University Press.

Bolino, M. C., & Turnley, W. H. (2008). Old faces, new places: Equity theory in cross-cultural contexts. *Journal of Organizational Behavior, 29,* 29–50.

Boll, T., Ferring, D., & Filipp, S. (2005). Effects of parental differential treatment on relationship quality with siblings and parents: Justice evaluations as mediators. *Social Justice Research, 18,* 155–182.

Bond, D., & Park, J. (1991). An empirical test of Rawls's theory of justice: A second approach, in Korea and the United States. *Simulation & Gaming, 22,* 443–462.

Boucher, D., & Kelly, P. (Eds.). (1998). *Social justice: From Hume to Walzer.* New York, NY: Routledge.

Bowie, N. E., & Simon, R. L. (2007). *The individual and the political order: An introduction to social and political philosophy* (4th ed.). New York, NY: Rowman & Littlefield.

Braithwaite, J. (1989). *Crime, shame, and reintegration.* New York, NY: Cambridge University Press.

Brickman, P. (1977). Preference for inequality. *Social Psychology Quarterly, 40,* 303–310.

Broadie, S. (2002). Philosophical introduction. In S. Broadie & C. Rowe (Eds.), *Aristotle, Nicomachean ethics: Translation, introduction, and commentary* (pp. 9–91). Oxford, UK: Oxford University Press.

Brockner, J., Heuer, L., Siegel, P. A., Wiesenfeld, B., Martin, C., Grover, S. et al. (1998). The moderating effect of self-esteem in reaction to voice: Converging evidence from five studies. *Journal of Personality and Social Psychology, 75,* 394–407.

Brockner, J., & Wiesenfeld, B. (1996). An integrative framework for explaining reactions to decisions: Interactive effects of outcomes and procedures. *Psychological Bulletin, 120,* 189–208.

Burke, E. (1987). Reflections on the revolution in France. In J. G. A. Pocock (Ed.), *Reflections on the revolution in France* (pp. 1–218). Indianapolis, IN: Hackett. (Original work published 1790).

Campbell, T. (2001). *Justice* (2nd ed.). New York, NY: St. Martin's Press.

Carlsmith, K. M., Darley, J. M., & Robinson, P. H. (2002). Why do we punish? Deterrence and just deserts as motives for punishment. *Journal of Personality and Social Psychology, 83,* 284–299.

Chen, E. S., & Tyler, T. R. (2001). Cloaking power: Legitimizing myths and the psychology of the advantaged. In A. Y. Lee-Chai & J. A. Bargh (Eds.), *The use and abuse of power: Multiple perspectives on the causes of corruption* (pp. 241–261). New York, NY: Psychology Press.

Christiansen, N. D., & Lavine, H. (1997). Need-efficiency trade-offs in the allocation of resources: Ideological and attributional differences in public aid decision making. *Social Justice Research, 10,* 289–310.

Clark, M. S., & Mills, J. (1979). Interpersonal attraction in exchange and communal relationships. *Journal of Personality and Social Psychology, 37,* 12–24.

Clayton, S., & Opotow, S. (2003). Justice and identity: Changing perspectives on what is fair. *Personality and Social Psychology Review, 7,* 298–310.

Cohen, R. L., & Greenberg, J. (1982). The justice concept in social psychology. In J. Greenberg & R. L. Cohen (Eds.), *Equity and justice in social behavior* (pp. 1–41). New York, NY: Academic Press.

Colquitt, J. A. (2001). On the dimensionality of organizational justice: A construct validation of a measure. *Journal of Applied Psychology, 86,* 386–400.

Colquitt, J. A., Greenberg, J., & Zapata-Phelan, C. P. (2005). What is organizational justice? A historical overview. In J. Greenberg & J. A. Colquitt (Eds.), *Handbook of organizational justice* (pp. 3–56). Mahwah, NJ: Erlbaum.

Crosby, F. (1984). Relative deprivation in organizational settings. In B. M. Staw & L. L. Cummings (Eds.), *Research in organizational behavior* (Vol. 6, pp. 51–93). Greenwich, CT: JAI Press.

Curtis, R. C. (1979). Effects of knowledge of self-interest and social relationship upon the use of equity, utilitarian, and Rawlsian principles of allocation. *European Journal of Social Psychology,* 9, 165–175.

Daniels, N. (1989). *Reading Rawls: Critical studies on Rawls' "A theory of justice."* Palo Alto, CA: Stanford University Press.

Deutsch, M. (1975). Equity, equality, and need: What determines which value will be used as the basis of distributive justice? *Journal of Social Issues, 31,* 137–149.

Deutsch, M. (1985). *Distributive justice: A social-psychological perspective.* New Haven, CT: Yale University Press.

Deutsch, M. (2006). Justice and conflict. In M. Deutsch, P. T. Coleman, & E. C. Marcus (Eds.), *The handbook of conflict resolution: Theory and practice* (2nd ed., pp. 43–68). San Francisco, CA: Jossey-Bass.

Doris, J. M. (2002). *Lack of character: Personality and moral behavior.* New York, NY: Cambridge University Press.

Dworkin, R. (1972). The original position. *The University of Chicago Law Review, 40,* 500.

Feinberg, J. (1973). *Social philosophy.* Englewood Cliffs, NJ: Prentice-Hall.

Femia, J. V. (1998). Pareto and the critique of justice. In D. Boucher & P. Kelly (Eds.), *Social justice: From Hume to Walzer* (pp. 67–79). London UK: Routledge.

Festinger, L. (1954). A theory of social comparison processes. *Human Relations, 7,* 117–140.

Fiske, A. P., & Tetlock, P. E. (1997). Taboo trade-offs: Reactions to transactions that transgress the spheres of justice. *Political Psychology, 18,* 255–297.

Flanagan, O. (1991). *Varieties of moral personality: Ethics and psychological realism.* Cambridge, MA: Harvard University Press.

Folger, R. (1977). Distributive and procedural justice: Combined impact of "voice" and improvement on experienced inequity. *Journal of Personality and Social Psychology, 35,* 108–119.

Folger, R., & Bies, R. J. (1989). Managerial responsibilities and procedural justice. *Employee Responsibilities and Rights Journal, 2,* 79–90.

Folger, R., Rosenfield, D., Grove, J., & Corkran, L. (1979). Effects of "voice" and peer opinions on responses to inequity. *Journal of Personality and Social Psychology, 37,* 2253–2261.

Fox, D. R. (1999). Psycholegal scholarship's contribution to false consciousness about injustice. *Law and Human Behavior, 23,* 9–30.

Frankena, W. K. (1962). The concept of social justice. In R. B. Brandt (Ed.), *Social justice* (pp. 1–29). Englewood Cliffs, NJ: Prentice-Hall.

Frankfurt, H. (1987). Equality as a moral ideal. *Ethics, 98,* 21–42.

Frohlich, N., & Oppenheimer, J. A. (1990). Choosing justice in experimental democracies with production. *American Political Science Review, 84,* 461–477.

Frohlich, N., & Oppenheimer, J. A. (1992). *Choosing justice: An experimental approach to ethical theory.* Berkeley: University of California Press.

Frohlich, N., Oppenheimer, J. A., & Eavey, C. L. (1987a). Choices of principles of distributive justice in experimental groups. *American Journal of Political Science, 31,* 606–636.

Frohlich, N., Oppenheimer, J. A., & Eavey, C. L. (1987b). Laboratory results on Rawls' principle of distributive justice. *British Journal of Political Science, 17,* 1–21.

Gamliel, E., & Peer, E. (2006). Positive versus negative framing affects justice judgments. *Social Justice Research, 19,* 307–322.

Gibson, J. L. (2008). Group identities and theories of justice: An experimental investigation into the justice and injustice of land squatting in South Africa. *The Journal of Politics, 70,* 700–716.

Gleason, M. E. J., Iida, M., Bolger, N., & Shrout, P. E. (2003). Daily supportive equity in close relationships. *Personality and Social Psychology Bulletin, 29,* 1036–1045.

Goldman, A. (1992). *Liaisons: Philosophy meets the cognitive and social sciences.* Cambridge: MIT Press.

Greenberg, J. (1980). Attentional focus and locus of performance causality as determinants of equity behavior. *Journal of Personality and Social Psychology, 38,* 579–585.

Greenberg, J. (1988). Equity and workplace status: A field experiment. *Journal of Applied Psychology, 73,* 606–613.

Greenberg, J. (1990). Employee theft as a reaction to underpayment inequity: The hidden cost of pay cuts. *Journal of Applied Psychology, 75,* 561–568.

Greenberg, J. (1993). Stealing in the name of justice: Informational and interpersonal moderators of theft reactions to underpayment inequity. *Organizational Behavior and Human Decision Processes, 54,* 81–103.

Greenberg, J., & Jonas, E. (2003). Psychological motives and political orientation—The left, the right, and the rigid: Comment on Jost et al. *Psychological Bulletin, 129,* 376–382.

Greene, J. D. (2003). From neural "is" to moral "ought": What are the moral implications of neuroscientific moral psychology? *Nature Reviews Neuroscience, 4,* 846–849.

Greene, J. D. (2007). Why are VMPFC patients more utilitarian? A dual-process theory of moral judgment explains. *Trends in Cognitive Sciences, 11,* 322–323.

Greene, J. D., & Cohen, J. (2004). For the law, neuroscience changes nothing and everything. *Philosophical Transactions of the Royal Society of London B, 359,* 1775–17785.

Greene, J. D., Morelli, S. A., Lowenberg, K., Nystrom, L. E., & Cohen, J. D. (2008). Cognitive load selectively interferes with utilitarian moral judgment. *Cognition, 107,* 1144–1154.

Gurr, T. (1970). *Why men rebel.* NJ: Princeton University Press.

Haidt, J. (2001). The emotional dog and its rational tail: A social intuitionist approach to moral judgment. *Psychological Review, 108,* 814–834.

Haidt, J., & Graham, J. (2007). When morality opposes justice: Conservatives have moral intuitions that liberals may not recognize. *Social Justice Research, 20,* 98–116.

Hare, R. M. (1981). *Moral thinking: Its levels, method, and point.* New York, NY: Clarendon Press.

Harman, G. (1999). Moral philosophy meets social psychology: Virtue ethics and the fundamental attribution error. *Proceedings of the Aristotelian Society, 99,* 315–331.

Hassebrauck, M. (1986). Ratings of distress as a function of degree and kind of inequity. *Journal of Social Psychology, 126,* 269–270.

Hatfield, E., & Sprecher, S. (1984). Equity theory and behavior in organizations. *Research in the Sociology of Organizations, 3,* 95–124.

Hayek, F. A. (1976). *The mirage of social justice: Law, legislation and liberty* (Vol. 2). Chicago, IL: University of Chicago Press.

Hegtvedt, K. A. (1990). The effects of relationship structure on emotional responses to inequity. *Social Psychology Quarterly, 53,* 214–228.

Homans, G. C. (1961). *Social behavior: Its elementary forms.* London UK: Routledge & Kegan Paul.

Hooker, B. (2011). Rule consequentialism. In E. N. Zalta (Ed.), *The Stanford encyclopedia of philosophy.* Retrieved from http://plato.stanford.edu/entries/consequentialism-rule

Houlden, P., LaTour, S., Walker, L., & Thibaut, J. (1978). Preference for modes of dispute resolution as a function of process and decision control. *Journal of Experimental Social Psychology, 14,* 13–30.

Husami, Z. (1980). Marx on distributive justice. In M. Cohen, T. Nagel, & T. Scanlon (Eds.), *Marx, justice, and history* (pp. 42–79). Princeton, NJ: Princeton University Press. (Original work published 1978).

Jasso, G. (1999). How much injustice is there in the world? Two new justice indexes. *American Sociological Review, 64,* 133–168.

Jost, J. T. (1995). Negative illusions: Conceptual clarification and psychological evidence concerning false consciousness. *Political Psychology, 16,* 397–424.

Jost, J. T. (2006). The end of the end of ideology. *American Psychologist, 61,* 651–670.

Jost, J. T. (2009). "Elective affinities": On the psychological bases of left-right differences. *Psychological Inquiry, 20,* 129–141.

Jost, J. T. (2012). Left and right, right and wrong. [Book review of J. Haidt, *The righteous mind: Why good people are divided by politics and religion.*] *Science, 337,* 525–526.

Jost, J. T., & Banaji, M. R. (1994). The role of stereotyping in system-justification and the production of false consciousness. *British Journal of Social Psychology, 33,* 1–27.

Jost, J. T., Banaji, M. R., & Nosek, B. A. (2004). A decade of system justification theory: Accumulated evidence of conscious and unconscious bolstering of the status quo. *Political Psychology, 25,* 881–920.

Jost, J. T., Glaser, J., Kruglanski, A. W., & Sulloway, F. J. (2003). Political conservatism as motivated social cognition. *Psychological Bulletin, 129,* 339–375.

Jost, J. T., & Kay, A. C. (2010). Social justice: History, theory, and research. In S. T. Fiske, D. Gilbert, & G. Lindzey (Eds.), *Handbook of social psychology* (5th ed., Vol. 2, pp. 1122–1165). Hoboken, NJ: Wiley.

Jost, J. T., Rudman, L. A., Blair, I. V., Carney, D., Dasgupta, N., Glaser, J., & Hardin, C. D. (2009). The existence of implicit bias is beyond reasonable doubt: A refutation of ideological and methodological objections and executive summary of ten studies that no manager should ignore. *Research in Organizational Behavior, 29,* 39–69.

Jost, J. T., & van der Toorn, J. (2012). System justification theory. In P. A. M. van Lange, A. W. Kruglanski, & E. T. Higgins (Eds.), *Handbook of theories of social psychology* (Vol. 2, pp. 313–343). London: Sage.

Jost, J. T., Wakslak, C., & Tyler, T. R. (2008). System Justification Theory and the alleviation of emotional distress: Palliative effects of ideology in an arbitrary social hierarchy and in society. In K. Hegtvedt & J. Clay-Warner (Eds.), *Justice: Advances in group processes* (Vol. 25, pp. 181–211). Bingley, United Kingdom: JAI/Emerald.

Jost, L. J., & Jost, J. T. (2007). Why Marx left philosophy for social science. *Theory & Psychology, 17,* 297–322.

Kahneman, D., Diener, E., & Schwarz, N. (Eds.). (1999). *Well-being: The foundations of a hedonic psychology.* New York, NY: Russell Sage Foundation.

Kahneman, D., Slovic, P., & Tversky, A. (Eds.). (1982). *Judgment under uncertainty: Heuristics and biases.* New York, NY: Cambridge University Press.

Kant, I. (2005). *Groundwork for the metaphysics of morals.* (T. K. Abbott, Trans.). L. Denis (Ed.). Toronto, Ontario: Broadview. (Original work published 1785).

Kelman, H. C. (1983). Creating the conditions for Israeli-Palestinian negotiations. *Journal of Conflict Resolution, 26,* 39–75.

Kelman, H. C. (2001). Reflections on the social and psychological processes of legitimization and delegitimization. In J. T. Jost, & B. Major (Eds.), *The psychology of legitimacy: Emerging perspectives on ideology, justice, and intergroup relations* (pp. 54–73). Cambridge, United Kingdom: Cambridge University Press.

Kelman, H. C., & Hamilton, V. L. (1989). *Crimes of obedience: Toward a social psychology of authority and responsibility.* New Haven, CT: Yale University Press.

Kohlberg, L. (1969). Stage and sequence: The cognitive-developmental approach to socialization. In D. Goslin (Ed.), *Handbook of socialization theory and research* (pp. 347–480). Chicago, IL: Rand-McNally.

Konow, J. (2003). Which is the fairest one of all? A positive analysis of justice theories. *Journal of Economic Literature, 41,* 1188–1239.

Kornblith, H. (Ed.). (1999). *Naturalizing epistemology.* Cambridge, MA: MIT Press.

Lamm, H., & Schwinger, T. (1980). Norms concerning distributive justice: Are needs taken into consideration in allocation decisions? *Social Psychology Quarterly, 4,* 425–429.

Lerner, M. J. (1974). The justice motive: "Equity" and "parity" among children. *Journal of Personality and Social Psychology, 29,* 539–550.

Lerner, M. J. (1980). *The belief in a just world: A fundamental delusion.* New York, NY: Plenum.

Lerner, M. J. (2003). The justice motive: Where social psychologists found it, how they lost it, and why they may not find it again. *Personality and Social Psychology Review, 7,* 388–399.

Leung, K., & Stephan, W. G. (2000). Conflict and injustice in intercultural relations: Insights from the Arab-Israeli and Sino-British disputes. In S. Renshon & J. Duckitt (Eds.), *Political psychology: Cultural and cross-cultural perspectives* (pp. 128–145). New York, NY: McMillan.

Leventhal, G. S. (1980). What should be done with equity theory? New approaches to the study of fairness in social relationships. In K. Gergen, M. Greenberg, & R. Willis (Eds.), *Social exchange* (pp. 27–55). New York: Plenum Press.

Leventhal, G. S., & Anderson, D. (1970). Self-interest and the maintenance of equity. *Journal of Personality and Social Psychology, 15,* 57–62.

Leventhal, G. S., Karuza, J., & Fry, W. R. (1980). Beyond fairness: A theory of allocation preferences. In G. Mikula (Ed.), *Justice and social interaction* (pp. 167–218). New York, NY: Springer-Verlag.

Lewin, K. (1948). Experiments in social space. In K. Lewin (Ed.), *Resolving social conflicts* (pp. 71–83). New York, NY: Harper. (Original work published 1939).

Lind, E. A., & Tyler, T. R. (1988). *The social psychology of procedural justice.* New York, NY: Plenum.

Loewenstein, G. F., Thompson, L., & Bazerman, M. H. (1989). Social utility and decision making in interpersonal contexts. *Journal of Personality and Social Psychology, 57,* 426–441.

Lupfer, M. B., Weeks, K. P., Doan, K. A., & Houston, D. A. (2000). Folk conceptions of fairness and unfairness. *European Journal of Social Psychology, 30,* 405–428.

Mansbridge, J. (2005). Cracking through hegemonic ideology: The logic of formal justice. *Social Justice Research, 18,* 335–347.

Markowski, B. (1988). Injustice and arousal. *Social Justice Research, 2,* 223–233.

Martin, J. (1986). The tolerance of injustice. In J. M. Olson, C. P. Herman, & M. P. Zanna (Eds.), *Relative deprivation and social comparison: The Ontario Symposium* (pp. 217–242). Hillsdale, NJ: Erlbaum.

Martin, J., Scully, M., & Levitt, B. (1990). Injustice and the legitimation of revolution: Damning the past, excusing the present, and neglecting the future. *Journal of Personality and Social Psychology, 59,* 281–290.

Marx, K. (2008). *Critique of the Gotha Program.* Rockville, MD: Wildside Press. (Original work written 1875).

Matania, E., & Yaniv, I. (2007). Resource priority, fairness, and equality-efficiency compromises. *Social Justice Research, 20,* 497–510.

Michelbach, P. A., Scott, J. T., Matland, R. E., & Bornstein, B. H. (2003). Doing Rawls justice: An experimental study of income distribution norms. *American Journal of Political Science, 47,* 523–539.

Mikula, G. (1984). Justice and fairness in interpersonal relations: Thoughts and suggestions. In H. Tajfel (Ed.), *The social dimension* (pp. 204–227). Cambridge, United Kingdom: Cambridge University Press.

Mikula, G., & Wenzel, M. (2000). Justice and social conflict. *International Journal of Psychology, 35,* 126–135.

Mill, J. S. (1910). *Utilitarianism, liberty and representation.* New York, NY: E.P. Dutton.

Miller, D. (1999). *Principles of social justice.* Cambridge, MA: Harvard University Press.

Miller, D. T. (2001). Disrespect and the experience of injustice. *Annual Review of Psychology, 52,* 527–553.

Mitchell, G., Tetlock, P. E., Mellers, B. A., & Ordóñez, L. D. (1993). Judgments of social justice: Compromises between equality and efficiency. *Journal of Personality and Social Psychology, 65,* 629–639.

Mitchell, G., Tetlock, P. E., Newman, D. G., & Lerner, J. S. (2003). Experiments behind the veil: Structural influences on judgments of social justice. *Political Psychology, 24,* 519–547.

Montada, L. (2003). Justice, equity, and fairness in human relations. In T. Millon & M. J. Lerner (Eds.), *Handbook of psychology: Personality and social psychology* (Vol. 5, pp. 532–568). Hoboken, NJ: John Wiley & Sons Inc.

Montada, L., & Schneider, A. (1989). Justice and emotional reactions to the disadvantaged. *Social Justice Research, 3,* 313–344.

Moore, B. (1978). *Injustice: The social bases of obedience and revolt.* White Plains, NY: Sharpe.

Mowday, R. T. (1991). Equity theory predictions of behavior in organizations. In R. M. Steers & L. W. Porter (Eds.), *Motivation and work behavior* (3rd ed., pp. 91–112). New York, NY: McGraw-Hill.

Nagel, T. (1991). *Equality and partiality.* New York, NY: Oxford University Press.

Napier, J. L., & Jost, J. T. (2008). Why are conservatives happier than liberals? *Psychological Science, 19,* 565–572.

Nielsen, K. (1985). *Equality and liberty: A defense of radical egalitarianism.* Totowa, NJ: Rowman & Allanheld.

Norton, M. I., & Ariely, D. (2011). Building a better America—One wealth quintile at a time. *Perspectives on Psychological Science, 6,* 9–12.

Nozick, R. (1974). *Anarchy, state and utopia.* New York, NY: Basic Books.

Parfit, D. (1998). Equality and priority. In A. Mason (Ed.), *Ideals of equality* (pp. 1–20). Oxford, United Kingdom: Blackwell.

Payne, B. K., & Cameron, C. D. (2010). Divided minds, divided morals: How implicit social cognition underpins and undermines our sense of social justice. In B. Gawronski & B. K. Payne (Eds.), *Handbook of implicit social cognition: Measurement, theory, and applications.* New York, NY: Guilford.

Peters, S. L., Van den Bos, K., & Bobocel, D. R. (2004). The moral superiority effect: Self versus other differences in satisfaction with being overpaid. *Social Justice Research, 17,* 257–273.

Piaget, J. (1965). *The moral judgment of the child.* New York, NY: Free Press. (Original work published 1932).

Rasinski, K. A. (1987). What's fair is fair—or is it? Value differences underlying public views about social justice. *Journal of Personality and Social Psychology, 53,* 201–211.

Rawls, J. (1971). *A theory of justice.* Oxford, United Kingdom: Oxford University Press.

Rawls, J. (1993). *Political liberalism.* New York, NY: Columbia University Press.

Reis, H. T. (1984). The multidimensionality of justice. In R. Folger (Ed.), *The sense of injustice: Social psychological perspectives* (pp. 25–61). New York, NY: Plenum Press.

Ring, K. (1967). Experimental social psychology: Some sober questions about some frivolous values. *Journal of Experimental Social Psychology, 3,* 113–123.

Rummel, R. J. (1997). *Death by government.* New Brunswick, NJ: Transactions.

Sampson, E. E., (1983). Deconstructing psychology's subject. *Journal of Mind and Behavior, 4,* 135–164.

Sandel, M. J. (1998). *Liberalism and the limits of justice* (2nd ed.). New York, NY: Cambridge University Press.

Sandel, M. J. (2005). *Public philosophy: Essays on morality in politics.* Cambridge, MA: Harvard University Press.

Schmitt, M., Behner, R., Montada, L., Müller, L., & Müller-Fohrbrodt, G. (2000). Gender, ethnicity, and education as privileges: Exploring the generalizability of the existential guilt reaction. *Social Justice Research, 13,* 313–337.

Schnall, S., Haidt, J., Clore, G. L., & Jordan, A. H. (2008). Disgust as embodied moral judgment. *Personality and Social Psychology Bulletin, 34,* 1096–1109.

Schulz, U., & May, T. (1989). The recording of social orientations with ranking and pair comparison procedures. *European Journal of Social Psychology, 19,* 41–59.

Schwinger, T. (1986). The need principle of distributive justice. In H. W. Bierhoff, R. L. Cohen, & J. Greenberg (Eds.), *Justice in social relations* (pp. 211–226). New York, NY: Plenum.

Scott, J. T., Matland, R. E., Michelbach, P. A., & Bornstein, B. H. (2001). Just deserts: An experimental study of distributive justice norms. *American Journal of Political Science, 45,* 749–767.

Sen, A. (1979). The welfare basis of real income comparisons. *Journal of Economic Literature, 17,* 1–45.

Shapiro, I. (2003). *The moral foundations of politics.* New Haven, CT: Yale University Press.

Sidanius, J., & Pratto, F. (1999). *Social dominance: An intergroup theory of social hierarchy and oppression.* New York, NY: Cambridge University Press.

Skitka, L. J. (2003). Of different minds: An accessible identity model of justice reasoning. *Personality and Social Psychology Review, 7,* 286–297.

Skitka, L. J., & Crosby, F. J. (2003). Trends in the social psychological study of justice. *Personality and Social Psychology Review, 7,* 282–285.

Skitka, L. J., & Tetlock, P. E. (1993). Providing public assistance: Cognitive and motivational processes underlying liberal and conservative policy preferences. *Journal of Personality and Social Psychology, 65,* 1205–1223.

Smith, A. (1776). *An inquiry into the nature and causes of the wealth of nations.* London, UK: Dent.

Solomon, R. C. (1990). *A passion for justice: Emotions and the origins of the social contract.* Reading, MA: Addison-Wesley.

Solomon, R. C., & Murphy, M. C. (Eds.). (2000). *What is justice? Classic and contemporary readings.* New York, NY: Oxford University Press.

Sprecher, S., & Schwartz, P. (1994). Equity and balance in the exchange of contributions in close relationships. In M. J. Lerner & G. Mikula (Eds.), *Entitlement and the affectional bond: Justice in close relationships* (pp. 11–41). New York, NY: Plenum Press.

Staub, E. (2011). *Overcoming evil: Genocide, violent conflict, and terrorism.* New York, NY: Oxford University Press.

Thaler, R. H. (1991). *Quasi rational economics.* New York, NY: Russell Sage Foundation.

Thibaut, J., & Walker, L. (1975). *Procedural justice.* Hillsdale, NJ: Erlbaum.

Törnblom, K. Y., & Foa, U. G. (1983). Choice of a distribution principle: Crosscultural evidence on the effects of resources. *Acta Sociologica, 26,* 161–173.

Toynbee, A. J. (1976). *Choose life: A dialogue between Arnold Toynbee and Daisaku Ikeda.* Oxford, UK: Oxford University Press. (Reprinted in 2007).

Tucker, R. (1969). *The Marxian revolutionary idea.* New York, NY: Norton.

Tyler, T. R. (2006). Psychological perspectives on legitimacy and legitimation. *Annual Review of Psychology, 57,* 375–400.

Tyler, T. R., & Bies, R. (1990). Interpersonal aspects of procedural justice. In J. S. Carroll (Ed.), *Applied social psychology in business settings* (pp. 77–98). Hillsdale, NJ: Erlbaum.

Tyler, T. R., & Jost, J. T. (2007). Psychology and the law: Reconciling normative and descriptive accounts of social justice and system legitimacy. In A. W. Kruglanski & E. T. Higgins (Eds.), *Social psychology: Handbook of basic principles* (pp. 807–825). New York, NY: Guilford.

Tyler, T. R., & Lind, E. A. (1992). A relational model of authority in groups. In M. P. Zanna (Ed.), *Advances in experimental social psychology* (Vol. 25, pp. 115–191). San Diego, CA: Academic Press.

Tyler, T. R., & McGraw, K. M. (1986). Ideology and the interpretation of personal experience: Procedural justice and political quiescence. *Journal of Social Issues, 42,* 115–128.

Tyler, T. R., & Smith, H. J. (1998). Social justice and social movements. In D. G. Gilbert, S. T. Fiske, & G. Lindzey (Eds.), *The handbook of social psychology* (4th ed., pp. 595–629). Boston, MA: McGraw-Hill.

Utne, M. K., Hatfield, E., Traupmann, J., & Greenberger, D. (1984). Equity, marital satisfaction, and stability. *Journal of Social and Personal Relationships, 1,* 323–332.

Van den Bos, K. (2005). What is responsible for the fair process effect? In J. Greenberg & J. A. Colquitt (Eds.), *Handbook of organizational justice* (pp. 273–300). Mahwah, NJ: Erlbaum.

Van Prooijen, J., Van den Bos, K., & Wilke, H. A. M. (2004). Group belongingness and procedural justice: Social inclusion and exclusion by peers affects the psychology of voice. *Journal of Personality and Social Psychology, 87,* 66–79.

Van Stekelenburg, J., & Klandermans, B. (2007). Individuals in movements: A social psychology of contention. In C. M. Roggeband & B. Klandermans (Eds.). *The handbook of social movements across disciplines* (pp. 157–204). New York, NY: Springer.

Van Yperen, N. W., & Buunk, B. P. (1990). A longitudinal study of equity and satisfaction in intimate relationships. *European Journal of Social Psychology, 20,* 287–309.

Van Zomeren, M., Postmes, T., & Spears, R. (2008). Toward an integrative social identity model of collective action: A quantitative research synthesis of three socio-psychological perspectives. *Psychological Bulletin, 134,* 504–535.

Vidmar, N. (2002). Retributive justice: Its social context. In M. Ross & D. T. Miller (Eds.), *The justice motive in everyday life* (pp. 291–313). New York, NY: Cambridge University Press.

Viereck, P. (1956). *Conservatism.* Princeton, NJ: D. Van Nostrand.

Vlastos, G. (1997). Justice and equality. In L. P. Pojman, & R. Westmoreland (Eds.), *Equality: Selected readings* (pp. 120–133). New York, NY: Oxford University Press. (Original work published 1962).

Wakslak, C. J., Jost, J. T., Tyler, T. R., & Chen, E. S. (2007). Moral outrage mediates the dampening effect of system justification on support for redistributive social policies. *Psychological Science, 18,* 267–274.

Walker, L., Lind, E. A., & Thibaut, J. (1979). The relation between procedural and distributive justice. *Virginia Law Review, 65,* 1401–1420.

Walster, E., Berscheid, E., & Walster, G. W. (1973). New directions in equity research. *Journal of Personality and Social Psychology, 25,* 151–176.

Walster, E. G., Walster, W., & Berscheid, E. (1978). *Equity: Theory and research.* Boston, MA: Allyn & Bacon.

Walzer, M. (1983). *Spheres of justice.* New York, NY: Basic Books.

Wenzel, M. (2000). Justice and identity: The significance of inclusion for perceptions of entitlement and the justice motive. *Personality and Social Psychology Bulletin, 26,* 157–176.

Wenzel, M. (2001). A social categorization approach to distributive justice: Social identity as the link between relevance of inputs and need for justice. *British Journal of Social Psychology, 40,* 315–335.

Wenzel, M. (2002). What is social about justice? Inclusive identity and group values as the basis of the justice motive. *Journal of Experimental Social Psychology, 38,* 205–218.

White, R. J. (1950). *The conservative tradition.* New York, NY: New York University Press.

Wildavsky, A. (1989). Choosing preferences by constructing institutions: A cultural theory of preference formation. In A. Berger (Ed.), *Political culture and public opinion* (pp. 21–46). New Brunswick, NJ: Transaction.

Wildavsky, A. (1991). *The rise of radical egalitarianism.* Washington, DC: American University Press.

Williams, B. (2000). Equality. In R. C. Solomon & M. C. Murphy (Eds.), *What is justice? Classic and contemporary readings* (pp. 188–194). New York, NY: Oxford University Press. (Original work published 1976).

Wood, A. W. (1980). The Marxian critique of justice. In M. Cohen, T. Nagel, & T. Scanlon (Eds.), *Marx, justice, and history* (pp. 3–41). Princeton, NJ: Princeton University Press. (Original work published 1972).

Chapter 2

A Psychological Framework for Social Justice Praxis

Jeannette Diaz

The integration of social justice perspectives within psychological research and theory is important for the discipline of psychology. Developing a psychological framework for social justice theory requires a critical and integrative understanding of the various dimensions and conceptualizations of social justice as reflected in key psychological traditions of research, theory, and praxis. This chapter provides this perspective through the synthesis of selected psychological literature on social justice. Given that social justice is an interdisciplinary venture, I also examine literature from other disciplines, most notably criminology and economics, as well as international frameworks of social justice as codified in documents such as the UN Universal Declaration of Human Rights and the UN Millennium Development Goals.

This chapter begins with an overview of existing conceptualizations and definitions of social justice in order to provide a common frame of understanding followed by a reframing of social justice within a global context and a broad-brush description of extant psychological social justice praxis. I then progress to a discussion of the socially constructed nature of social justice and the role of empathy and empowerment in social justice. Drawing from these deliberations, I frame social justice as a relational process founded upon empathy and empowerment, rather than an idealized outcome state. I offer implications of this understanding of social justice for teaching, practice, and research in psychology.

DIMENSIONS OF SOCIAL JUSTICE

Distributive Justice

Distributive justice focuses primarily on the manner in which resources are distributed within a society. As discussed by Jost and Kay (2010), contemporary theories on distributive justice find their roots in the early writings of Aristotle who discussed the distribution of resources in society as linked to issues of equity and merit, a conception of justice that emphasizes equity and proportionality vis-à-vis an individual's disposition, behavior, and effort. In their nuanced discussion of Aristotelian notions of justice, Jost and Kay examine the extent to which political and ideological differences hinder the ability to reach agreement on equity, merit, and the most beneficial structure for society (see also Jost, 2009). Such differences are oftentimes at the heart of political disputes and even violent conflict, and distinctions between governance models (i.e. statist, communist, socialist, democratic, democratic socialism) are commonly based on philosophical differences regarding the distribution of social and material goods in a society. Does a government institutionalize a safety net for its citizens that may result in people receiving benefits they do not deserve? Does the practice of distributive justice follow the principle of "each according to his/her need" or that of "each according to what he/she deserves?" and, in either one of these cases, who decides what constitutes need or deserving behavior/effort? Both the UN Universal Declaration of Human Rights (United Nations, 2012) and the UN Millennium Development Goals (United Nations, 2012) take a position on distributive justice based on basic human need: all living beings, simply by virtue of being human, have the right to food, clean water, health, gender equality, primary education. Yet other forms of social structure, for example, those based on aristocracy and lineage, may hold that class position is what defines merit and access to resources. In a world that is far from equitable, ideological differences regarding equity versus system justification (Blasi & Jost, 2006) make it very difficult to agree whether or not, or the process by which, humans should achieve the ideals of distributive justice.

Procedural Justice

In the 1970s Thibaut and Walker (1978) drew attention to aspects of justice inherent within the decision-making process itself, pointing out that human beings are process-driven as well as outcome-driven. Thibaut and Walker's work, which focused primarily on the resolution of conflict, helped clarify the extent to which the justice "litmus test" of legal proceedings is the extent to which egotistical concerns are mitigated through a decision-making process that equally distributes procedural control among the parties involved.

As outlined by Jost and Kay (2012), the body of empirical literature in the area of procedural justice suggests that control, the opportunity to express one's views and feelings, and perceptions regarding process characteristics (consistency, neutrality, accuracy, self-correction, and ethical behavior) are all grounded in perceptions of procedural justice. When people are aware that they have input into, and some form of control over, the procedures and processes involved in justice-based decisions, they tend to be more satisfied with these decisions and outcomes (Thibaut & Walker, 1975). Thibaut and Walkers' seminal ideas, and the subsequent research these ideas spawned (Lind & Tyler, 1988), situated social justice within the context of psychological processes of perceptions, cognition, agency, and affect.

Achieving the ideals of procedural justice is complicated by the same psychological dynamics that problematize distributive justice; who is permitted agency and awarded a voice in the decision-making processes of justice is typically decided by those in power through the systems they have created. Does an inter-sexed baby have voice regarding sex assignment decisions made on his or her behalf? Is a woman, by virtue of the fact that she is born in a society that devalues women, worthy or unworthy of procedural justice? To what extent does a person suffering from a mental illness have the right to express his or her opinion regarding institutionalization? Who ensures that the governing bodies of the poorest and least developed countries have a fair say in the framing of global trade agreements? Within the sphere of ecological and animal rights movements, who gives voice to living beings that are voiceless? As with distributive justice, the answers to these questions rest upon decisions regarding merit and, in a broader sense, perceptions of morality.

Interactional and Relational Justice

Bies (2001), drawing from narrative data that focused on people's experience of injustice, came to the conclusion that people care not only about the procedural aspects of justice-oriented decision making but also about the manner in which they are treated by others. He writes: "people possess a view of the self as 'sacred,' and a violation of that sacred self arouses the sense of injustice" (p. 90). Steeped in the context of the organizational setting, Bies astutely noted that worker satisfaction is related to a sense of being valued by an organization; this sense of value emerges from interactions that are respectful, truthful, proprietary, and fair (see also Colquitt, Conlon, Wesson, Porter, & Ng, 2001). For Bies, justice arises within the interpersonal realm of relationship.

This interpretation of justice is similar to that discussed by Gilligan (1982) who viewed justice as emergent from the context of relationship as opposed to a logical process of evaluating inputs to outputs. Posing the classic Heinz dilemma to both girls and boys, Gilligan discovered that the responses provided by girls indicated that, for them, justice was epiphenomenal to relationship. This moral dilemma places the need for a husband (Heinz) to save his wife's life in juxtaposition to the rights of a pharmacist to charge a price for a life-saving medicine, albeit an exorbitant price. Should Heinz steal the drug to save his wife's life? Gilligan's young participant Amy believed that if the pharmacist is simply made to see the impact of his actions (charging too much for the drug) then surely he will change his position and reach an agreement with the dying woman's husband (p. 29). Amy's position vis-à-vis this dilemma was consonant with those of the other girls and young women interviewed by Gilligan. Within this relational framework, justice arises from the web of relationships of care and meaning, a web that sensitizes individuals to the implications of their actions for another human being.

Restorative Justice

As discussed by Cordella (2008), typical notions of justice are inherently exclusionary in that certain individuals or groups are perceived as not having the capacity to engage in dialogues of justice. As he astutely points out, within the context of the criminal justice system transgressors are viewed in one of three ways: psychologically deficient and in need of therapeutic intervention, morally deficient and in need of punishment, rationally deficient and therefore not capable of contributing to the overall happiness and well-being of a society. In each of these views, fault lies within the boundaries of the individual rather than in the reciprocal relationship between the offender and the systems that govern that individual. Restorative justice approaches move away from this deficit model of the individual to view each person as fully capable of engaging, as an equal, in dialogues of justice and healing. The assumption of restorative justice is that relationships are "set right" when the person responsible for inflicting harm or damage is able to confront the person he or she harmed and acknowledge his or her misconduct. The ontogenetic assumption of restorative justice is that human beings are all linked to one another: harm to one individual results in harm to all individuals (Sullivan & Tifft, 2008).

Although similar to the procedural justice approach in its focus on voice and empowerment, the desired outcomes of a restorative justice approach are no less than the creation of a participatory civil society where each person, without exception, is included in the process of participation, thereby creating connections between individuals and the larger community and creating a space for empathy, mutual understanding, restitution, and accountability (Braithwhaite, 2006; Pranis, 2007).

The most well-known example of restorative justice is that of the South African Government of Reconciliation where perpetrators and victims of the system of apartheid were brought together to hear each other's stories in the hopes of contributing to a national process of healing and forgiveness. Less well known are projects such as healing circles in New Zealand (Maxwell & Morris, 2006); Victim Offender Mediation (VOM) programs in Europe (Pelikan & Trenczek, 2006); Victim Offender Reconciliation Programs (VORP) in the United States (Bradshaw & Roseborough, 2005); the use of restorative justice circles in the classroom

(Stuart & Pranis, 2007); and various interventions in prisons, courtrooms, church halls, and community centers in countries and communities throughout the world (www.restorativejustice.org).

Although the widespread appeal of restorative justice is clear, the approach is not without criticism. As discussed by Daly (2007), restorative justice processes are successful only to the extent that perpetrators are truly able to apologize and victims are truly able to forgive. Williams and Arrigo (2001) critique the highly structured and scripted nature of VOM programs that dictate how participants must behave and constrain the outcomes that can be reached. Additionally, there is concern that restorative justice does not address the larger structural issues that may give rise to criminal behavior, thereby falling short of its goal of social transformation (Gil, 2007; Sullivan & Tifft, 2007).

Retributive Justice

Retributive justice focuses on how individuals respond when they view a person (or a group) inflicting harm upon another and is, essentially, focused on moral intuitions that everyday people hold (Darley & Pittman, 2003). Research in this domain explores the attributions individuals make regarding wrongdoing. If, for example, individual A harms individual B purely by accident (i.e., with no malicious intent), then the interpretation of individual A's behavior would be different from if individual A harmed individual B through malicious intent. People also make attributions regarding whether or not individual B deserved to be harmed by individual A (as in the case of the death penalty).

The role of emotion in the enactment of justice is readily seen in the domain of retributive justice. For example, historically in the United States the punishment administered to a Black person who killed a White person was much harsher than that administered to a White person who killed a Black person. The difference was not the crime itself, but the differential value placed upon the life of a White person versus that of a Black person and the differential emotion experienced by White jurors vis-à-vis a White victim and Black perpetrator versus a Black victim and White perpetrator (Gross & Mauro, 1989). More recently, Demuth (2003) documented the "triple burden" that Latino defendants undergo at pre-trial stages, being the one group more likely to be required to pay bail and to receive the highest bail amounts, despite the fact that they are the group least able to pay bail. Unnever and Cullen (2007) show the extent to which White racism, in their survey of White and Black Americans, was the strongest predictor of support for the death penalty. These studies point out the social-cognitive underpinnings of justice.

Social Justice as Human Development

Gould (2008) defines social justice as equal access to the conditions required for self-transformation and/or self-development; essentially, social justice across the life span results in human flourishing across the life span. Economists have also developed theoretical frameworks for understanding the optimum conditions under which humans flourish. Most notable of these is the work of Sen (1999) who articulates economic development as improvements that eliminate major sources of "unfreedom"—poverty, tyranny, social deprivation, neglect of public facilities and resources, political repression. The notion of human rights codified in the UN Universal Declaration of Human Rights was created in the hope of institutionalizing norms of distributive and procedural justice in a manner that ultimately results in ensuring equal access to the conditions required for humans to flourish.

Nussbaum (2003) critiqued the UN notion of human rights as limited by a legalistic, individualistic, and culturally bound understanding of human rights. In its stead, Nussbaum proposed a capabilities approach to human rights that focuses on what people are actually capable of doing and what people value doing. Nussbaum's approach is in contrast to a normative notion of what people need and parallels the critiques that standard developmental approaches in psychology offer a prescriptive "one sides fits all" understanding of human development and flourishing (Jensen, 2011b). Nussbaum's idea of human capability provides a culturally sensitized way of implementing Gould's idea of social justice as human development and converges with psychology's recent understanding of the importance of cross-cultural variations in development (Arnett, 2012; Jensen, 2011a).

Global Social Justice

Capeheart and Milavonavic (2007) astutely point out that social justice is fluid and dynamic, and changes as a result of variations in the political, cultural, and social climate. A historical and temporal framing of social justice requires embedding notions of social justice into a newly contextualized awareness of global socioeconomic and sociopolitical relations (Diaz & Zirkel, 2012; Marsella, 2012). Extant understandings of poverty, for example, reflect awareness that the processes that mitigate or exacerbate poverty are cross-national and multinational in nature and scope. These processes involve integrated global systems of production and distribution that link producers and consumers, customers and service providers in intricate webs of production that are at any one time exploitative or beneficial depending upon where one is situated in this global web (i.e., Aneesh, 2006; Harrison, 2006; Parrenas, 2001; Shiva, 2000). In various countries throughout the world, poverty is the result of decisions made by distant agents of international financial institutions on the part of developing countries through decision-making processes that are distinctly void of procedural justice (Diaz, Schneider, & Pwogwam Sante Mantal, 2012; Dollar, 2001).

Robinson (2005), in articulating a vision for global social justice, pointed out the difficulties of limiting a discussion of social justice to the boundaries of the nation-state. The interdependence that is a defining characteristic of globalization highlights the false dichotomy between the "local" and the "global"; conversations about "us" and "them" ring hollow in an era where each person's material and nutritional life-world is linked to the lives and hands of thousands of people throughout the globe. As with Gilligan (1982), Robinson speaks of the interdependent nature of morality and of the basic human need for care, which, in her analysis, is as much a moral prescription for global relations as it is a moral orientation for interpersonal relations. Her discussion of global justice as global care brings to mind the wizened faces of the elderly people of the small island nation of Tuvalu, a nation-state slowly inundated by the rising tides of the world's seas and oceans. In a world where refugees are legally defined as political refugees and where immigration criteria are often decided through merit, the elderly grandmothers of Tuvalu are left to fend for themselves (Nash, 2010): a global ethic of care makes their fate our fate.

An understanding of the globally integrated nature of humanity requires an expansive reconceptualization of traditional notions of social justice: resource distribution not just for citizens within a reified notion of the nation-state, but for citizens throughout the world; engagement of all human beings in the decision-making processes that impact their livelihood (e.g., the engagement of the small farmer in trade decisions); the creation of forums for dialogue through which perpetrators and victims at the global level sit face-to-face (e.g., the CEOs of multinational corporations and international financial institutions and the villagers left homeless or unemployed because of global trade agreements or damaging environmental practices); and fair labor and employment for all individuals regardless of age or nationality (International Labour Organization, 2008). As discussed by Scott et al. (2011), the global marketplace requires an inclusive notion of social justice that incorporates analyses of consumption patterns and their relationship to a global capacity to maximize human capability. The global ethics of care discussed by Robinson (2005) require shifting the I-It nature of the relationship between producer and consumer to an I-Thou relationship (Buber, 1937).

Psychology and Social Justice

Decades ago, in an article in *The American Psychologist*, George Albee created a vision and plan for how psychology could realize a just society (Albee, 1982, 1986; Pachter & De Leon, 2006). He defined a just society as "a world in which preventable stress has been reduced for the majority of people"; and one "in which everyone has the opportunity to maximize his or her potential as long as such behavior does not infringe on the rights of others" (1986, p. 896). Further, he defined specific conditions and activities that would lead to a just world—safe water, immunization programs, adequate sewer systems, equitable food distribution, fast-growing trees for fuel, safe farming practices, empowerment for those who are disenfranchised and the elimination of child abuse, sexual abuse, involuntary unemployment, discrimination, racism, and sexism. In short, Albee viewed societal inequality and concomitant powerless and exploitation as the nomothetic underpinnings of ill health and psychopathology for human beings throughout the world. Albee's view of social justice is reflected in Goodman et al.'s (2004) more recent discussion of social justice in counseling psychology where they, again, discuss social justice as existing when each person has access to food, safety, education, health care, child care, sleep and freedom from slavery, exploitation, terrorism, and more. These authors develop a framework for how counseling psychologists can engage in the work of providing disadvantaged individuals and groups with access to all the conditions required for justice. As an institution, the American Psychological Association (APA) has embraced social justice as a worthy goal of the discipline writ large. This commitment is evidenced by the APA Resolution on Poverty and Socioeconomic Status (APA, 2000), the APA Statement on Reforming the Juvenile Justice System (APA, 2010), various statements and policy positions regarding LGBT concerns, and specific statements developed by individual APA divisions (e.g., Ellsworth, Haney, & Costanzo, 2001).

Most recently, Vasquez (2012), in her APA presidential address, drew attention to the fact that many subdisciplines of psychology, most notably, community, social, and counseling, have made specific commitments to social justice through focusing on the elimination of human suffering and the promotion of equality. She also illuminated the various ways in which other subdisciplines in psychology (e.g., cognitive, developmental) provide important insights into the psychological dynamics of social justice and reveal the psychological underpinnings of beliefs such as racism or behaviors such as violence. In her presidential address Vasquez defined social justice as: " 'fairness,' behaving toward others in an impartial manner with the goal of treating others equally" (p. 338). She goes on to state that in situations of inequality, treating others "fairly" may mean treating others unequally in order to rectify historical situations of inequality. Her recapitulation of social justice, similar to the definition of social justice offered by Albee (1982, 1986), reflects common definitions of social justice as the equitable distribution of resources, the elimination of oppression, and the implementation of norms of fairness.

For psychologists, advocating socially just systems, relationships, and processes is increasingly an outcome of empirical evidence demonstrating the importance of social justice to human health and well-being. Such research emanates from, and resonates with, ecological and bio-psychosocial models of analysis that posit that any one person's developmental trajectory can be fully understood only through a systematic understanding of the systems within which he or she is embedded (Biglan Flay, Embry, & Sandler, 2012; Bronfrenbrenner, 1977; Kenny, Horne, Orpinas, & Reese, 2009; Nelson & Prilleltensky, 2005). Psychologists know that inequity results in differential access to resources and, as a result, differential capacity to flourish throughout the lifespan (Bullock & Lott, 2001). Patel (2007) discussed the cyclical relationship between economic underdevelopment and poor mental health; Prilleltensky and Prilleltensky (2006) discussed the relationship between societal inequity and poor psychosocial well-being; Beard (2003) explored how inadequate nutrition can lead to permanent loss of cognitive developmental capacity; Pieterse, Neville, Todd, and Carter (2012) examined how perceptions of racism are negatively associated with mental health. In psychology the praxis of social justice typically involves promoting psychosocial well-being through directly addressing systems and practices of injustice or through empowering and healing at the individual level.

WHERE IS SOCIAL JUSTICE LOCATED?

A central difference across conceptualizations of social justice is where social justice is located. In the distributive and procedural dimensions of social justice, justice lies in the hands of those who have resources and those who make decisions. Jost and Kay (2010) state that justice is a property of social systems and the capacity of systems to foster psychosocial well-being, empowerment, inclusion, democratic decision making, and flourishing. The ecological and bio-psychosocial perspectives of psychology discussed also situate social justice within systems. The codification of social justice in documents such as the UN Universal Declaration of Human Rights or the International Rights of the Child are exemplars of the notion of social justice as a system characteristic. In the relational and restorative aspects of social justice, justice lies within persons themselves and varies according to individual capacity to shift relational communication patterns and psychological responses to the other. As evidenced by the intense practices of restorative justice, these shifts oftentimes occur only through mediated face-to-face meetings that allow each person to glimpse through veils of information and/or prejudice to see the other as a vulnerable human being.

Upon closer inspection, the distinction between system and individual presents a false dichotomy. As argued by Halliburton (2004), for example, changing the system or legal structure does not guarantee social justice. His analysis demonstrates that although previous civil decisions in the United States such as *Brown vs. the Board of Education* (1954) sought to eliminate racial bias from systems of procedural justice, such laws have not changed the racial biases that exist within the hearts and minds of the people entrusted to enact these laws. As such, individual acts of racial bias result in the perpetuation of institutionally racialized systems that, in turn, perpetuate procedural and distributive injustice. Halliburton's analysis requires linking the thoughts and feelings of individuals to the day-to-day functioning of the systems that they create and enact.

SOCIAL JUSTICE AS SOCIAL CONSTRUCTION

A common theme across all dimensions of social justice discussed thus far is the socially constructed nature of social justice—an act, event, or institution is defined as just if most people believe it to be so (Colquitt et al., 2001); individual understandings of merit, morality, and equity, shape individual and system responses to justice. Complicating a social constructivist notion of justice are studies that demonstrate the existence of perceptions of fairness in nonhuman primates as well as in domesticated dogs and certain fish species (Brosnan & de Waal, 2012). Such studies elucidate the extent to which responses to perceptions of fairness and equity may be an evolutionarily selected for and essential component of what it means to be human. At the same time, it is difficult to negate the role of social-perception in human understandings of and responses to fairness and equity. Although conceptualizations of social justice typically ignore or underplay the role of prejudice in the maintenance of systems of oppression (Scott et al., 2011), it is these fundamentally psychological aspects of social justice, shared beliefs of who is and is not worthy, that determine our capacity to realize social justice.

Social Justice and Moral Exclusion

As considered within moral exclusion theory (Opotow, Gerson, & Woodside, 2005), each person has a scope of justice—the psychological boundary that surrounds those individuals whom one believes are deserving of moral treatment. Those who fall outside this boundary are morally excluded from just and fair treatment, and subsequently deemed eligible or deserving of deprivation, exploitation, or other harmful behavior. As discussed by Woolf and MacCartney (2014), in many parts of the world people who are not self-identified as heterosexual fall outside the boundaries of moral inclusion and are thereby perceived as deserving of harassment, discrimination, and violence. During times of war, entire nations fall outside the zone of moral inclusion. Within business and organizational practices, undocumented workers or workers who labor in sweatshop conditions also fall outside the moral scope of inclusion, and are deemed to be unworthy of fair labor practices. People with mental illnesses oftentimes fall outside of the zone of moral inclusion, as is the case of forced institutionalization, imprisonment, or abusive treatment (Drew, Funk, Pathare, & Swartz, 2005). Who falls in and outside of a zone of moral inclusion changes according to the demographics of who (e.g., sex, ethnicity, age) is involved, as well as when and where an individual lives. As such, social justice perceptions are contextual and historical.

Social Justice as Emotion

The link between cognition and emotion within the context of social justice is amplified by research documenting the emotional catalysts of perceptions of justice and injustice. As discussed by Miller (2001), perceptions of injustice are oftentimes triggered by the sense that one is being treated disrespectfully, an assessment that often leads to, or is linked to, anger. When a person pairs this anger with an assessment that the treatment he or she receives is unfair, then the individual is more likely to take action against a believed transgressor. Leach, Snyder, and Iyer (2002) discussed guilt as a prominent emotion that motivates people to act in favor of equalizing unjust distribution of resources. Feelings of guilt, however, are mediated by the perceptions one has of why resources are unequally distributed. If one feels that he or she was entitled to such resources or that people on the short end of the stick deserve what they get, then feelings of guilt are mitigated.

Empathy as a Social Justice Catalyst

As outlined by the principles and practice of restorative justice, the potential for social justice is activated through the feelings that develop in the context of relationships; when the offender meets the person he or she has offended and sees firsthand the damage caused by his or her actions, behavioral change and remorse are more likely. Similarly, when the offender meets the perpetrator and sees him or her as a fellow human being, forgiveness is more likely. The judgment errors people make due to fundamental attribution errors break down when they get to know someone and are able to see the environmental presses on his or her life. An empathic response to the other creates the emotional space for compassion and the realization that all human beings have similar needs, desires, and fears.

Neuropsychological research in the area of mirror neurons corroborates the neural foundations for empathy; as Rifkin (2009) and others (de Waal, 2009) have discussed, it is the human capacity for empathy that will, ultimately, propel our species to develop less destructive and more just systems. Recent debates in the United States regarding changes to U.S. immigration law highlight the importance of the relational and empathic element of justice. In a discussion of undocumented immigrants in the United States, a prominent Republican politician stated

> You know this is not a statistic. You know them as a human being, a walking, talking person who is in pain, and who came here because they were hungry and because their kids were starving and their family was hurting, and they did what any parent would do when faced with that circumstance. They did whatever they had to do to provide for them. And you have to always remember that when you talk about this. (*Huffington Post Politics*, November 15, 2012)

Empathic human connection can shift ideology.

Within the context of globalization, there are similar examples in documentaries such as *Mardi Gras Made in China* (Redmon, Smith, Smith, & Sabin, 2008) or *Bling: A Planet Rock* (Cepeda & Bozotti, 2007). In *Mardi Gras Made in China* video footage brings together revelers in New Orleans and young women factory workers in China: the former become aware of the unhealthy working conditions of these young woman, their longs hours, and abysmal pay, and the latter become aware of how much people pay for the beads they themselves are paid so little to make and are shocked at how their products are used. In *Bling: A Planet Rock*, hip-hop artists travel to Sierra Leone to see firsthand the human misery caused by the diamond trade that produced the diamonds used in the signature "bling" they wear. The artists also become aware of how the violence of hip-hop lyrics provided some of the cultural scaffolding for the violence of the civil war. As depicted in both films, contact with the other increased the consumers' capacity for empathy and their ability to understand their role in typically invisible systems of production and consumption.

Empathy, however, is not immune from the social construction of the other. Avenanti, Sirigu, and Aglioti (2010) demonstrate the degree to which racial bias, as assessed by the Implicit Association Test (IAT), mediates the magnitude of the vicarious mapping of pain experienced by another, thereby impacting empathic reactivity. Their use of an anatomically correct human hand colored violet as a stimulus condition, revealed that differences in empathic reactivity were not due to perceptions of physical difference, but rather to the socially constructed meaning of physical differences. Lamm, Batson, and Decety (2007) showed that perspective taking and cognitive appraisal impact the specific neural underpinnings of empathic response, with different brain structures stimulated by "imagining the other" versus "imagining myself" or, in the case of cognitive appraisal, believing that an intervention is or is not successful in alleviating the pain of the other.

Social Justice and Empowerment

Empathy is important to a discussion of social justice to the extent that empathic concern is translated into a behavioral response, a process that links information, emotion, cognition, and behavior. A crucial element in this process is that of empowerment. As discussed by Cattaneou and Chapman (2010), empowerment is a process whereby an individual is able to articulate a particular goal as well as the steps through which he or she will achieve that goal. According to these authors, empowerment is not something that accidentally "happens" to a person (or to a group) but rather the result of a thoughtful and conscious approach to understanding goals, objectives, pathways, and obstructions. Within the context of social justice, such goals and objectives may differ according to how one is situated within systems of power. For those at the bottom rung of the social justice ladder, empowerment may mean developing the skills and creating the alliances required for one to progress beyond poverty and discrimination so as to affect policy change. For those at the top of the ladder of privilege, empowerment may mean discovering ways to use one's privilege to create privileges for others, at either the local or global level. New models of capitalism and business, such as Mohammad Yunus' (2007) idea of social entrepreneurship, provide a method of empowerment both for individuals in poverty (e.g., the women who form the community of the Grameen bank in Bangladesh) or for those with capital (e.g., the budding social entrepreneurs of our planet).

Social Justice and the Role of Information

A defining characteristic of globalization is the spatial and temporal integration of systems of communication (Aneesh, 2006). This level of communicative integration enables individuals to learn about the lives of people throughout the world in the space of time that it takes to tweet a message, check a Facebook page, or input an Internet search term. The global integration of communication allows for a sophisticated understanding of how any one person is linked to countless numbers of people throughout the world, thereby creating the potential to create a world propelled by empathy (Rifkin, 2009). Knowing about the other creates the opportunity for empathy, and empathy when linked with empowerment creates the opportunity for transformation. It is these webs of communication, empathy, and empowerment that allow for social movements such as that of *alterglobalization* (Pleyers, 2010).

SOCIAL JUSTICE AS CONTINUOUS AND UNBOUNDED RELATIONSHIP

An assumption underlying nearly all of the discussion thus far is that social justice is an idealized end state in which a world exists where poverty, inequality, and violence (both direct and indirect) are but painful memories of an earlier civilization. An understanding of social justice as socially constructed might lead us to the conclusion that humanity will never be able to reach such an idealized end state since it is unlikely that all human beings will ever be able to agree on issues of merit and morality. Or, that if such an agreement is reached, it will slip through our collective fingers as larger system changes (e.g., environmental) alter the fiber of human existence. Understanding social justice as an idealized outcome state may lead one to agree with Derrida (2002) when he offered the opinion that social justice is an exemplar of *aporia*—a puzzle that cannot be solved—or, as he wrote, "the experience of the impossible" (p. 244). Conceptualizing social justice as an outcome also demands embracing a dichotomized view of reality that separates process from outcome. At its most extreme, an outcome-based understanding of social justice requires a belief in the linear assumptions of social positivism—the ability to marshal human science and human intelligence for the goal of advancing humanity toward a progressively better and more advanced future (Comte, 1957).

At its essence, though, social justice is a relational construct; it is epiphenomenal to the web of relationships within which individuals are immersed, be it the school, the church, larger political and socioeconomic systems, or the intimate relations of friends and family. Essentially, the concept of social justice is meaningless in a world of one isolated human being. The relational nature of social justice, in combination with the deep emotional and cognitive elements of social justice, suggests that social justice is less an end state than it is a mode of being that must be created and re-created from one moment to the next and from one relational experience to the next. As such, social justice is not achieved at any one point in time (e.g., through reaching the Millennium Development Goals by 2015), but is the infinite and regenerative process of being informed, empathic, and empowered human beings; of meeting the other through an empathic awareness of who he or she is (Hecker, 2010).

Opotow et al. (2005) listed the following as the emotional and cognitive building blocks of social justice: tolerance, minimal cooperation, sharing resources, making sacrifices, engaging in dialogue, sharing personal narratives. Adams (2000) listed the following as some of the characteristics of a peace culture: democratic participation, tolerance and understanding, free flow and sharing of information, dialogue and negotiation, sustainable development. Deutsch, Marcus, and Brazaitis (2012) discussed the following prerequisites to building global community: using communication to interconnect people through the use of social networking sites, imagining the possibilities of a global community, and the development of action steps that can bring into fruition collective imagination. A psychological approach to social justice is therefore one that places preeminence on the development of relationships that are characterized by empathy, compassion, forgiveness, empowerment, dialogue, and cooperation within a context of local and global awareness.

The pedagogical practice of social justice is effectively outlined by Prilleltensky and Prilleltensky (2006) in their elucidation of critical consciousness, characterized by an increased capacity for compassion in combination with an understanding that individuals have the capacity to change systems (see also Diaz, 2012). The research associated with an understanding of social justice as grounded in empathy and empowerment might focus on understanding the conditions and mechanisms by which human beings increase their capacity for both, and how individuals can expand boundaries of moral inclusion. Recent work on mindfulness and empathy point to an important avenue for future research and practice (Block-Lerner, Plumb, Rhatigan, & Orsillo, 2007; Greason & Cashwell, 2009; Krasner et al. 2009). The classic social psychological work of contact theory (Allport, 1954), cooperative learning (Sharon, 1980), and of problem solving (Kelman & Cohen, 1976) also come to mind, but re-conceptualized for a socially and globally networked age. Understanding empathy as a building block of social justice points to the importance of the everyday praxis of being informed of local and global situations of injustice and then engaging with injustice by building relationships etched in empathy, compassion, and empowerment. This is not an easy task, as it requires one to remain steadfastly rooted in the moment and to view all relationships as worthy of justice—worthy of empathy.

When people disabuse themselves of the belief that social justice is an arrival at a certain end point, they also disabuse themselves of disappointment that society has not yet arrived. As the world enters into yet another era of drastic changes in human and natural environments, it may be psychology's unique role to help us increase our local and global relational and behavioral capacities for empathy and caring.

REFERENCES

Adams, D. (2000). Toward a global movement for a culture of peace. *Peace and Conflict: Journal of Peace Psychology, 6*(3), 259–266.

Albee, G. W. (1982). Preventing psychopathology and promoting human potential. *American Psychologist, 37*(9), 1043–1050.

Albee, G. W. (1986). Toward a just society. *American Psychologist, 41*(8), 891–898.

Allport, G. (1954). *The nature of prejudice*, Reading, MA: Addison-Wesley.

American Psychology Association (2000). *Resolution on poverty and socioeconomic status.* Retrieved from http://www.apa.org/about/policy/poverty-resolution.aspx

American Psychology Association (2010). *APA statement on reforming the juvenile justice system to improve children's lives and public safety.* Retrieved from http://www.apa.org/news/press/statements/juvenile-justice.aspx

Aneesh, A. (2006). *Virtual migration.* London, UK: Duke University.

Arnett, J. J. (2012). *Human development: A cultural approach.* New York, NY: Pearson.

Avenanti, A., Sirigu, A., & Aglioti, S. M. (2010). Racial bias reduces empathic sensorimotor resonance with other-race pain. *Current Biology, 20*(11), 1018–1022.

Beard, J. (2003). Iron deficiency alters brain development and functioning. *The Journal of Nutrition, 133* (5), 14685–14725.

Bies, R. J. (2001). Interactional (in)justice: The sacred and the profane. In J. S. Greenberg, and R. Cropanzano (Eds.), *Advances in organizational justice* (pp. 89–118). Palo Alto, CA: Stanford University.

Biglan, A., Flay, B. R., Embry, D. D., & Sanler, I. N. (2012). The critical role of nurturing environments for promoting human well-being. *American Psychologist, 67*(4), 257–271.

Blasi, G., & Jost, J. T. (2006). System justification theory and research: Implications for law, legal advocacy and social justice. *California Law Review, 94*(4), 1119–1168.

Block-Lerner, J., Adair, C., Plumb, J. C., Rhatigan, D. L., & Orsillo, S. M. (2007). The case for mindfulness-based approaches in the cultivation of empathy: Does nonjudgmental, present-moment awareness increase capacity for perspective-taking and empathic concern? *Journal of Marital and Family Therapy, 33*(4), 501–516.

Bradshaw, W., & Roseborough, D. (2005). Restorative justice dialogue: The impact of mediation and conferencing on juvenile recidivism: A meta-analysis. *Conflict Resolution Quarterly,* 24(1), 87–98.

Braithwaite, J. (2006). Doing justice intelligently in civil society. *Journal of Social Issues, 62*(2), 393–409.

Bronfrenbrenner, U. (1977). Toward an experimental ecology of human development. *American Psychologist,* 513–531.

Brosnan, S. F., & de Waal, F. B. M. (2012). Fairness in animals: Where to from here? *Social Justice Research, 25,* 336–351.

Buber, M. (1937). *I and Thou.* London, UK: T&T Clark Ltd.

Bullock, H. E., & Lott, B. (2001). Building a research and advocacy agenda on issues of economic justice. *Analysis of Social Issues and Public Policy,* 147–162.

Capehart, L., & Milavanovic, D. (2007). *Social justice, theories, issues, and movements.* New York, NY: Rutgers University.

Cattaneou, L. B., & Chapman, A. R. (2010). The process of empowerment. *American Psychologist, 65*(7), 646–659.

Cepeda, R., & Bozotti, F. (2007). *Bling: A planet rock* [Motion Picture]. United States: Image Entertainment.

Colquitt, J. A., Conlon, D. E., Wesson, M. J., Porter, C. O. L. H., & Ng, K. Y. (2001). Justice at the millennium: A meta-analytic review of 25 years of organizational justice research. *Journal of Applied Psychology, 86*(3), 425–445.

Comte, A. (1957). *A general view of positivism.* New York, NY: Robert Speller and Sons.

Cordella, P. (2008). Sanctuary as a refuge from state justice. In D. Sullivan & L. Tifft (Eds.), *Handbook of restorative justice* (pp. 198–206). New York, NY: Routledge.

Daly, K. (2007). The limits of restorative justice. In G. Johnstone & D. W. Van Ness (Eds.), *Handbook of restorative justice* (pp. 134–146). Portland, OR: Willan Publishing.

Darley, J. M., & Pittman, T. S. (2003). The psychology of compensatory and retributive justice. *Personality and Social Psychology Review, 7*(4), 324–336.

de Waal, F. (2009). *The age of empathy*. New York, NY: Three Rivers Press.

Demuth, S. (2003). Racial and ethnic differences in pretrial release decisions and outcomes: A comparison of Hispanic, Black, and White felony arrestees. *Criminology, 41*(3), 873–907.

Derrida, J. (2002). *Acts of religion*. New York, NY: Routledge.

Deutsch, M., Marcus, E. C., & Brazaitis, S. (2012). A framework for thinking about developing a global community. In P. T. Coleman & M. Deutsch (Eds.), *The psychological components of sustainable peace* (pp. 299–324). New York, NY: Springer.

Diaz, J. (2012). Developing critical global consciousness in the psychology classroom. *Psychology Learning and Teaching, 11*(3), 388–395.

Diaz, J., Schneider, R., & Pwogwam Sante Mantal. (2012). Globalization a re-traumatization: Rebuilding Haiti from the spirit up. *Journal of Social Issues, 68*(3), 493–593.

Diaz, J., & Zirkel, S. (2012). Globalization, psychology, and social issues research: An introduction and conceptual framework. *Journal of Social Issues, 68*(3), 439–453.

Dollar, D. (2001). Is globalization good for your health? *Bulletin of the World Health Organization, 79*(9), 827–833.

Drew, N., Funk, M., Pathare, S., & Swartz, L. (2005). Mental health and human rights. In World Health Organization, *Promoting mental health* (Ch. 7, pp. 81–88).

Ellsworth, P., Haney, C., & Costanzo, J. (2001). *SPSSI Statement on the Death Penalty*. Retrieved from http://www.spssi.org/index.cfm?fuseaction=page.viewpage&pageid=1461

Gil, D. (2007). Toward a "radical" paradigm of restorative justice. In G. Johnstone & D. W. Van Ness (Eds.), *Handbook of restorative justice* (pp. 499–511). Portland, OR: Willan Publishing.

Gilligan, C. (1982). *In a different voice*. Cambridge, MA: Harvard University.

Goodman, L. A., Liang, B., Helms, J. E., Latta, R. E., Sparks, E., & Weintraub, S. R. (2004). Training counseling psychologists as social justice agents: Feminist and multicultural principles in action. *The Counseling Psychologist, 32*(6) 793–837.

Gould, C. C. (2008). Recognition *in* redistribution: Care and diversity in global justice. *The Southern Journal of Philosophy, XLVI*, 91–103.

Greason, P. B., & Cashwell, C. S. (2009). Mindfulness and counseling self-efficacy: The mediating role of attention and empathy. *Counselor Education and Supervision, 49*, 2–19.

Gross, S. F., & Mauro, R. (1989). *Death and discrimination: Racial disparities in capital sentencing*. Chicago, IL: Northeastern University.

Halliburton, C. (2004). Neither separate nor equal how race-sensitive enforcement of criminal laws threatens to undo *Brown v. Board of education*. *Seattle Journal for Social Justice, 3* (1), 45–71.

Harrison, S. (2006). Globalization and poverty. Working Paper 12347 National Bureau of Economic Research. Retrieved from http://www.nber.org/papers/w12347

Hecker, J. (2012). Relating differently. *Sexualities, 13* (4), 403–411.

Huffington Post Politics (2012). 2016 Republican nomination race, step one: Reject Romney. Retrieved from http://www.huffingtonpost.com/2012/11/15/2016-republican-romney_n_2138091.html

International Labor Organization (2008). *ILO Declaration on social justice for a fair globalization*. Geneva, Switzerland: ILO.

Jensen, L. A. (2011a). *Bridging cultural and developmental approaches to psychology*. New York, NY: Oxford University.

Jensen, L. A. (2011b). Introduction: Changing our scholarship for a changing world. In L. Jensen (Ed.), *Bridging cultural and developmental approaches to psychology* (pp. xxi–xxvi). New York, NY: Oxford University.

Jost, J. T. (2009). "Elective affinities": On the psychological bases of left-right differences. *Psychological Inquiry, 20,* 129–141.

Jost, J. T., & Kay, A. C. (2010). Social justice: History, theory and research. In S. T. Fiske, G. Lindzey, & D. T. Gilbert (Eds.) *Handbook of social psychology* (pp. 1122–1165). Hoboken, NJ: Wiley & Sons.

Kelman, H., & Cohen, L. (1976). The problem-solving workshop: A social psychological contribution to the resolution of international conflicts. *Journal of Peace Research, 2*(8), 79–90.

Kenny, M. E., Horne, A.M., Orpinas, P. E., & Reese, L. R. E. (2009). *Realizing social justice: The challenge of preventive interventions.* Washington, DC: American Psychological Association.

Krasner, M. S., Epstein, R. M., Beckman, H., Suchman, A., Chapman, B., Mooney, C. J., & Quill, T. E. (2009). Association of an educational program in mindful communication with burnout, empathy, and attitudes among primary care physicians. *The Journal of the American Medical Association, 302*(12), 1284–1293. doi: 10.1001/jama.2009.1384

Lamm, C., Batson, C. D., & Decety, J. (2007). The neural substrate of human empathy: Effects of perspective-taking and cognitive appraisal. *Journal of Cognitive Neuroscience, 19* (1), 42–58.

Leach, C. W., Snider, N., & Iyer, A. (2002). "Poisoning the consciences of the fortunate": The experience of relative advantage and support for social equality. In I. Walker & H. J. Smith (Eds.), *Relative deprivation specification, development and integration,* Chapter 7 (pp. 136–163). Boston, MA: Cambridge University.

Lind, E A., & Tyler T. R. (1988). *The social psychology of procedural justice.* New York, NY: Plenum.

Marsella, A. (2012). Psychology and globalization: Understanding a complex relationship. *Journal of Social Issues, 68*(3), 454–427.

Maxwell, G., & Morris, A. (2006). Youth justice in New Zealand: Restorative justice in practice? *Journal of Social Issues, 62*(2), 239–258.

Miller, D. T. (2001). Disrespect and the experience of injustice. *Annual Review of Psychology, 52,* 527–553.

Nash, D. (2010). *Climate refugees* [Motion Picture]. United States: PMG Platform Group.

Nelson, G., & Prilleltenksy, I. (2005). *Community psychology in pursuit of liberation and well-being.* New York, NY: Palgrave MacMillan.

Nussbaum, M. C. (2003). Capabilities as fundamental entitlements: Sen and social justice. *Feminist Economics, 9*(2–3), 33–59.

Opotow, J., Gerson, J., & Woodside, S. (2005). From moral exclusion to moral inclusion: Theory for teaching peace. *Theory into Practice, 44*(4), 303–318.

Pachter, W. S., & DeLeon, P. H. (2007). Reflections on George Albee's legacy of promoting human potential and social justice. *The Journal of Primary Prevention, 28*(1), 45–53.

Parrenas, S. (2001). *Servants of globalization.* Palo Alto, CA: Stanford University.

Patel, V. (2007). Mental health in low and middle-income countries. *British Medical Bulletin, 81 and 82,* 81–96.

Pelikan, C., & Trenczek, T. (2006). Victim offender mediation and restorative justice: The European landscape. In G. Johnstone & D. W. Van Ness (Eds.), *Handbook of restorative justice* (pp. 63–90). Portland, OR: Willan.

Pieterse, A. L, Todd, N. R., Neville, H. A., & Carter, R. T. (2012). Perceived racism and mental health among Black American adults: A meta-analytic review. *Journal of Counseling Psychology, 59*(1), 1–9.

Pleyers, G. (2010). *Alterglobalization.* Cambridge, MA: Polity.

Pranis, K. (2007). Restorative values. In G. Johnstone & D. W. Van Ness (Eds.), *Handbook of restorative justice* (pp. 59–74). Portland, OR: Willan.

Prilleltensky, I., & Prilleltensky, O. (2006). *Promoting well being: Linking personal, organizational and community change.* Hoboken, NJ: Wiley.

Redmon, D., Smith, D., Smith, D., & Sabin, A. (2008). *Mardi Gras made in China* [Motion Picture]. United States: Carnivalesque Films.

Rifkin, J. (2009). *The empathic civilization.* New York, NY: Penguin Group.

Robinson, F. (2005). Care, gender and global social justice: Towards a moral framework for ethical globalization. Downloaded February 12, 2013, from http://www.cpsa-acsp.ca/papers-2005/Robinson.pdf

Scott, L., Williams, J. D., Baker, S. M, Brace-Govan, J., Downey, H., Hakstian, A., Henderson, G. R., Loroz, P. S., & Webb, D. (2011). Beyond poverty: Social justice in a global marketplace. *Journal of Public Policy & Marketing, 30*(1), 39–46.

Sen, A. (1999). *Development as freedom.* New, York, NY: Anchor Books.

Sharon, S. (1980). Cooperative learning in small groups: Recent methods and effects on achievement, attitudes, and ethnic relations. *Review of Educational Research, 50*(2), 241–271.

Shiva, V. (2000). *Stolen harvest: The hijacking of the global food supply.* Cambridge, MA: South End.

Stuart, B., & Pranis, K. (2007). Peacemaking circles: Reflections on principal features and primary outcomes. In G. Johnstone & D. W. Van Ness (Eds.), *Handbook of restorative justice* (pp. 121–133). Portland, OR: Willan.

Sullivan, D., & Tifft, L. (2007). Introduction: The healing dimensions of restorative justice: A one-world body. In D. Sullivan & L. Tifft (Eds.), *Handbook of restorative justice* (pp. 1–16). New York, NY: Routledge.

Thibaut, J., & Walker, L. (1975). *Procedural justice: A psychological analysis.* New York, NY: L. Erlbaum Associates.

Thibaut, J., & Walker, L. (1978). A theory of procedure. *California Law Review, 66*(3), 541–566.

United Nations (2012). *The millennium development goals report.* New York, NY: United Nations.

Unnever, J. D., & Cullen, F. T. (2007). The racial divide in support for the death penalty: Does white racism matter? *Social Forces, 85*(3), 1281–1301.

Vasquez, M. J. T. (2012). Psychology and social justice: Why we do what we do. *American Psychologist, 67*(5) 337–346.

Williams, C. R., & Arrigo, B. A. (2001). Anarchaos and order: On the emergence of social justice. *Theoretical Criminology, 5,* 223–252.

Woolf, L. M., & MacCartney, D. (2014). Sexual and gender minorities. In C. Johnson, H. Friedman, J. Diaz, Z. Franco, & B. Nastasi (Eds.). *Praeger handbook of social justice and psychology.* Westport, CT: Praeger.

Yunus, M. (2007). *Creating a world without poverty.* Philadelphia, PA: Perseus Books.

Chapter 3

A Critical Look at Social Justice Ideology in Counseling and Psychotherapy[1]

Jonathan D. Raskin

In her forceful and passionate book on psychology, poverty, and social exclusion, Laura Smith (2010) argues that the duties of practicing psychologists and counselors include patronizing companies with fair trade policies, speaking out in favor of unions, supporting health care and prison reform, demanding smaller class sizes in schools, fighting environmental injustice, resisting unfairness in the judicial system, and standing up for a living wage. Her premise is, in many respects, a compelling one. In anticipating potential critics, she remarks:

> Why don't we stick to mental health? Well, pardon me—this *is* mental health. Contributing our work toward the evolution of a more just society where all families have enough, toward a more democratic society where every person has a voice, and toward a more humane society where no one is kept on the outside looking in, is promoting mental health. . . . Through our practice, theory, research, and advocacy, we have a unique role to play in ending social exclusion. (p. 146)

In other words, psychotherapists are obliged to advance *social justice*, defined as "the full and equal participation of all groups in a society . . . where resources are equitably distributed, and all members are physically and psychologically safe" (Vasquez, 2012, p. 76). From a social justice perspective, instead of restricting their clinical attention to peoples' inner lives, psychologists and counselors have a professional responsibility to redress oppressive social conditions (Aldarondo, 2007; Chung & Bemak, 2012; Fouad, Gerstein, & Toporek, 2006; Goodman et al., 2004; Lee & Walz, 1998; Prilleltensky & Nelson, 2002; Rubel & Ratts, 2011; L. Smith, 2010; Speight & Vera, 2004; Toporek, Gerstein, Fouad, Roysircar, & Israel, 2006; Vasquez, 2012; Vera & Speight, 2003). As L. Smith (2010) puts it, a "social justice psychological perspective" requires a "willingness to address oppression beyond the traditional individualistic purview of applied psychology and an expanded notion of ethical duty that incorporates a responsibility to work for the liberation of oppressed peoples" (p. 25). By implication, a social justice perspective needs to be infused into psychotherapeutic training, research, and practice because psychologists and counselors "are situated in an optimal position to help society's inhabitants understand the undue effects of social injustices for the well-being of the larger society" (Constantine, Hage, Kindaichi, & Bryant, 2007, p. 28).

At a surface level, this call for psychotherapists to take up the mantle of social justice sounds wonderful. However, although everyone may be for social justice in the abstract, making it central to applied psychology and professional counseling raises a number of thorny issues that have not been adequately addressed. Defining, implementing, and grappling with the ethical implications of a social justice orientation is a more nuanced and complex task than its adherents often acknowledge. This chapter critically examines the move toward social justice in psychotherapy and counseling.

NEED FOR THEORY DEVELOPMENT

Herein social justice is treated as a theoretical approach to psychotherapy rather than a discipline-wide imperative because framing it as the former clears space for one to use it when desired (S. D. Smith, Reynolds, & Rovnak, 2009), but also to critique it without falling prey to accusations of immorality or professional disloyalty (Raskin, 2010). That said, despite declaring themselves the "fifth force" (Chung & Bemak, 2012; Lee, 2012), social justice counselors have a long way to go when it comes to fully articulating their theoretical perspective. As it stands, a social justice orientation remains underdeveloped and therefore is incapable of providing an adequate social-psychological model to guide the provision of clinical services. Goodman et al.'s (2004) seminal article on social justice in counseling psychology exemplifies this deficiency. Six principles of a social justice orientation are presented: *ongoing self-examination*, *sharing power*, *giving voice*, *facilitating consciousness-raising*, *building on strengths*, and *leaving clients tools to work toward social change*. However, it is necessary to flesh these principles out into a comprehensive theory that can guide applied practice. As Thompson and Shermis (2004) noted, Goodman et al.'s principles are more intuitive than theoretical. They wonder what theoretical basis Goodman et al. (2004) encourage their students to use when judging what is or is not socially just: Egalitarianism? Socialism? Democratic theory? Without clarification, the implication is that what constitutes social justice is readily apparent, and this is not always the case.

Without a better-developed theoretical foundation, the principles Goodman et al. (2004) present become vague generalities offering little that is new. For example, "ongoing self-examination" and "building on strengths" are principles found in most every counseling theory. "Sharing power" holds a bit more promise as a guiding principle, but without a fuller theoretical articulation, it is difficult to know what this principle means for clinicians because the concept of power needs to be further unpacked and, likewise, its operational elements further discussed. Thus, it is important not only to assert that sharing power enhances personal growth but also to provide a theoretical underpinning for the assertion.

Interestingly, it is common for social justice practitioners to stress the importance of equalizing power differentials (Chung & Bemak, 2012; Goodman et al., 2004; L. Smith, 2010; Vera & Speight, 2003). Power—even when not explicitly defined—is something social justice psychologists are confident should be given away. Yet there is something paradoxical about the notion that social justice psychologists should relinquish power to their clients. If it is theirs to relinquish (and, ostensibly, reclaim when necessary), then are they not the ones in the power position to begin with? Perhaps it is the lack of theoretical rigor that causes such questions to arise, but can power between client and therapist ever really be equal? Their very roles empower each of them in different ways, but if equal means "the same," then the answer is no. Being comfortable with power and attempting to use it wisely seem preferable to paternalistically pretending that the therapist can grant power to the client. Clients know better and so should their therapists.

For example, clients realize that they have limited (and often no) say in where sessions take place, how long sessions last, how much services cost, and what theoretical strategies their counselors will be using. The counselor determines most of the basic ground rules. Therapists have power over aspects of the process that clients simply do not—and arguably should not—have. There is nothing necessarily oppressive about this. Again, if social justice psychologists offered a more carefully articulated theoretical definition of power, confusion around what they mean by "power sharing" might be easier to resolve.

Not only is power vaguely delineated, but also the very definition of social justice often remains unclear. For example, the Social Justice and Ethics Social Action Group at the 2001 National Counseling Psychology conference in Houston defined social justice as

> a concept that advocates engaging individuals as co-participants in decisions that directly affect their lives; it involves taking some action, and educating individuals in order to open possibilities, and to act with value and respect for individuals and their group identities, considering power differentials in all areas of counseling practice and research. (Fouad et al., 2004, pp. 42–43)

This definition is extremely hazy. What precisely does it mean to "co-participate" with clients? (And does this mean that traditional therapists are somehow doing therapy without client participation?) Does any action count as taking "some action"? What exactly should therapists be educating people about? When they consider power differentials, does that mean they need to go back and reexamine whether "educating" constitutes the exercise—or even misuse—of clinician power? The Houston Conference definition of social justice cries out for clarification.

Unfortunately, other definitions do not fare much better. Goodman et al. (2004) characterize social justice as "scholarship and professional action designed to change societal values, structures, policies, and practices, such that disadvantaged or marginalized groups gain increased access to these tools of self-determination" (p. 795). This definition is consistent with that of Chung and Bemak (2012), who contend that from a social justice perspective "all people, not just a privileged few, receive an equal distribution of resources" and "are psychologically and physically safe and secure" (p. 36). Speight and Vera (2004) describe social justice as involving "the promotion of the values of self-development and self-determination for everyone" (p. 111), while Vasquez (2012) contends that social justice "implies that people come together to work for the common good by transforming the social organizations and processes that contribute to power inequalities, oppression, and marginalization" (p. 76).

In many respects, it is their very fuzziness that makes all of these definitions sound good. Absent deeper reflection, there is little to oppose in such broad generalities. We all likely agree that oppression should be eliminated and the common good advanced. It is only as we get into the specifics that disagreements emerge. What is the common good? What constitutes self-development and self-determination? What must be provided for one to feel psychologically and physically secure? Which social values, policies, and practices warrant change? How should they be changed? By what means? Who gets to decide? These questions beg two broader ones, namely what exactly does it mean to combat oppression, and are there proper and improper ways for psychologists and counselors to do so?

Failing to clearly operationalize social justice results in its implications being so vague that no reasonable person has grounds for dissent. Claiming that social justice is fighting for the common good or empowering people or combating oppression or redistributing advantages and disadvantages more fairly provides little more than comforting platitudes. What is needed is a much more detailed psychosocial theory for conceptualizing and guiding how social justice practice is supposed to be carried out. Otherwise, counselors and psychologists are simply relying on their personal beliefs about justice as their primary guide. As discussed next, psychologists and counselors should be careful about this because it potentially leads them to think they know better than others what justice is.

PSYCHOLOGISTS AND COUNSELORS DO NOT KNOW BEST WHAT JUSTICE IS

Social justice practitioners often critique their more traditional peers for espousing a "neutral" logical positivist view of psychotherapy (Prilleltensky & Nelson, 2002). They are skeptical of a "just the facts" approach because it overlooks the socially constructed nature of inquiry, thereby ignoring how power and privilege impact what psychotherapists do, how they research it, and what counts as clinical knowledge (Prilleltensky & Nelson, 2002; L. Smith, 2010). Social justice psychologists astutely note that the science and practice of psychotherapy are always conducted from a particular point of view (Prilleltensky & Nelson, 2002; L. Smith, 2010). Findings about counseling and therapy are inevitably a socially constructed product of discourses and relationships that legitimize particular perspectives and methods, yielding socially negotiated conclusions that then tend to be taken as everlasting truths (Burr, 2003; Gergen, 1994, 2009). According to social justice advocates, when clinicians see themselves as dispassionate investigators whose purpose is merely to tell clients and the public how things are (as opposed to make them what they should be), they unwittingly maintain the status quo (Chung & Bemak, 2012; Prilleltensky & Nelson, 2002; L. Smith, 2010; Vera & Speight, 2003). As Payton (1984) famously put it, "doing nothing *is* taking action" (p. 395, italics in original). Therefore, neutrality is not an option. From a social justice perspective, psychologists and counselors must change dominant and oppressive social constructions, not uphold them as timeless truths revealed through beneficent science (Morrow, Hawxhurst, Montes de Vegas, Abousleman, & Castañeda, 2006; Prilletensky & Nelson, 2002; Roy, 2007; L. Smith, 2010; Vera & Speight, 2003; Waldegrave, 2005).

Paradoxically, the socially constructed nature of knowledge does not seem to apply to these practitioners' own visions of social justice. On the contrary, they tend to treat their assessments as the very kind of universal truths they warn others to avoid. Nowhere is this more apparent than when they positively connote and recommend *consciousness-raising* (Goodman et al., 2004; Morrow et al., 2006; Toporek & Williams, 2006). Under the banner of consciousness-raising, social justice counselors help "clients understand the extent to which individual and private difficulties are rooted in larger historical, social, and political forces" (Goodman et al., 2004, p. 804). This presumably liberates clients from a state of *false consciousness* (Prilleltensky & Fox, 1997). Despite multicultural concerns about imposing hegemonic beliefs on others, psychologists and counselors operating from a social justice orientation continue to speak of consciousness-raising as a means to educate clients about the ways in which they are oppressed (Crethar, Torres Rivera, & Nash, 2008). In so doing, they claim to combat "political illiteracy" (Prilleltensky, Dokecki, Frieden, & Ota Wang, 2007, p. 24; Prilleltensky & Nelson, 2002, p. 44). Said another way, they assume there is a real state of societal affairs and it is the social justice psychologist's purpose to educate people about it. After all, "if there was a test about what constitutes the public good, most of us would fail miserably, including those of us with university degrees" (Prilleltensky & Nelson, 2002, p. 44). We need social justice psychologists to set us straight.

The contradiction here is readily apparent: mainstream psychologists oppress people by treating their socially constructed theories and research findings about psychotherapy as universal truths, but social justice psychologists liberate people by raising consciousness about how things really are. When people disagree with the social justice view that emotional and psychological suffering is primarily caused by oppressive social forces, they are living in a state of false consciousness. That is, they are wrong. Although adopting such a definitive stance is one way to counter traditionalists (who seem equally confident that human suffering is traceable to individual character flaws and psychopathology), it may be that those on both sides of this conceptual divide end up as victims of their own righteous certitude. Previously, I suggested that social justice counselors might inoculate themselves against this sort of worrisome self-assurance and more consistently sustain their purported social constructionism by reframing consciousness-raising as *consciousness-raising within a tradition* (Raskin, 2010). Instead of viewing themselves as revealing ultimate truths to the masses of ignorant oppressed people, they merely become advocates for particular moral discourses, which their clients are free to entertain or dismiss. With this shift, social justice psychologists keep in mind that every discourse has the potential to both liberate and oppress—even those marketed under a social justice banner (Foucault, 1980).

IMPOSING VALUES

The idea that all views have the potential to oppress raises the related issue of imposing values. It feels good to fight for truth and justice. Believing that one is raising the consciousness of oppressed people and—by alerting them to the sad realities of life—liberating them to recast society in a new and fairer mold is indeed a heroic undertaking. However, with strong conviction comes high risk. Seeing truth as on one's side potentially leads to righteously imposing one's values on others (Butt, 2000; Gergen, 1994; Raskin, 2001). Social justice psychologists need to be careful that they do not become so enamored of their own sociopolitical moral beliefs that they unfairly force them on people. After all, is this not precisely what they accuse oppressive status quo upholders of doing?

The danger here can be seen in some of the more vigorous assertions of those operating from a social justice orientation. For example, Speight and Vera (2004, p. 114) suggest that psychologists are ethically obligated to use the "transformative potential of psychology" to work toward liberating the oppressed. They go so far as to suggest that those who fail to do so should be sanctioned. Brown (1997) expresses a similar sentiment and argues that psychologists are ethical only if they fight against racism, sexism, and other forms of oppression. This is because a social justice perspective holds that "oppression significantly affects the lives of many diverse clients" and therefore demands "that counselors must go outside the boundaries of traditional counseling technique and theory to serve these clients" (Rubel & Ratts, 2011, p. 33).

Again, it is easy to agree with these sentiments, so long as they remain vaguely defined. But what exactly must a psychologist do to avoid being accused of ethically ignoring the imperatives of social justice? Are there particular political positions that must be adopted? Candidates supported? Policy statements subscribed to? Must a socially just psychologist or counselor be pro-choice? In favor of prescription privileges for psychologists? Against treatment manuals? Or, as those from a social justice orientation often imply, must ethical psychologists and counselors support unions and the 99% against the 1%, while opposing consumerism and individualism (Chung & Bemak, 2012; Prilleltensky & Nelson, 2002; L. Smith, 2010)? There seems to be tension within the social justice counseling literature, with it sometimes stressing how important it is to listen to clients when it comes to deciding where injustice resides (Chung & Bemak, 2012; Goodman et al., 2004) and other times contending that being socially just requires psychologists and counselors to endorse a specific politics, typically some version of communitarianism (Chung & Bemak, 2012; Prilleltensky & Nelson, 2002; L. Smith, 2010). Implying that psychologists and counselors can be "socially just" only by adopting "correct" political viewpoints is a rather chilling proposition. It requires that everyone affirm the political ideology of social justice psychologists or be considered collaborators with unethical oppressors. Those pushing a social justice agenda need to be careful that they not censor or condemn those with divergent opinions (S. D. Smith et al., 2009). Even when agreeing with some of their specific political views, it seems appropriate to remain worried about the righteous tendency of some social justice counselors to treat their vision of justice as revealed truth. Once this occurs, all competing perspectives become false, unethical, and—most concerning of all—officially illegitimate.

PROFESSIONAL HUBRIS

Imposing values is often a product of professional hubris. The very act of calling ourselves social justice agents smacks of such hubris. Doing so makes one right and those who disagree wrong (Raskin, 2010). If we are for social justice, then those who oppose us are against it. In this regard, there is a great deal of power and privilege to be gained by identifying as social justice advocates because any time we are able to convince others that we stand on the side of justice while our adversaries are on the side of oppression, we have scored a rhetorical victory, casting ourselves as moral exemplars and justifying the silencing of those who do not share our views (S. D. Smith et al., 2009; Raskin, 2010). The resulting self-importance may lead us to decide that all of our colleagues must believe as we do. If individualism and capitalism are the fundamental causes of client problems and psychologists and counselors have an ethical duty to resist them (as social justice practitioners typically claim; Chung & Bemak, 2012; A. G. Johnson, 2001; Prilletensky & Nelson, 2002; L. Smith, 2010), then it is reasonable to assume that those who disagree with such an analysis are unethical and must either have their consciousness raised or be removed from the profession.

When social justice psychologists declare that they wish all dissenting voices to be heard, does this include, for instance, those who strongly defend free markets, such as conservative Republicans? Conservative Republicans tend to consider the things social justice counselors believe—such as involving government in the allocation of resources—to be unfair, unjust, and counterproductive. For instance, they often contend that minimum wage laws decrease employment opportunities for entry-level workers, thus making the plight of the poor that much worse. Even if we do not accept this assessment, is it not reasonable to feel uncomfortable casting all those who do as oppressors? It is important to remember that power and privilege vary by context and, in some areas of professional psychology and counseling today, it ironically may be that conservative voices are the ones lacking a space to be heard. Although social justice practitioners warrant praise for presenting a theoretical perspective that examines oppression and discrimination, in situations where they hold all the positions of power and privilege (e.g., when they are the majority of faculty in a department, staff in a facility, or officers in a professional organization), they run the risk of unwittingly imposing their views on others in the same way they purportedly decry (S. D. Smith et al., 2009; Raskin, 2010). Social justice psychologists court danger when,

> holding the majority of positions that warrant voice in professional circles, they work to make their brand of social justice the categorical imperative for the field. We may wish to acknowledge that invoking social justice is a way of warranting voice for our own preferred agenda while undermining the discursive power of those with whom we disagree. (Raskin, 2010, p. 261)

That is to say, there is

> the potential for the oppressed to become the oppressor, wherein the oppressed use the strategies of the oppressor, such as labeling, personalization, isolation, and rigid adherence to one particular stance against another, rather than engage in thoughtful counter dialogue. (S. D. Smith et al., 2009, p. 488)

As an illustration, social justice counselors Bemak and Chung (2008) diagnose colleagues who seem less inclined than they are to raise a ruckus when faced with perceived injustices as suffering from NCS, or "Nice Counselor Syndrome." This syndrome is characterized by, among other things, "taking a neutral stance in an attempt to avoid upsetting others," trying to maintain "harmony with coworkers, supervisors, and organizations," and avoiding "conflict or unpleasant realities by giving positive reinforcement and feedback even when the situation warrants criticism, challenges, and confrontation" (Chung & Bemak, 2012, p. 70). Those who suffer from NCS "demonstrate a willingness to help perpetuate the status quo"

(Bemak & Chung, 2008, p. 374). Apparently, Chung and Bemak know better than the rest of us when and where confrontation is called for. There is something remarkable about social justice counselors like Chung and Bemak invoking a facsimile of the medical model—which elsewhere they make clear is a form of oppressive and imperial Western individualism (Chung & Bemak, 2012, p. 57)—to cut down those who might not share their political fervor.

My concern is that those espousing a social justice orientation often fail to acknowledge the possibility of genuine differences of opinion (Harrist & Richardson, 2012; Raskin, 2010). They tend to believe that all rational actors—and certainly all fellow psychologists and counselors—share their ideas of what justice is and how it should be implemented. When they push their colleagues to adopt a social justice perspective, they seem to assume that all counselors and psychologists have an identical view of justice. But why would this be so? Psychologists and counselors are a diverse group of people. They come from different religious, political, and ethnic backgrounds—which likely shape their views about justice as much (if not more!) than psychology or counseling ever could. It seems naïve to take it for granted that all psychologists and counselors share attitudes about social justice simply based on their choice of profession (Raskin, 2010).

Why would anyone presume such a high degree of professional consensus? Think about how many issues psychologists disagree about—for example, prescription privileges, treatment guidelines, and the proper role of psychologists in eliciting confessions from alleged terrorists. When the Society for Humanistic Psychology (2011) published its "Open Letter to the DSM" criticizing proposed changes to psychiatry's *Diagnostic and Statistical Manual of Mental Disorders*, psychologists were divided over the right thing to do. Some American Psychological Association divisions signed the accompanying petition, others did not, and numerous internal debates occurred over whether APA, as an organization, should or should not endorse the letter. Any of those involved could quite easily have claimed that their view best represented the interest of social justice. Many psychologists who favored the letter stood opposed to what they saw as the expansion of a medical model that blames individuals, rather than social structures, for human suffering; as such, signing the letter could have been framed as an act of justice. At the same time, psychologists who declined to sign the letter likely felt that changes expanding the scope and number of DSM disorders would allow more people to receive much-needed services; for them, not signing the letter served the cause of justice. My point is that how one defines justice varies across persons and contexts. Simply being psychologists does not guarantee that we all see things the same way. Just like any group of people, psychologists and counselors are not of one mind when it comes to defining and implementing ideas about social justice.

What's more, psychologists and counselors who hold themselves up as exemplars of morality should remember that being a psychologist or counselor does not make one more ethically upstanding or sophisticated than anyone else (Raskin, 2010). Yet it is common to implicitly assume that it does. For instance, some psychologists (who likely thought they were acting in the name of social justice) argued vociferously in recent years that psychologists must be present during interrogations seeking information from suspected terrorists (Pope, 2011). Their argument seemed based on the belief that psychologists are somehow more morally advanced than other professionals and therefore if they were present, they would stop others from abusing prisoners. This ignored unfortunate instances when psychologists did indeed engage in unethical behaviors that harmed people, not to mention extensive social psychology data indicating that the power of the situation typically trumps the power of the person (Benjamin & Simpson, 2009; Burger, 2009; Latane & Darley, 1968; Milgram, 1963). The presumptuousness of the position that psychologists were somehow in a privileged position to educate people about and prevent mistreatment was borne out when it was later revealed that it was actually two psychologists who talked the CIA into using harsh interrogation techniques (Shane & Mazzetti, 2009). Indeed, it is dangerous to suppose that psychologists are trained authorities in the domain of social justice and are inherently more moral than others. Such righteous certainty potentially makes one believe anything one does is just. The two psychologists who advocated torturing prisoners likely felt they were advancing the public good and serving the cause of justice.

Even if psychologists and counselors were somehow more ethically responsible than others, they would still face another dilemma, namely that there is no politics unique to psychology or counseling. That is, social justice may be defensible as a theoretical orientation, but not as a profession-wide imperative because, though we might wish it to be otherwise, "*there is nothing in the science or practice of psychology that demands loyalty to a particular political ideology*" (Raskin, 2010, p. 265, italics in original). Social justice practitioners need to tread more carefully when they claim that it is a psychologist or counselor's professional duty to support unions, resist venture capitalism, demand a living wage, and insist on health care reform. While any individual psychologist or counselor (and often many of them) might find some of these causes to be worthwhile, there should be no political litmus test one must pass in order to be a member in good standing of the psychology and counseling professions.

CONCLUSION

I am not arguing that psychologists and counselors can be neutral. Nor am I advocating for the status quo. What I am suggesting is that justice is a complicated concept and that some of the personal, professional, and political boundaries that professionals have erected may be worth retaining. Why retain them? Namely, because practitioners are not always going to agree on what justice is, nor should they be expected to. Demanding that psychologists and counselors import all their political views into their professional work is unreasonable. Yes, the personal may be political, but just because one can never truly be neutral does not mean that actively encouraging people to introduce their political beliefs into their professional work is the wisest option. People have not necessarily erected professional boundaries to maintain the status quo, but to protect people from righteous crusaders who believe they know best how others should live and how society should be structured. Stated more succinctly, what one psychologist or counselor sees as an act of justice, another sees as oppressive or unethical. By representing their new and potentially generative theoretical orientation as a discipline-wide imperative, social justice therapists unfairly impose their beliefs on clients and colleagues alike.

Finally, by framing the everyday activities of psychotherapists as acts of justice or oppression, social justice counselors run the risk of not just professional hubris, but grandiosity. By this I mean that social justice counselors often inflate the importance of what they do by portraying their everyday counseling interventions as global acts of political and social significance. A recent email I received touted the importance of advocating for clients. It used the example of counselors educating poor clients who are being discriminated against by their landlords. It encouraged counselors to actively intervene by doing things such as calling around to find these clients subsidized housing or going with them to public meetings to confront their landlords. Some psychologists might approve of such therapeutic strategies, whereas others might not. However, by framing these strategies as acts of justice rather than simply counseling informed by a liberal progressive theoretical ideology, a sense of grandiosity creeps into the proceedings. In some respects, those calling themselves social justice counselors would be better to rename their approach "liberal progressive counseling" because this would more honestly communicate their perspective without the aggrandizement that implies that only their brand of counseling has proprietorship over social justice and the public good.

The kind of grandiosity that often permeates a social justice orientation leads to what Scott Johnson (2001) dubbed a "messianic view" in which helping professionals come to believe it is their mission "to end, in some way or another, social injustice and save humanity" (p. 4). When articulating such a view, it is not enough for psychologists and counselors to provide clinical services. They must save the world. Therapy becomes "less an effort to improve human relationships than a holy crusade" (S. Johnson, 2001, p. 10). Yet each of us works for justice in our own way. Some of us do so through professional activities, while others do so on our own time. Social justice counselors and psychologists are encouraged to continue developing their theoretical perspective, offering both evidence and argument in its favor. However, as with any theoretical orientation, clinicians should remain free to adopt it or discard it without having their morality or professional legitimacy called into question. To do otherwise seems an injustice in and of itself.

NOTE

1. Some of this chapter's content is drawn from Raskin, J. D. (2010). Constructing and deconstructing social justice counseling. In J. D. Raskin, S. K. Bridges, & R. A. Neimeyer (Eds.), *Studies in meaning 4: Constructivist perspectives on theory, practice, and social justice* (pp. 247–276). New York, NY: Pace University Press.

REFERENCES

Aldarondo, E. (Ed.). (2007). *Advancing social justice through clinical practice.* Mahwah, NJ: Lawrence Erlbaum.

Bemak, F., & Chung, R. C.-Y. (2008). New professional roles and advocacy strategies for school counselors: A multicultural/social justice perspective to move beyond the nice counselor syndrome. *Journal of Counseling & Development, 86,* 372–381. doi: 10.1002/j.1556-6678.2008.tb00522.x

Benjamin, L. T., Jr., & Simpson, J. A. (2009). The power of the situation: The impact of Milgram's obedience studies on personality and social psychology. *American Psychologist, 64,* 12–19. doi: 10.1037/a0014077

Brown, L. S. (1997). Ethics in psychology: *Cui bono?* In I. Prilleltensky & D. Fox (Eds.), *Critical psychology: An introduction* (pp. 51–67). London, UK: Sage.

Burger, J. M. (2009). Replicating Milgram: Would people still obey today? *American Psychologist, 64,* 1–11. doi: 10.1037/a0010932

Burr, V. (2003). *Social constructionism* (2nd ed.). London, UK: Routledge.

Butt, T. (2000). Pragmatism, constructivism, and ethics. *Journal of Constructivist Psychology, 13,* 85–101. doi: 10.1080/107205300265892

Chung, R. C.-Y., & Bemak, F. P. (2012). *Social justice counseling: The next steps beyond multiculturalism.* Thousand Oaks, CA: Sage.

Constantine, M. G., Hage, S. M., Kindaichi, M. M., & Bryant, R. M. (2007). Social justice and multicultural issues: Implications for the practice and training of counselors and counseling psychologists. *Journal of Counseling and Development, 85,* 24–29. doi: 10.1002/j.1556-6678.2007.tb00440.x

Crethar, H. C., Torres Rivera, E., & Nash, S. (2008). In search of common threads: Linking multicultural, feminist, and social justice counseling paradigms. *Journal of Counseling and Development, 86,* 269–278. doi: 10.1002/j.1556-6678.2008.tb00509.x

Fouad, N. A., Gerstein, L. H., & Toporek, R. L. (2006). Social justice and counseling psychology in context. In R. L. Toporek, L. H. Gerstein, N. A. Fouad, G. Roysircar, & T. Israel (Eds.), *Handbook for social justice in counseling psychology: Leadership, vision, and action* (pp. 1–16). Thousand Oaks, CA: Sage.

Fouad, N. A., McPherson, R. H., Gerstein, L., Blustein, D. L., Elman, N., Helledy, K., & Metz, A. J. (2004). Houston, 2001: Context and legacy. *The Counseling Psychologist, 32*(1), 15–77. doi: 10.1177/0011000003259943

Foucault, M. (1980). *Power/knowledge: Selected interviews and other writings, 1972–1977* (C. Gordon, Ed.; C. Gordon, L. Marshall, J. Mepham, & K. Soper, Trans.). New York, NY: Pantheon Books.

Gergen, K. J. (1994). *Realities and relationships: Soundings in social construction.* Cambridge, MA: Harvard University Press.

Gergen, K. J. (2009). *An invitation to social constructionism* (2nd ed.). London, UK: Sage.

Goodman, L. A., Liang, B., Helms, J. E., Latta, R. E., Sparks, E., & Weintraub, S. R. (2004). Training counseling psychologists as social justice agents: Feminist and multicultural principles in action. *The Counseling Psychologist, 32,* 793–837. doi: 10.1177/0011000004268802

Harrist, S., & Richardson, F. C. (2012). Disguised ideologies in counseling and social justice work. *Counseling and Values, 57,* 38–44. doi: 10.1002/j.2161-007X.2012.00006.x

Johnson, A. G. (2001). *Privilege, power, and difference.* Boston: McGraw-Hill.

Johnson, S. (2001). Family therapy saves the planet: Messianic tendencies in the family systems literature. *Journal of Marital and Family Therapy, 27*(1), 3–11. doi: 10.1111/j.1752-0606.2001.tb01132.x

Latane, B., & Darley, J. M. (1968). Group inhibition of bystander intervention in emergencies. *Journal of Personality and Social Psychology, 10*(3), 215–221. doi: 10.1037/h0026570

Lee, C. C. (2012). Social justice as the fifth force in counseling. In C. Y. Chang, C. A. Barrio Minton, A. L. Dixon, J. E. Myers & T. J. Sweeney (Eds.), *Professional counseling excellence through leadership and advocacy* (pp. 109–120). New York, NY: Routledge.

Lee, C. C., & Walz, G. R. (Eds.). (1998). *Social action: A mandate for counselors.* Alexandria, VA & Greensboro, NC: American Counseling Association & ERIC Counseling and Student Services Clearinghouse.

Milgram, S. (1963). Behavioral study of obedience. *Journal of Abnormal and Social Psychology, 67*(4), 371–378. doi: 10.1037/h0040525

Morrow, S. L., Hawxhurst, D. M., Montes de Vegas, A. Y., Abousleman, T. M., & Castañeda, C. L. (2006). Toward a radical feminist multicultural therapy: Renewing a commitment to activism. In R. L. Toporek, L. H. Gerstein, N. Fouad, G. Roysircar, & T. Israel (Eds.), *Handbook for social justice in counseling psychology: Leadership, vision, and action* (pp. 231–247). Thousand Oaks, CA: Sage.

Payton, C. R. (1984). Who must do the hard things? *American Psychologist, 39,* 391–397. doi: 10.1037/0003-066X.39.4.391

Pope, K. S. (2011). Are the American Psychological Association's detainee interrogation policies ethical and effective? Key claims, documents, and results. *Zeitschrift Für Psychologie/Journal of Psychology, 219*(3), 150–158. doi: 10.1027/2151-2604/a000062

Prilleltensky, I., Dokecki, P., Frieden, G., & Ota Wang, V. (2007). Counseling for wellness and justice: Foundations and ethical dilemmas. In E. Aldarondo (Ed.), *Advancing social justice through clinical practice* (pp. 19–42). Mahwah, NJ: Lawrence Erlbaum.

Prilleltensky, I., & Fox, D. (1997). Introducing critical psychology: Values, assumptions, and the status quo. In I. Prilleltensky & D. Fox (Eds.), *Critical psychology: An introduction* (pp. 3–20). London, UK: Sage.

Prilleltensky, I., & Nelson, G. (2002). *Doing psychology critically: Making a difference in diverse settings.* New York, NY: Palgrave Macmillan.

Raskin, J. D. (2001). On relativism in constructivist psychology. *Journal of Constructivist Psychology, 14,* 285–313. doi: 10.1080/107205301750433414

Raskin, J. D. (2010). Constructing and deconstructing social justice counseling. In J. D. Raskin, S. K. Bridges & R. A. Neimeyer (Eds.), *Studies in meaning 4: Constructivist perspectives on theory, practice, and social justice* (pp. 247–276). New York, NY: Pace University Press.

Roy, B. (2007). Radical psychiatry: An approach to personal and political change. In E. Aldarondo (Ed.), *Advancing social justice through clinical practice* (pp. 65–90). Mahwah, NJ: Lawrence Erlbaum.

Rubel, D. J., & Ratts, M. J. (2011). Diversity and social justice issues in counseling and psychotherapy. In D. Capuzzi & D. R. Gross (Eds.), *Counseling and psychotherapy: Theories and interventions* (5th ed., pp. 29–51). Alexandria, VA: American Counseling Association.

Shane, S., & Mazzetti, M. (2009, April 21). In adopting harsh tactics, no inquiry into their past use. *The New York Times.* Retrieved from http://www.nytimes.com

Smith, L. (2010). *Psychology, poverty, and the end of social exclusion*. New York, NY: Teachers College Press.

Smith, S. D., Reynolds, C. A., & Rovnak, A. (2009). A critical analysis of the social advocacy movement in counseling. *Journal of Counseling & Development, 87*, 483–491. doi: 10.1002/j.1556-6678.2009.tb00133.x

Society for Humanistic Psychology (2011). *Open letter to the DSM-5*. Retrieved from http://dsm5-reform.com

Speight, S. L., & Vera, E. M. (2004). A social justice agenda: Ready or not? *The Counseling Psychologist, 32*, 109–118. doi: 10.1177/0011000003260005

Thompson, C. E., & Shermis, S. S. (2004). Tapping the talents within: A reaction to Goodman, Liang, Helms, Latta, Sparks, and Weintraub. *The Counseling Psychologist, 32*, 866–878. doi: 10.1177/0011000004269277

Toporek, R. L., Gerstein, L. H., Fouad, N., Roysircar, G., & Israel, T. (Eds.). (2006). *Handbook for social justice in counseling psychology: Leadership, vision, and action*. Thousand Oaks, CA: Sage.

Toporek, R. L., & Williams, R. A. (2006). Ethics and professional issues related to the practice of social justice in counseling psychology. In R. L. Toporek, L. H. Gerstein, N. Fouad, G. Roysircar, & T. Israel (Eds.), *Handbook for social justice in counseling psychology: Leadership, vision, and action* (pp. 17–34). Thousand Oaks, CA: Sage.

Vasquez, M. (2012). Social justice and civic virtue. In S. J. Knapp, M. C. Gottlieb & L. D. Vande-Creek (Eds.), *APA handbook of ethics in psychology: Vol. 1. Moral foundations and common themes* (pp. 75–97). Washington, DC: American Psychological Association.

Vera, E. M., & Speight, S. L. (2003). Multicultural competence, social justice, and counseling psychology: Expanding our roles. *The Counseling Psychologist, 31*(3), 253–272. doi: 10.1177/0011000003031003001

Waldegrave, C. (2005). "Just therapy" with families on low incomes. *Child Welfare, 84*, 265–276.

Chapter 4

Philosophical Reflexivity in Social Justice Work

Thomas Teo, Zhipeng Gao, and Raha Sheivari

Critical and nontraditional researchers and practitioners in the human sciences have emphasized for some time the importance of reflexivity in the production of social and psychological knowledge (Finlay & Gough, 2003; Morawski, 2005; Parker, 2005). But in critical work, including social justice work (theory and practice), the call for reflexivity has been in conflict with the demand for praxis. Marx (1845/2000) famously suggested in his 11th thesis on Feuerbach that "the philosophers have only interpreted the world, in various ways; the point is to change it" (p. 173). This argument has been interpreted to suggest that there is no need for further armchair talk but rather that action and radical transformation of society should be the primary goal. Particularly in contexts of massive oppression the notion that "true practice has primacy of over true theory" (Martín-Baró, 1994, p. 26) has been very strong—justifiably.

However, in recent decades reflexivity has experienced an upsurge. The call for reflexivity in the social sciences and in psychology has led to various criticisms from radical points of view (e.g., Burman, 2006) as well as academic perspectives (Lynch, 2000). According to Maton (2003), a process of "narcissistic reflexivity" (p. 54) may paralyze action and prevent an analysis of the social consequences of research and practice. Burman (2006) connects the call for reflexivity with the neo-liberal, therapeutic society where attention toward emotions is understood as progressive in itself. Indeed, as soon as reflexivity becomes an institutionalized routine for research, it converts into a new self-surveillance technology that normalizes particular subjective accounts while pathologizing others. A reflexive focus that urges researchers to work on themselves may substitute for participation and radical collaborative action. Thus, following Burman, reflexivity may contribute to reducing structural problems to personal ones, enhance the process of individualization, and transform reflexivity into a methodological intervention.

We propose a philosophical attitude toward reflexivity that avoids self-surveillance, individualization, or a confessional attitude, but rather is intended to inspire informed action in social justice work. This perspective follows Parker (1999) who offered a reminder "to look at how the subjectivity of the researcher affects and interconnects with that of the researched, and, in particular, what forms of agency are facilitated or blocked in the process" (pp. 32–33). Such a critical attitude toward reflexivity provides the conditions for the possibility of reflexivity to challenge the status quo. We attempt to provide a useful heuristic when dividing reflexivity into ontological, epistemological, and ethical dimensions, and when applying these dimensions, as interconnected as they are, to reflect upon social justice work (theoretical, academic, practical, or political). We also propose that reflexivity is a first-person psychological concept, meaning that it should be applied to oneself, that is, to one's own theories and practices, before it is applied to the *other*. This entails an understanding of the reasonable perspective of the other as legitimate as one's own view (even if these perspectives disagree).

ONTOLOGICAL REFLEXIVITY

Ontological questions in philosophy concern the being and nature of *things* and *events*. When it comes to social justice work, we suggest discussing assumptions about the nature of social justice phenomena, the nature of social justice theories and concepts, and the nature of social justice work itself. This ontological reflexivity includes a consideration of the implicit assumptions about the nature of humans and human activity. The hermeneutic philosopher Gadamer (1960/1997) suggested that the essence of the hermeneutic experience can be found in an open dialogue. Thus, although reflexivity is a first-person process, it always includes the other in an intersubjective exchange. Because for Gadamer, "the logic of the human sciences is a logic of the question" (p. 370), we express entry points for reflexivity in the form of questions.

What Is the Nature of Humans?

Most social justice work (it does not matter whether it is located within a Catholic or radical tradition) begins with the assumption that humans are not just isolated individuals. We trace this idea in the Western world to G. Vico (1668–1744), G. Hegel (1770–1831), but particularly to K. Marx (1818–1883). Marx argued that people are individuals only to the degree that history and society enables them to be individuals because human consciousness is sublated in the history and society we live in (Teo, 2011). Mental life is socially embedded; there is no unsocialized self. Marx argued, providing an entry point for reflexivity, that perceptions about human nature are influenced by one's own societal position and by an ideological understanding of social reality. Marx also provided a solution to such misrepresentations that have influenced radical social justice work: praxis allows one to do something about societal dependencies, injustices, and intellectual misrepresentations.

Following Marx, critical thinkers have suggested that human existence takes place within a societal context, that society is not an external environment or an external variable, but rather an active agent that constitutes the self even if one is not determined by it (Holzkamp, 1983). However, one of the main problems stems from the question of how one should understand *society* and which categories social justice workers should privilege. This problem is an important site for ontological reflexivity because it determines which social justice goal "I" will focus on. For instance, how can one describe contemporary Western society? One might describe it as developed, industrialized, secular, democratic, liberal, neo-liberal, multicultural, open, advanced; or as patriarchal, neo-colonial, capitalist; or as consumerist, leisure-oriented, communicative, information-based, technological, modern or postmodern; or as combinations thereof. Descriptions can be based on the economy, political system, industry, technology, knowledge production, and so on.

Derived from such theoretical preferences emerges the reflexive question of whether society is, for instance, something holistic and positive or divided into antagonistic interests and negative. Social justice work may differ based on such theoretical choices. Can justice be reached for an individual or a community or society with or without addressing basic antagonisms in society? For the radical thinker Žižek (1989) "society is always traversed by an antagonistic split which cannot be integrated into symbolic order" (p. 126). He argued that ideological fantasy needs to construct "a society in which the relation between its parts is organic and complementary" (p. 126) while denying this antagonistic division. On the other side is Martín-Baró (1994), who drew on Marxist and Catholic roots, and who understands the injustice of poverty less as a result of class divisions but as a form of "sin" (p. 26). Sin is something that contradicts God's will—a concept that does not make much intellectual sense for atheist social justice workers. Can social justice workers operate with concepts in which they do not believe, but which may motivate large groups?

The notion of a societal nature of humans (Holzkamp, 1983) involves a discussion about human nature in which way human life takes place in society and history, and suggests that it may be problematic to abstract the individual from society (as is done in most of mainstream psychology). This notion includes reflexivity about society, about how one conceptualizes it, but also about the nature of concepts addressing human nature, society, and social justice concepts (e.g., the concept of class has a different history and meaning from the concept of sin).

What Is the Nature of Social Justice Concepts?

Researchers such as Gergen (2001) and Danziger (1997) in psychology, or Hacking (1986, 1995) in philosophy, have asked whether the concepts that are used in the social sciences represent an external world or whether they contribute to the construction of the social world. Martin and Sugarman (2009) summarized such discussions by arguing that concepts in the human science as *socially constituted* do not exist in a separate form before they are introduced in social life (e.g., IQ); moreover, human kind concepts are subject to *looping effects* (Hacking, 1995), meaning that there is an interaction between humans and the classes to which they have been assigned (people understand themselves through psychological concepts, which then suggests the reality of these concepts); finally, psychological kinds are value-laden (having a low IQ entails something negative in Western society).

Similar arguments could apply to concepts used in social justice research as they have a history and a social background. Philosophers and psychologists have looked at the various meanings of social justice (e.g., Prilleltensky & Nelson, 2009), but this examination needs to be accompanied by an analysis of the nature of the concept of social justice itself: Where does this concept come from? Who used it within which political and philosophical background? How did it become part of "my" identity? What positive and negative values are assigned to it within a particular culture? For example, the concept of social justice has religious Christian backgrounds, and roots in the French revolution, but is also inspired by socialist and radical traditions. What is it about "my" own cultural and political background that makes certain traditions more palatable to "me" than to others and what are the action consequences that these traditions bring with them?

If social justice is socially, historically, and culturally constituted, then does this entail that social justice is relative? Not necessarily! The historicity of concepts does not imply that there is no progress concerning concepts (however, progress is a historical assumption that requires its own justification). Yet, historicity can explain why great thinkers such as Aristotle (384–322 BCE), who developed sophisticated ethical systems, did not think about social justice for slaves. It can explain why Immanuel Kant (1724–1804), who suggested never treating humans as means but always as ends could provide "racist" constructions of "blackness" (Bernasconi, 2001). Reflexivity in this context means deciding on the possibly valid, yet historically limited, meanings of social justice.

Another example of ontological reflections in this area concerns the nature of the concept of difference versus the nature of the concept of inequality. At first sight, it might seem that *difference* is a concept that refers to natural kinds whereas *inequality* refers to social kinds. A closer look reveals that difference is never difference for itself—it is always difference for "us." One might have different ear sizes but this difference is not meaningful to us although it might have been (Teo, 2010). Difference can be real or imagined but difference is made real through social constructions, actions, and structures. Inequality is clearly a social kind and has major ramifications for social life, including health, crime, and so on (Wilkinson & Pickett, 2009). However, inequality demonstrates historical and cultural trajectories and takes on different shapes in different countries. The reconstruction of the nature of those differences should be part of ontological reflections.

What Is the Nature of Social Justice Work?

It is evident throughout history that social justice work need not be a unified program, and that diverse approaches exist that reflect particular contexts. Thus, totalizing ideas about the true meaning of social justice work might run counter to the complexity of this endeavor. For example, in Europe more radical initiatives have been proposed, often in the context of political programs, whereas in English-speaking North America reformist approaches have been seen as appropriate and legitimate. The point here is to understand one's own location and the choices one prefers as reflecting one's own societal embeddedness, which may influence the assessment of the possibilities and limitations of particular approaches. A broad definition of social justice work may provide the conditions for the possibility of working together on a larger scale (if one thinks this is important).

EPISTEMOLOGICAL REFLEXIVITY

Social justice work produces, distributes, and consumes knowledge. Epistemological reflexivity challenges one's knowledge, one's assumptions about knowledge, and one's practice of knowledge. Academics have argued that epistemological reflexivity needs to be applied at all stages of research (Finlay, 2002; Guillemin & Gillam, 2004; Parker, 2005; Peshkin, 1988), including "the selection of problems, the formation of hypotheses, the design of research (including the organization of research communities), the collection of data, the interpretation and sorting of data, decisions about when to stop research, the way results of research are reported, and so on" (Harding, 1992, p. 69).

Differences between the researcher (this may include practitioners) and the participant or client (the other) in terms of gender, ethnicity, class, age, experience, and so on, come into play in the production and dissemination of knowledge. These social labels may reflect different rationalities, values, languages, and norms that can be traced to cultural or subcultural contexts. The researcher, informed by his or her particular cultural assumptions, may prefer particular research topics, methodologies, interpretations, interventions, and so on, that neglect or even violate the participant's unique subjectivity and life conditions. The social justice worker may impose his or her own version of health, empowerment, and resistance onto the other, a rationality that is shaped under the influence of existing power relations.

Are Power and Knowledge Related?

There is no way around it: research contexts are laden with power, and a power differential exists in the researcher-participant relationship. Traditional researchers are less concerned with this issue, partly because the power imbalance actually helps to control the variables under investigation and to promote certain interventions. Social justice workers, in contrast, may intend to empower the other but may find themselves occupying a position that is reinforced by professional status, expertise, class, educational background, institutional support, to a certain degree, interpersonal expertise, and by the relational structure of research as it is conducted in our societies. With such a privileged position, the researcher can easily, in spite of best intentions, produce, disseminate, and reify cultural assumptions, visions of self-realization, and social utopias (Siraj-Blatchford & Siraj-Blatchford, 1997).

Feminists, postcolonial theorists, and historians have shown that the production and dissemination of knowledge is susceptible to power, money, and social relationships. In this context it is important that researchers reflect on whether or in what ways they perpetuate and reproduce the political, economic, patriarchal, and racialized status quo. This may require relativizing and contextualizing in front of the other the power of the psychologist, revealing the historical-cultural positioning of knowledge, and explicating the influence of power and money on social justice work. In that sense, epistemological reflexivity is not oriented toward "ourselves" as an inner monologue, but rather as a dialogue with the other. Parker (2005) phrased it so aptly when he suggested that people should not consider themselves as "the bedrock of experience but as something that is crystallized from historical and institutional structures" (p. 29).

Bourdieu (1988) conceptualized researchers as social actors who tend to struggle for status and resources. While doubting Bourdieu's concept of an absolute "will to power" in social justice work, social justice workers should reflect on motivations for research and practice. Does one research and practice for the sake of social justice, and what is the role of publications, grants, promotions, and reputation? Although critical social justice researchers align themselves with the marginalized instead of with the governmental, industrial, or corporate bodies that provide resources, the continuation and actualization of many projects often cannot be carried out without financial resources and institutional support. A reflection on issues of power in the "game of knowledge" can help to trace institutional and discursive inequalities (Parker, 1999, 2005). Social justice workers who are unreflexive about power, knowledge, and their own subjectivities (as taking place in a social context) may perpetuate the status quo and colonize the other.

How Do We Understand the Other?

It should be mentioned that the term *Other* is problematic and requires some ontological reflection itself. In a phenomenology of the *Other* one would quickly understand that "my" husband as the other is different from "my" neighbor as the other, is different from the homeless person on the streets as the Other, and is different from the aboriginal activist as the Other. We do not discuss these differences here but consider, for reflexive reasons, the participant in our research as the Other and the "client" in social justice practice as the Other.

Considering the Other in research and taking the Other into account in our practices means that one challenges an egological approach to the Other (Lévinas, 1961/1969). With R. Descartes (1596–1650) one could argue that "I am the source of knowledge," with K. Marx (1818–1883) that "We are the source of knowledge," and with E. Lévinas (1906–1995) that "You are the source of knowledge." Epistemological reflexivity means to take the other's experiences radically into account and not to transform them into "my" framework (Kögler, 1999). One's own knowledge of the Other needs be transformed from within the standpoint of the Other in a way that it changes and extends "our" horizons. Again, we emphasize: although reflexivity is a first-person concept, it needs to be articulated under the guidance (not dominance) of the Other whereby the Other is recognized as someone who can speak for himself or herself.

A radical first-person psychology involves the perspective of the other in a way that may be uncomfortable. Holzkamp (1984) argued, using the example of an alcoholic, that if a researcher or therapist already knows at the beginning of an intervention with an alcoholic that drinking must end, subjectivity, the Other's standpoint, is excluded. It might turn out, after a thorough analysis of the person's situation, that drinking alcohol is the best solution for this specific individual. A first-person psychology accepts the Other's perspective even if one disagrees completely with the Other. Thus, people need to ask, what are they willing to do if a victim of oppression does not want social justice the way he or she conceptualizes it?

The commitment to the Other needs to be expressed when working with the Other. On the one hand, any research participant should have the opportunity to express his or her experiential situation as well as context, to discuss his or her intentional horizon, and to voice his or her value system and vision of existence (Kögler, 1999). On the other hand, the researcher possesses conceptual and methodological training and has the opportunity to address the dynamics between participant and researcher as well as the dynamics between the participant's life and the social-political context. The researcher might question his or her status as a researcher and actually change the roles of researcher-participant as is done in some participatory action research. Epistemological reflexivity means having awareness of one's own intellectual and practical traditions and of how cultural assumptions can hinder or foster social justice work.

Social justice psychologists could even go further and use Lacanian ideas to emphasize the point of radical reflexivity. Nobus and Quinn (2005) argued that, "in Lacanian psychoanalysis the analysand (i.e., client) is guided not towards a moment of (self) recognition, as the culmination of a Socratic 'know thyself,' but towards a practice of non-recognition in which knowledge appears as a foreign substance" (p. 111). Taking the Other into account could lead one in the process of epistemological reflexivity to a trauma "whereby theories collapse, beliefs fall apart and that which we thought we knew is revealed as deception and sham" (p. 111).

It is clear at this point that epistemology and ethics interact. Considering the Other as an end and not as a means in social justice work is not only an epistemological stance but also an ethical position (Kögler, 2005). This puts social justice psychologists outside the standards of the discipline of psychology. As Richardson and Slife (2011) summarize this situation aptly: "Academic or professional psychologists with a social justice orientation are commonly viewed as arbitrarily injecting their preferred moral outlook into their work rather than remaining appropriately value-neutral, or at least tolerant and nonjudgmental" (p. 169). They recommend not cordoning off ethical commitments but rather acknowledging moral choices, virtues, and goods.

Is Social Justice Knowledge Universal or Particular?

Claims to universality in the human sciences appear to be problematic. Indeed, history has established an "acute consciousness . . . of the inescapabilities and particularities of places, characters, historical trajectories, and fate" (Rabinow, 1996, p. 56). In order to deal with such situations we emphasize the position that reflexivity requires more than listening and engaging with the Other. Perhaps the most important epistemological part is not to assume universality of "my" ideas, but to show *epistemological modesty* by assuming the local nature of "my" knowledge. It may turn out that "my" knowledge is more culturally transcendent than "I" assume; yet it should not be the starting point for knowledge practices.

ETHICAL REFLEXIVITY

We suggest that any kind of social or psychological activity is inherently a moral project because it engages with persons, communities, or cultures. Ontological and epistemological decisions have ethical dimensions. The conducting of research has a moral dimension as has the presentation of research and the practice of social justice work. Given the huge amount of literature on ethics that indicates the complexity of the debates, we present only some examples that intend to represent ethical dilemmas and issues that social justice workers might encounter or that they need to reflect upon.

Are "My" Self-Evident Ethics Arrogant?

Sati (widow burning) is a ritual wherein the Hindu widow joins the pyre of a dead husband and immolates herself (Spivak, 1988). The British annulled this practice as illegal and as a crime. Sati seems to be a case for self-evident ethics, but may reflect a Western approach to the problem. According to the postcolonial thinker, Spivak (1988), the act of the criminalization of Sati can be understood as a case of "white men saving brown women from brown men" (p. 297). Spivak asks, if given a voice, how would a subaltern subject, in this case, an Indian widowed woman, speak for her condition?

According to Spivak (1988), Sati is not considered a suicide in Hinduism. It is a sacred ritual in which all members of the religion, including women, understand death as a signifier of free will. The practice of Sati symbolizes a woman's choice. When the woman is burned in the fire, she becomes free from her body for the entire cycle of birth. According to Spivak, the abolition of widow burning imposed a greater ideological constriction on Hindu women than before and deprived them from exercising their freedom. However, Western ideals of modernity have contempt for this type of courage and for such ideals of womanly conduct. Spivak then contrasts her understanding of Sati with ideals of sacrifice in the West: "Perhaps Sati should have been read with martyrdom, with the defunct husband standing in for the transcendental One; or with war, with the husband standing in for sovereign or state, for whose sake an intoxicating ideology of self-sacrifice can be mobilized" (p. 302).

Spivak does not advocate the killing of widows nor do we. The ethical problem arises when the social justice workers already know what is best for the Other, but neglects the voice and the standpoint of the Other. Social justice workers need to be reflexive of the history and contexts of activities that may diametrically oppose their own values. They need to ask, especially in contexts that are dissimilar to their own, whether the subaltern subject or the victim of social injustice is given voice to speak and how it is possible to recover his or her subjectivity without constructing his or her wishes as inferior, problematic, or stupid. One might even ask whether social justice work is required in contexts, in which the subject does not perceive a problem to act upon.

Does "My" Social Justice Work Problematize the Other?

The history of psychology and social research shows that summaries and interpretations (in books, journal articles, chapters, presentations, etc.) often present the Other as a problem or as inferior. Although most current social justice work does not invoke notions of natural inferiority, "we" need to be aware and reflexive in not portraying participants as problems. The interpretation of data always contains a *hermeneutic surplus* (interpretations of data contain more than data), as well as a *hermeneutic deficit* (interpretations are deficient because they contain elements of speculation) (Teo, 2008). But interpretations that suggest that the Other is a problem (e.g., based on race, class, gender, disability, sexual preference, age) are not just epistemologically limited but are also a form of violence. The presentation of knowledge through interpretations is not only an epistemological but also an ethical issue and may have a harmful impact on people (as epistemological violence).

The term *epistemological violence* is closer to personal violence than to structural violence because it has a subject, an object, and an action, even if the violent act is indirect and nonphysical. In the social sciences, the subject of violence is the researcher (or researchers), the object is the Other, and the action is the interpretation of data that is presented as knowledge. Epistemological violence is executed in empirical work, when theoretical interpretations of empirical results implicitly or explicitly construct the Other as inferior or problematic, despite the fact that alternative interpretations, equally viable based on the data, are available. From that perspective social justice needs an inclusion of epistemological justice (i.e., doing justice to individuals and groups in the knowledge of the social sciences and psychology). Instead of making the Other into a problem social justice workers need to work on the problems that the Other encounters.

Does "My" Social Justice Work Idealize the Other?

The other side of problematization is idealization, which follows the same *ego-logic* in that it begins with "me" and not with the Other. There exists a dialectical relationship between problematization and idealization in that idealization can move to its opposite quickly and vice versa. What happens if a person experiencing social injustice, a person who one may idealize for that reason, expresses and enacts racist or sexist beliefs? What if a victim of racism is racist toward another person or group? This situation requires reflection about one's own ethical compass and practices, and might require an understanding that the victim or object of racism needs to be supported regardless of his or her attitudes, while at the same time challenging the racism that he or she expresses. It also might require an ontological and epistemological reflection of racism as something less personal and more structural, applying analyses that are able to address the structural nature of injustice. This may prevent an idealization and problematization of subjects of social injustice.

In this context, value clarifications might be useful as well. Prilleltensky (2008) has argued that the values of the French revolution ("liberty, equality and fraternity") that can be understood as attending to personal (liberty), collective (equality), and relational (fraternity) needs require a balance. These principles can also be used to reflect on one's own societies and on the values they endorse. For example, how important is liberty versus equality in the United States, France, or China? Do the values that a nation endorses influence the values that "my" social justice work supports? Is there a better balance in Europe than in the United States? Is fraternity (solidarity) a form of social justice that demands, for instance, a national health care or publicly funded system, as practiced in most European countries?

What about Violence?

The issue of violence appears on several levels: we have pointed out that academic interpretations of empirical data can assume the form of violence. A research interpretation that is underdetermined by data and that leads to a construction of inferiority or problematization of the Other is a form of violence. Ethical and epistemological reflexivities need to attend to this issue. Another level of violence is structural violence, which Galtung (1969) differentiated from personal violence. Galtung argued convincingly that a structure such as social injustice should be understood as a form of violence. A different form of violence is expressed in the question of whether violence is a legitimate means of social justice work.

What if individuals find themselves in a society with extreme inequality? In such a context the master does not care at all about the slave. The slave is neglected, not cared for, exposed to a variety of forms of violence and injustice, and disposed like trash if no longer needed. Would one be surprised to see that the slave strikes back in a manner that appears incomprehensible to an outside observer and that the slave in turn does not care at all about what happens to the master? Unfortunately, in some countries violence has become a pervasive reality and extreme forms of criminality have taken over the quest for justice. We believe that a social justice analysis of violence should not begin with an analysis of personal psychological problems, but with an analysis of structure. As studies have shown, greater inequality is associated with greater criminal outcomes (Fajnzlber, Lederman, & Loayza, 2002; Wilkinson & Pickett, 2009). Yet, one also needs to be reflexive that social justice is primarily not about reducing crime but about taking care of the Other.

But is violence a means to fight social injustice? For most Western social justice workers violence is no longer an option, nor is it for us. But what if conditions are so horrendous that violence appears as a viable option to those experiencing extreme social injustice? History has a long list of violent actions that overcame horrendous injustices, from Spartacus (c. 109–71 BCE) to World War II, so should activists automatically discount the option of violence? What if, from the standpoint of the object of extreme social injustice, violence appears as the only option for restructuring society?

There has been much debate about Fanon's (1963) stance toward violence. But one can read Fanon in a way such that violence is the objective outcome of a violent situation (colonialism). Instead of attempting to moralize the violent actions of colonizer and colonized, he described in a neutral manner of fact the consequences of violence on victims and perpetrators. His avoidance of psychologization in the context of colonial violence appears to support violence. Because his psychological project did not subjugate his political program, violence is a factual political outcome, a *historical* reality that social justice work should not dismiss *a priori*. Both proponents and opponents of violence need to ask: What are the political and psychological reasons for promoting or avoiding violence when it comes to social justice?

CONCLUSION

Smith (2005) summarized the current status quo on the issue very well: "[T]here is the reflexivity of academics in a particular field, say social theory, interested in persuading colleagues to examine the taken-for-granted concepts, values and practices of the field" (p. 3). The question is what this reflexivity embellishes. We think that Maton (2003) makes valid points when discussing the attitude that might emerge from reflexivity: "[I]t has now become a sin to not be reflexive. The term is used as a marker of proclaimed distinction and originality, with position-takings effectively claiming, 'I am a reflexive actor producing reflexive accounts of reflexive modernity, while you are unreflexive and inadequate, an outdated relic of a bygone era' " (p. 54).

Yet, reflexivity, the way we understand it, includes respect for the research intentions of the Other, which should prevent such sentiments, or at least allow one to work on such sentiments. Reflexivity is not a monological endeavor but includes the participation of Others. It involves an understanding of the societal nature of humans, the historicity of social concepts, and the disunified reality of much of social justice work. It means discussing the role of the Other, which includes a discussion of the role of "me," that research needs to be with and for the Other and not merely about the Other, or that social justice research and practice is an ethical project. Such reflexivity may allow the conditions for avoiding the narcissistic trap of adoring reflexivity for its own sake while engendering social justice work and informed action that is aware of its limitations as well as its possibilities in the here and now.

REFERENCES

Bernasconi, R. (2001). Who invented the concept of race? Kant's role in the Enlightenment construction of race. In R. Bernasconi (Ed.), *Race* (pp. 11–36). Malden, MA: Blackwell.

Bourdieu, P. (1988). *Homo academicus*. (P. Collier, Trans.). Stanford, CA: Stanford University Press.

Burman, E. (2006). Emotions and reflexivity in feminised education action research. *Educational Action Research, 14*(3), 315–332.

Danziger, K. (1997). *Naming the mind: How psychology found its language*. Thousand Oaks, CA: Sage.

Fajnzlber, P., Lederman, D., & Loayza, N. (2002). Inequality and violent crime. *Journal of Law & Economics, 45,* 1.

Fanon, F. (1963). *The Wretched of the earth* (C. Farrington, Trans.). New York, NY: Grove Press.

Finlay, L. (2002). "Outing" the researcher: The provenance, process, and practice of reflexivity. *Qualitative Health Research, 12*(4), 531–545. doi: 10.1177/104973202129120052

Finlay, L., & Gough, B. (Eds.). (2003). *Reflexivity: A practical guide for researchers in health and social sciences*. Oxford, UK: Blackwell.

Gadamer, H.-G. (1997). *Truth and method* (J. Weinsheimer & D. G. Marshall, Trans.). New York, NY: Continuum. (Original work published 1960).

Galtung, J. (1969). Violence, peace, and peace research. *Journal of Peace Research, 3,* 167–191.

Gergen, K. J. (2001). Psychological science in a postmodern context. *American Psychologist, 56*(10), 803.

Guillemin, M., & Gillam, L. (2004). Ethics, reflexivity, and "ethically important moments" in research. *Qualitative Inquiry, 10*(2), 261.

Hacking, I. (1986). Making up people. In T. C. Heller, M. Sosna, & D. Wellbery (Eds.), *Reconstructing individualism: Autonomy, individuality, and the self in Western thought* (pp. 222–236). Stanford, CA: Stanford University Press.

Hacking, I. (1995). The looping effects of human kinds. In D. Sperber, D. Premack, & A. J. Premack (Eds.), *Causal cognition: A multidisciplinary debate* (pp. 351–383). New York, NY: Oxford University Press.

Harding, S. (1992). Rethinking standpoint epistemology: What is "strong objectivity"? *The Centennial Review, 36*(3), 437–470.

Holzkamp, K. (1983). *Grundlegung der Psychologie [Laying the foundations for psychology].* Frankfurt am Main: Campus.

Holzkamp, K. (1984). Die Menschen sitzen nicht im Kapitalismus wie in einem Kaefig [Interview] [Humans are not trapped in capitalism as in a cage]. *Psychologie Heute, 11,* 29–37.

Kögler, H.-H. (1999). *The power of dialogue: Critical hermeneutics after Gadamer and Foucault.* (P. Hendrickson, Trans.). Cambridge, MA: MIT Press.

Kögler, H.-H. (2005). Recognition and difference: The power of perspectives in interpretive dialogue. *Social Identities, 11*(3), 247–269.

Lévinas, E. (1969). Totality and infinity: An *essay on exteriority* (A. Lingis, Trans.). Pittsburgh, PA: Duquesne University Press. (Original work published 1961).

Lynch, M. (2000). Against reflexivity as an academic virtue and source of privileged knowledge. *Theory, Culture & Society, 17*(3), 26–54. doi: 10.1177/02632760022051202

Martin, J., & Sugarman, J. (2009). Does interpretation in psychology differ from interpretation in natural science? *Journal for the Theory of Social Behaviour, 39*(1), 19–37.

Martín-Baró, I. (1994). *Writings for a liberation psychology.* (A. Aron & S. Corne, Eds.). Cambridge, MA: Harvard University Press.

Marx, K. (2000). Theses on Feuerbach. In D. McLellan (Ed.), *Karl Marx: Selected writings.* New York, NY: Oxford University Press. (Original work written in 1845).

Maton, K. (2003). Reflexivity, relationism, & research: Pierre Bourdieu and the epistemic conditions of social scientific knowledge. *Space and Culture, 6*(1), 52–65.

Morawski, J. G. (2005). Reflexivity and the psychologist. *History of the Human Sciences, 18*(4), 77.

Nobus, D., Quinn, M. (2005). *Knowing nothing, staying stupid: Elements for a psychoanalytic epistemology.* New York, NY: Routledge.

Parker, I. (1999). Critical reflexive humanism and critical constructionist psychology. In D. J. Nightingale & J. Cromby (Eds.), *Social constructionist psychology: A critical analysis of theory and practice* (pp. 23–36). Buckingham, UK: Open University Press.

Parker, I. (2005). *Qualitative psychology: Introducing radical research.* Buckingham, UK: Open University Press.

Peshkin, A. (1988). In search of subjectivity—One's own. *Educational Researcher, 17*(7), 17–21.

Prilleltensky, I. (2008). The role of power in wellness, oppression, and liberation: The promise of psychopolitical validity. *Journal of Community Psychology, 36*(2), 116–136.

Prilleltensky, I., & Nelson, G. (2009). Community psychology: Advancing social justice. In D. Fox, I. Prilleltensky & S. Austin (Eds.), *Critical psychology: An introduction (2nd ed.)* (pp. 126–143). London, UK: Sage.

Rabinow, P. (1996). *The anthropology of reason.* Princeton, NJ: Princeton University Press.

Richardson, F. C., & Slife, B. D. (2011). Critical thinking in social and psychological inquiry. *Journal of Theoretical and Philosophical Psychology, 31*(3), 165.

Siraj-Blatchford, I., & Siraj-Blatchford, J. (1997). Reflexivity, social justice and educational research. *Cambridge Journal of Education, 27*(2), 235–248.

Smith, R. (2005). Does reflexivity separate the human sciences from the natural sciences? *History of the Human Sciences, 18*(4), 1–25.

Spivak, G. C. (1988). Can the subaltern speak? In C. Nelson & L. Grossberg (Eds.), *Marxism and the interpretation of culture* (pp. 271–313). Urbana, IL: University of Illinois Press.

Teo, T. (2008). From speculation to epistemological violence in psychology: A critical-hermeneutic reconstruction. *Theory & Psychology, 18*(1), 47–67.

Teo, T. (2010). What is epistemological violence in the empirical social sciences? *Social and Personality Psychology Compass, 4*(5), 295–303.

Teo, T. (2011). Radical philosophical critique and critical thinking in psychology. *Journal of Theoretical and Philosophical Psychology, 31*(3), 193–199. doi: 10.1037/a0024708

Wilkinson, R. G., & Pickett, K. (2009). *The spirit level: Why more equal societies almost always do better.* London, UK: Allen Lane.

Žižek, S. (1989). *The sublime object of ideology.* New York, NY: Verso.

Chapter 5

Ideology and the Role of Dialogue in Political Mobilization

William R. Earnest and Tod S. Sloan

Why are nonelite citizens of nominally democratic societies unlikely to act to mobilize for social arrangements more aligned with their interests? When poverty and unemployment rates are high, when cuts are made to public services, when young people are sent to fight in questionable wars, when the environment is destroyed in the interest of corporate profit, and when the rich accumulate unprecedented wealth, why are there not more widespread social unrest, organized protest, and resistance? Where are the movements to construct alternative economies and communities? Many factors account for the general absence of mass mobilization, including poor education, lack of information, distraction by the media, fear of reprisal, policing, propaganda, exclusion from decision-making arenas, and so forth. Yet, one concept is especially handy in accounting for conformity to the status quo, and it tends to be ignored especially in psychological accounts of social behavior: the concept of ideology.

In critical sociology, the concept of ideology is usually introduced to answer the questions posed earlier. Related terms such as false consciousness (Engels, 1893/1968) or hegemony (Gramsci, 1971) might also be referenced. At the outset, it is important to distinguish critical uses of the concept of ideology from its usual meaning. Ideology is commonly understood simply as a set of beliefs or ideas, such as conservatism or communism. In critical scholarship, however, it refers to a matrix of representations of social reality that is interwoven with institutional practices and social structures in a way that implies the impossibility of improvement (Lukács, 1919–23/1971). Critical scholars call social behavior ideological, rather than simply cultural, when its effects are such that a given social order is reproduced systematically and when alternatives to it are made to appear impossible and, at the extreme, literally unthinkable. The principal argument in what follows is that the processes subsumed under the concept of ideology entail subjective moments about which critical psychology and psychoanalysis provide important insights. It is essential for psychologists to take these insights into account in waging struggles for social justice, and particularly in understanding the role of dialogic practices in political mobilization and in deepening democratic control of workplaces and governments.

As critical psychologists have often pointed out (Parker, 2007; Prilleltensky, 1994; Sloan, 1996), the individualism inherent in scientific psychology has led to ignorance of both history and societal context among psychologists. Psychology and psychologists thus contribute to the reproduction of the societal status quo. To counter this, in assessing possible courses of action for social justice in contemporary societies, it is essential to review the major global trends of the past few centuries for a refreshed sense of the objective context of the ideological processes that block action. Part of the effectiveness of advanced psychological training in conjunction with status-quo maintenance is the abstraction of human behavior from historical and political contexts. We seek, in contrast, to point out how they are related. Obviously, there are endless debates about how history may best be characterized (Jameson, 2002; Wallerstein, 2004), but something along the lines of the next few paragraphs would be generally accepted by progressive scholars.

A BRIEF OVERVIEW OF THE WORLD-SYSTEM CONTEXT

Following the rise of scientific thinking during the Renaissance, advances in material and social technologies harnessed natural resources and concentrated labor power for increasingly rapid industrialization. In Western Europe over the next few centuries, the economic arrangements associated with industrialization were such that the owners of land and factories, in their drive to accumulate capital, developed productive capacities at hitherto unimaginable rates, driving a search for natural resources and labor, and eventually for new product markets. As power became concentrated in the new capitalist class, tensions with feudal and monarchical elites grew, eventually giving rise to *bourgeois revolutions*—reorderings of societies to make them more compatible with the capitalist economic order. As part of these transformations, agrarian working people were displaced by foreclosure and mechanization. Cities swelled as these landless laborers found work in factories; this process is still underway today across large areas of the developing world. Management of these urban masses became a problem for the emerging nation-states.

Previous colonization of the globe by European (and later, American) powers seeking slaves, gold, spices, and other resources valued by mercantile economies laid pathways for later imperialist expansion driven by the needs of industrialization. This continued almost unchecked even after colonies gained their independence in the wave of post–World War II liberation struggles. Attempts by the former colonies to augment their political independence with economic independence by import substitution development strategies yielded only mixed results (e.g., Pollin, 2005). Eventually all developing countries, most spectacularly the Soviet Union and the People's Republic of China (PRC), successively came to accept positions in an international division of labor determined by globe-spanning capitalist institutions centered first in EuroAmerica, but eventually including Japan, then so-called Asian Tigers (principally South Korea and Taiwan), and finally the PRC.

Resistance to this capitalist-directed division of labor has taken a myriad of forms. The most ambitious and explicit alternatives, powerfully embodied in the social experiments of the Soviet Union and the PRC, failed due to a combination of having been carried out in agrarian countries, external pressures, and internal bureaucratic ossification. Both social formations proved incapable of providing much beyond a modest standard of living for their populations and a concomitant capacity for defensive war.

Nevertheless, the threat of an international alternative to capitalism served to intimidate capitalist elites, during the middle 50 years of the 20th century, bolstering the efforts of domestic labor unions and civil rights organizations in Europe and the Americas to claim a larger share of economic output, and to guarantee acceptable living conditions.

The erosion and collapse of the alternatives to capitalist models has, since the 1970s, unfettered capitalism's coercive genius at minimizing production costs to maximize profit. One result has been incredible gaps between wealthy and poor, both within societies, and especially between the societies of the North and those in the global South.

Another direct result of industrialization has been the degradation of the natural environment through deforestation, mining, industrial agriculture, pollution of air, water, and soil, carbon emissions producing climate change, to the point of threatening all life on earth, not to mention the ongoing extinction of millions of species. Despite urgent warnings from scientists for several decades now, corporate and political leaders have been unwilling to protect the basis for life if doing so requires giving up opportunities for continued capital accumulation.

In advanced capitalist societies, multinational corporations and the national governments they increasingly control quite effectively mobilize or constrain citizen behavior as needed to ensure elites' continuing accumulation of capital. Advertising steadily generates illusory needs that consumers rush to satisfy, even as real wages and job security erode. Police surveillance and welfare systems monitor deviance and quickly incarcerate or reduce to penury those who do not conform.

A booming culture industry keeps the general population glued to TVs and computer monitors. Meanwhile, symptoms of depression and anxiety stemming from alienation and social disconnection are medicated. This array of measures implemented under capitalist consumerist regimes to address crises and maintain stability has been described by the German social philosopher Jürgen Habermas (1987) as the *colonization of the lifeworld*, a concept seeking to register social psychological dimensions not included in economistic accounts of social control. The lifeworld consists of communicative interactions that sustain meanings related to ethics, aesthetics, and lived experience separate from the demands of the economic and bureaucratic systems.

IDEOLOGY, COMPROMISE FORMATION, AND DESYMBOLIZATION

These realities are of interest to psychologists not only because of the unnecessary physical and emotional suffering that accompanies labor exploitation, poverty, and the destruction of the environment, but because viable and necessary alternatives to existing power structures and irrational social systems are rarely considered and even more rarely taken seriously. This quiescence poses a range of questions involving a psychological aspect: How do those who benefit from global capitalist arrangements contain social tensions and ensure the reproduction of the social order? What happens to notions of a better world that people may entertain? How do people formulate and address problems and situations where their sense of justice is violated? Why do citizens behave in ways that fail to reflect plausible formulations of their individual or collective best interest, and instead contribute to the maintenance of a social order that exploits them? Why do citizens have trouble moving beyond individualistic lifestyle solutions to social and environmental problems? Clearly, the term *colonization of the lifeworld* applies to such situations wherein resistance is cut short, voices are silenced, and control is exerted in the service of distant beneficiaries.

To begin to answer such questions, we explain the subjective or psychological substrate of ideology with reference to basic psychoanalytic concepts and core elements of critical social theory as developed by the Frankfurt School (Held, 1980). Understanding this substrate is a key component in dialogic practices that aim toward the decolonization of psyches and everyday lives.

The concept of ideology has been used in a variety of ways since its appearance in the 16th century. Readers are likely most familiar with a connotation implying an elaborated system of thought that is rigidly adhered to, typically by members of a politically active group, in contrast to a flexible, pragmatic orientation to political questions. To reiterate, here we differ from that connotation by drawing on one that orients readers to the process by which a critical perspective about dominant institutions is denied plausibility, or even possibility. As developed by the Frankfurt School (Held, 1980), the concept drew on the work of Georg Lukács, a Marxist critic who sought to understand how capitalist society comes to appear naturalized, to be seen as second nature, to its members. Lukács placed great emphasis on the universal commodification carried out by capitalism (Lukács, 1971). Under capitalism, everything becomes marketable, including the labor power of individuals, and submission to this reality and to the concomitant market-driven fluctuations in the value of their labor contributes to a stance of *passive acceptance.* The Frankfurt School accepted this analysis, but sought to deepen it by critically culling through social science concepts, particularly those of psychoanalysis, in order to explain this passivity.

Following their lead, we start by emphasizing how—far from being a collection of ideas that are more or less logically organized, for example, as one might read in a political pamphlet—ideology can be thought of as a process of containment of thoughts and emotions associated with criticism of core institutions. By institutions, we mean practices and related assumptions that are essential to the functioning of the current social order, such as the assumption that massive, socially essential production facilities should be privately controlled, that owners of these means of production may keep surpluses generated by workers, that one must obey the boss or risk being fired, that hard work is essential to self-respect, and so on (Weeks, 2011). People live within interpersonal fields that register the rules governing social reality as well as more personal, biographically grounded understandings of that reality. As they negotiate their lives, they try to reconcile both internal and external pressures, and it is in the process of this reconciliation that ideology transpires. Some of those thoughts and emotions take conscious, explicit forms but, to give due recognition to the layered complexity of human experience, it is necessary to acknowledge the place of pre- and unconscious thought and its impact on the development of a critical stance (Shevrin, Bond, Brakel, Hertel, & William, 1996).

To develop this psychoanalytic dimension of ideology, the concept of a *compromise formation* is pertinent (Abend, 2005; Rothstein, 2005). Within psychoanalysis, the concept refers to how a symptom reflects a solution made up of a balanced mixture of gratification, displeasure, defensive operations, and the oversight of the superego. For example, a patient who becomes angry with his or her therapist over a perceived slight may find himself or herself instead complaining about a brusque storekeeper the patient encountered earlier in the day in a way that airs some of his or her objection to the therapist's behavior but is safely directed at a different person. Simultaneously, in his or her presentation to the therapist the patient is gratified by being listened to sympathetically. The patient is inclined to this maneuver because in managing his or her relationship with the therapist he or she draws on models derived from the way he or she came to manage relationships with, in this case, his or her father (i.e., avoiding direct conflict and passively fabricating a sense of being cared for). The real opportunity to discuss the slight directly with the therapist is not actualized, and the patient's handling of the situation is crucially directed by defense mechanisms that give the compromise formation a reflex-like, automatic quality.

Especially when framed in object relational terms (Kernberg, 1988), the psychoanalytic concept of the compromise formation is quite congruent with the social processes that we are analyzing.[1] Societies impose frameworks of obligations and rewards on their members, the open-ended exchange of labor power for a wage being the most obvious example. Beginning in the first days of childhood, individuals learn routines of self-restraint and gratification that, although they occur within the sphere of the family, anticipate the more elaborate and institutionally specific schemata they will encounter as adults (Earnest, 1992). As part of this learning, they not only come to know situations in the sense that they have information about them. They also internalize them as object-relational schemas: scenarios involving self, other, and linking affects that progressively become part of an identity grounded in experience of others.

As development proceeds, the subject's capacity to reflect on these schemata, to reflectively evaluate them in imagined trial actions, progresses unevenly. Drawing on the work of the psychoanalyst Lorenzer (1970) regarding a process he calls *desymbolization*, we hold that the subject's ability to fully consider schemas depends on his or her ability to represent them as *symbols*, with complex conscious meanings, as opposed to more limited and one-sided *stereotypes*. To refer to the preceding example, a subject's symbolized representations of his or her father attain a degree of synthesis and integration—for example, the father who steadily supported the family and the father who was never sick is thought of alongside the father who could be irritable and frightening—composing a multi-sided and differentiated image of the father and of the history of their relationship. But, in the case of stereotyped representations, the father's remembered image is divided up into disconnected elements, each ultimately corresponding to the way the father appeared to the child at a particular conjuncture in their relationship—here, the father who would fly into a rage if criticized. Thus stereotypically represented scenes are, compared with symbolized relationships, only one-sided fragments of a subject's relationship with an object, cordoned off from other fragments. The patient thereby preserves a one-sidedly affirmative, idealized view of the father, and maintains a way of evacuating, through defenses such as splitting and displacement, any negative feelings and the scenes associated with them.

In the course of psychotherapy, these stereotyped fragments may be integrated with other stereotypes and memories, allowing the patient to gradually establish a more complete, multivalent, symbolized understanding of the object (i.e., the father). But before that, the stereotype is not subject to reflective appraisal and cannot be evoked as a memory that can be consciously synthesized with other memories and perceptions. Instead, the stereotype is triggered automatically as affect and behavior within contexts reminiscent of the original scene. Thus, in dealings with the therapist—as possibly in dealings with other authorities—the patient avoids mentioning the slight by the therapist and can only complain about the storekeeper.[2]

This is the most important feature of the stereotyped object-relation: in contrast to symbolized, composite representations of relations with an object or other, which may be explored consciously through trial-action and imaginative playing with reality (Ogden, 1985), the stereotyped object relation in effect presents itself to the subject as an action imperative or, to draw on Lukács, it becomes "second nature" to the subject (Lukács, 1919–23/1971, p. 86).

Put succinctly, the promulgation of social ideology is supported by stereotyped features of the compromise formations that people bring to the management of their lives in dominant institutions. These compromise formations are the unquestionable, and in important respects unthinkable, personal components that undergird and rigidify social thought. From the discussion so far it might be assumed that we see one source of stereotyped, ideological understanding as residing in an individual's idiosyncratic psychic reality. This is correct: we are maintaining that, for example, positions of institutional authority are the heirs to patterns of adaptation to childhood authority, and that stereotyped, automatic patterns of deference can become active in people's handling of their hierarchical relationships (cf. Adorno, Frenkel-Brunswik, Levinson, & Sanford, 1950).

But this social psychoanalytic perspective on limited capacities for representation and critical thought is only part of the picture. It is a common experience that role relations in dominant institutions are coercively presented in daily life as beyond consideration, as a second nature to which people must adapt. For example, in the workplace employees are expected, in return for a wage, to do what their employer tells them to do; if they challenge this they are fired and free to go to another job, albeit with a questionable resume. Alternative ways of organizing the workplace are not to be discussed at work. This silencing at an institutional level sets up a second phase of desymbolization. In other words, coercive exclusion from the universe of public discourse prompts the subject to experience these core role relations at work in ways that trigger personal stereotypes grounded in individual psychic reality and life experience (Luke, 2004; Marcuse, 1964; Padavic & Earnest, 1994). An artifactual institutional practice thus becomes enshrined within a taboo—the intersection of socially grounded fear and intrapsychic anxiety.

Since work relations are core to capitalism, we will pursue this example a bit further. This is not a process that involves repression in technical psychoanalytic terms and so the full excommunication from consciousness that is crucially associated with a stereotype does not prevail. After all, people working in a factory, in retail, or in service industries might well be conscious of alternative organizations of work (having seen them discussed in their local paper or over a beer after work) and could have decided they are not interested. They may simply weigh the costs and benefits of opposing a supervisor's authority at their job and decide to maintain the status quo.

However, this nominally rational adjustment to oppressive situations is actually more complex. This complexity is evident, for example, in analyses of life history interviews with factory workers that include questions about the possibilities for improved working conditions (Earnest, 1992). Typically, when they are given the opportunity to talk about their adjustment in an open-ended interview, employees will express what amounts to a compromise formation regulating everyday work life, a bricolage of anticipated gratifications, frustrations, displacements of anger onto others, identifications with the aggressor (their employer), identifications with the interests of those depending on them, and so forth. As one listens to them, it becomes apparent that the interview session is in some ways akin to a psychoanalytic session, especially in the sense that it presupposes the relaxation of the everyday constraints of the workplace. Freer to speak of their experience, the various components of the compromise formation are given a more full-throated representation. In effect, the listener is invited into a theater of object relations in which the speakers endeavor to reconcile competing pressures (McDougall, 1991). As one listens, one is less likely to encounter the wholesale repression of unpleasant aspects of the relationship with the employer. Instead, these unpleasant aspects may be acknowledged, but in a routinized way, as "the way the world works." In other words, the employee will draw on a culturally available *cliché*—akin to what Lorenzer (1970, p. 125) would call a *sign* (*Zeiche*)—to refer to the conflicts with the employer in a purely descriptive mode, drained of potentially inflammatory emotions and critical ideas and instead integrated into a web of compensations: the wage, a hope for promotions or, given the increasingly contingent nature of work, a hope of a better job in the future.

An essay by British theorist Raymond Williams, "Base and Superstructure in Marxist Cultural Theory" (1973), is helpful in conceiving of the social pressures shaping the desymbolization process we are outlining and advocating as key to decolonization. Williams wanted to revise the crudely mechanistic notion in some formulations of Marxist theory that economic relationships, the *base*, determine a society's culture, its *superstructure*. Thus, for example, trends in philosophy directly mirror changes in production systems and the social relations immediately linked to them. He proposed that the interaction between economy and culture instead could be thought of as involving selective incorporation and suppression of practices arising in the culture. That is, preservation of the core economic relationships, those having to do with control over the processes of production and distribution, would serve as a touchstone for assessing the worth of, or threat posed by, particular forms of thought and behavior. The suppressive side of this process would be carried out in a fashion distributed across a number of institutions, under various rubrics, such as anticommunism, affirmation of the right to work in a narrowly anti-union form, wars on crime, welfare cheating, and so on. Likewise, incorporative efforts would be broadly distributed and thematically diverse; for example, leisure would be equated with consumption to fortify demand for commodities, whereas critical, countercultural trends would be co-opted as fashionable ways of expressing a sexy edginess. Thus, in contrast to the original Marxist framework that in at least some renderings seemed to arbitrarily prioritize labor relations over all other human interactions, Williams proposed a framework embodying agency, monitoring, suppression, and synthesis.

Williams's thesis can be summarized as presenting a notion of socially distributed agency. For our purposes, it usefully highlights a stance expected of members of any society: that they monitor their actual performance as well as their internal dispositions, in light of role requirements and group expectations that are related to requirements of the social system. Responding to a cascade of pressures encountered throughout development, members of society are expected to carry out a process of culling, suppression, and incorporation internally that parallels what an array of institutions carries out externally. In other words, they are enlisted to maintain a consonance between their personal compromise formations and institutional arrangements, doing their part in sustaining the colonization of the lifeworld. How tightly maintained this consonance is can vary widely depending on life histories and institutional conditions.

In making this claim we wish to avoid recapitulating the mechanistic Marxist error in another form, as a rigid theory of socialization. We do not mean that individuals are simply products of institutional templates, as was the case with some critical socio-psychoanalytic models, such as those formulated by Erich Fromm and, to a certain extent, Theodor Adorno (Adorno et al., 1950; Fromm, 1978). Rather, it means that individuals, at both conscious and unconscious levels, are aware of what Hobbes, putting it in terms reflecting one notion of the proper mission of elites, called the building of "hedges and fencerows" of a social order and of a mandate for others to live within the pasture they demarcate (Hobbes, 1660/2012). At times reckoning with these limits may mean an emphasis on rejecting certain thoughts or associating them with a certain kind of person, as when a demand for a shorter working day is associated with laziness, whereas at other times it might be a matter of imagining one's future in a way that conforms to established status hierarchies.

Because we started from a psychoanalytic standpoint linked to an individual analysis, to this point we have tended to portray compromise formations as useful for managing limited, individual-level grievances. But Williams's level of analysis alerts us to larger tensions. In capitalist societies different core institutions embody and legitimate different object relational schemata, and these exist in tension with each other. For example, the capitalist workplace is characteristically hierarchically ordered, whereas political institutions at least nominally observe democratic forms. The clash of contradictory institutional logics and statuses encourages system-critical thinking, which achieves additional impetus when crises develop that threaten expected levels of rewards for compliance. In short, endemic to the capitalist social order are crisis tendencies that strain compromise formations and generate ways of thinking that threaten to transcend capitalism.[3]

Moreover, because capitalist elites themselves operate within the ideology promulgated to maintain the system, their ability to address system problems generated by its faulty presuppositions is significantly limited (Lukács, 1919–23/1971; Habermas, 1975). Nothing demonstrates the limits of elite rationality better than the ongoing despoliation of the environment, treated as an external cost that should not constrain the system imperative to accumulate profit. Increasingly apparent in this period of global warming, the Fukushima meltdown and fracking for oil, the impact of cost externalization delegitimizes elites and over time compels individuals to reconsider their compromise formation-based habits of self-suppression in deference to elite control of problem definition and resolution. Increasingly, the vast majorities of the world are in a situation that recalls the much-ridiculed Marxist idea of the working class' role in history being forced upon it because only the working class can think outside of a suffocating ideological box.

RESYMBOLIZATION: UNRAVELING THE IDEOLOGICAL COMPROMISE FORMATION VIA DIALOGUE-IN-ACTION

To this point, we have emphasized how ideological compromise formations operate to defuse individual and collective action against social injustice. As noted, however, system contradictions and crises set up situations in which these compromise formations begin to unravel, and subjects are moved to seriously consider alternatives and begin to act to construct them. Since hegemonic control is not absolute, social spaces in which cultures of resistance are sustained can be found almost everywhere, and actors within these spaces nourish ideas and organize projects related to the establishment of an alternative social order.

Resymbolization linked to decolonization transpires through an interplay of imagined and actual interpersonal experience. Talking with others about one's institutionally situated grievances asserts a more complete representation of the range of one's experience, including an insistence on the reality of suffering that is denied representation in ideological discourse. Doing so reanimates supportive relational forms that begin to develop in the earliest years of life, and those models of interactions with parents are gradually supplemented and superseded by models that are not grounded in the family but in the community. Talking with others works to both define—quite literally, the individual is hearing what is on his or her own mind and asserting it publicly—and refine a grievance as others bring out their own experience and points of agreement and degrees of urgency are worked out. Simultaneously, new dialogic parameters, the rules of expression and recognition, develop. Depending on the nature of the conversation, its to and fro allows the discovery of more facets of the problem as experienced by the individual, establishes the outlines of alliance, and perpetually affirms a model of speaking and listening. "My experience" becomes "our experience," and a new way of being with others takes shape. The emergence of interpersonal solidarity remediates prior experience of social suppression, and the developing contrast between receptive listeners and a suppressive social surround helps reinforce the importance of the emerging group. Just as in psychotherapy, resymbolization contra ideology is alliance-based, an act of assertion with others (Greenson, 1965). And, just as in psychotherapy, this act of assertion can become internalized so that, even without the tangible support of others, they are still present and sustaining in both fantasy and action.

The object-relational coordinates of this emerging solidarity are often recognized in a semi-formal fashion as identities: the "citizen" of the French Revolution, the "sister" of the women's movement, the "comrade" of international socialism, and so on. These concepts varyingly draw upon relational forms of everyday life—often explicitly from the family—and rework them to affirm a countersuppressive identity-in-solidarity.

This sketch of mobilization defines a progressive movement pitted against the ideological process we have described. In conversations with family, friends, and newly made allies, the limits of the existing ideological compromise formation are pushed back and a new compromise formation takes shape, one guided by principled and, indeed, theory-guided agreements addressing a more adequately symbolized reality. For example, working people may not only demand higher wages but also come to feel justified in extending democratic control over production processes that have been heretofore thought of as the prerogative of owners.

However, the new form is tentative, stalked by an interplay of relatively realistic fears—threats from elites and their allies who benefit from the status quo—and anxieties associated with disrupting the old compromise formation as well as regressive reactions to those anxieties. Even though the new compromise formation may be guided by internal critique, by an extrapolation from familiar, legitimized practices and ways of thinking about self and other that lend it a certain gut-level legitimacy (Geuss, 2008; Kauppinen, 2002), a potential to experience doubt and transgressive guilt can nonetheless arise. Outright fear, disputes over strategy and tactics, worries expressed by family and friends and guilt over time lost with them, associations to past fears and anxieties, and others merge in a confusing mass that can only with difficulty be sorted out in the heat of practice.

Earlier we emphasized how the expression of a demand draws on early models of support, perhaps from loving parents, but obviously models of suppression are evoked as well. Even apparently well-demarcated issues that appear to have institutional sanction—for example, a demand to increase wages within the context of routine labor negotiations—can for some people evoke the most profound anxieties. For them, any challenge to authority threatens anarchy, a breakdown of an order conceived in terms of absolute parental authority. As one moves to consider less-structured demands and more global changes in a social order, the potential for anxiety increases. It is not just a matter of the increasing possibility of state repression that one must face, but also the way in which making demands recalls and reignites much earlier personal struggles.

Archaic roles are part of these archaic anxieties. The idealized models of citizen, sister, or comrade carry with them role prescriptions that ensure respect and caring. They affirm mutual recognition and stand against both relatively well-defined hierarchical relational models—master-slave, technocrat-mass public, and so on—and intimations of bad behavior that reflect the activation of stereotyped, archaic responses to the conflicts associated with demanding expressive freedom. As in the preceding therapeutic example, wherein the patient's response to the relative freedom of the therapy session was both to dare to voice complaints but also turn the therapist into a forbidding parent, so, too, life in oppositional groups is often beset by transference. The inherently open-ended and ambiguous nature of political action, when the hitherto impossible may be demanded and may indeed happen, holds tremendous potential for emotional regression, both with respect to triggering myriad forms of conflict—distrust, intolerance of different analyses, fear of manipulation, and so on—and with respect to regressive solutions, running the range from helpless renunciation and withdrawal to reliance on charismatic leaders who essentially re-establish a parental order (Freud, 1921).

For example, an activist recalled that during a union organizing drive she found herself much less inclined to criticize the U.S. president than she usually was. She felt that the pressures of organizing made her want to avoid pissing everybody off and so somehow she let the president off the hook. Psychologically astute, she realized that her psychological move likely represented a displacement from her relationship with her intimidating, conservative father, but this awareness didn't completely eliminate the symptom. She realized that, in effect, she was striking a kind of tactical compromise, mediated by an internal fantasy, that left her feeling a little more secure. But, she also knew that, this paternalized conciliatory impulse might infiltrate her current political efforts and possibly muddy her analysis of prospective compromises with management as well as make her alliances with other activists unsteadier. For our purposes here, it is reasonable to extrapolate and imagine everyone around her engaged in their own private equilibrations, constantly generating stereotyped overlays to the immediate social conflict.

We caution against simplistically interpreting political mobilization and action along the lines of something like Habermas' ideal speech situation, as the achievement of an open organization of individuals in which unpressured reflection allows the formation of demands that are regarded as truth claims, fully voiced and analyzed in light of empirical investigation (Habermas, 1987; Sloan, 1996). Such a formal model, strongly implying a distrust of stereotype-infused thinking, misses how stereotypes are arguably an important component of encouragement and inspiration, which we conceive of as hinging on some degree of identification with certain group members, or ideals associated with lauded, charismatic figures. Stereotypes often contribute to a radically revised self-conception, in which prior concerns, embedded in a life structure consonant with the prior ideological compromise formation, are transcended: a new sense of self in relation to others becomes salient. Paradoxically, what may begin as articulation of immediate grievances interpreted prosaically—for example, higher wages—can transform into a sense of profound identification with and commitment to others, both living, dead, and yet to be born. The experience of greater freedom of self-expression leads to insight into what is necessary for that self-expression to be generalized. In an important respect, this new orientation corresponds to the current psychoanalytic understandings of love: instead of it crucially involving a discharge of somatic excitation, the self transcends a narrow individualistic hedonism and is enhanced through identification with the object of their love (Kernberg, 2011).

POSSIBILITIES FOR DIALOGIC PRACTICE

We now explore contrasting models of dialogic practice in light of our critical psychoanalytic perspective. The first model we consider is that of decision-oriented public dialogue such as the kind one encounters in town hall gatherings. We then consider the dynamics of explicitly nonhierarchical spaces such as those associated with the Occupy movement that started in the United States in 2011, inspired by uprisings in Greece, Spain, and the Middle East. In both cases, we focus on how possibilities for resymbolization are shaped by dialogic frameworks experienced by participants.

A bit of background on a particular connotation of the term *dialogue* is necessary. In progressive community, academic, or political settings in North America, a dialogue usually implies a facilitated (moderated) discussion with several to 30 or more participants. Ground rules for the discussion emphasize not only the rather unremarkable guarantee of an opportunity to speak, but also to be heard, with the theme of discovering difference, conveying a pact to remain open to opposing analyses and to avoid preemptive devaluation of disagreeing speakers and their ideas. The aim is to foster understanding across differences so as to generate the basis for cooperation through a mobilized collective wisdom (Atlee, 2002). Participants are encouraged to speak from their hearts and from personal experience rather than cite authorities, a strategy that can preclude respectful listening by justifying devaluation of different views (cf. the work of the Public Conversations Project, publicconversations.org).

Clearly, these ideas are consonant with the town hall democratic model, wherein citizens come together, offer and listen to a range of alternatives, refine their opinions in light of their interests and newly available information, deliberate, urge the adoption of rational policies, and support representatives who will enact them. From our perspective, this process reflects an attempt to suspend established conceptions of interest and the alliances and divisions prescribed by them and, instead, to demonstrate to participants that, if the all too easily mobilized prejudices of everyday life can be restrained, fresh perspectives and alliances are possible. However, in actual practice these town-hall norms are hard to follow and the feared outcomes—seemingly unproductive debates, authoritative posturing, discouraged withdrawal, and so on—play out. In response, dialogue practitioners call for better meeting design and stronger facilitation to create safe spaces for all voices to be heard. Others would point to the importance of taking into account distorting factors such as agenda-setting power, rhetorical style, access to relevant information, and so forth, in order to equalize power differentials (cf. the work represented at the National Council for Dialogue and Deliberation at ncdd.org).

It is possible to dismiss these attempts at dialogue as naively idealistic, vain bids to get participants to leap out of their social skins and become dialogic angels, unfettered by material interests (Mannheim, 1968). We believe, however, that writing off dialogic-based opportunities for change misses an important counter-ideological dimension to this effort, and we now turn to consider the Occupy movement as an example of how group process can register counter-ideological intent.

What we are terming the dialogic practice of Occupy emerged with the 15-M movement in response to austerity measures in Spain in 2011 and with the Occupy movement in the United States. In these societies, the accentuation of social contradictions has revealed existing democratic institutions incapable of countervailing the power of wealthy national and international elites. In response, citizens have come together in urban centers and, in effect, are beginning democracy afresh. One by one, they stand up and are recognized by their fellow citizens. They are recognized as they speak the truth of the exploitation, alienation, exclusion, or discrimination that they have each suffered. They feel heard, perhaps for the first time, especially when participants implement the exercise known as the *human microphone* to echo each person's words to a large crowd. People in the front rows repeat each sentence they hear and the rows behind them repeat in turn until everyone has heard. This practice retrieves and powerfully enacts a practice at the core of democratic aspirations, that of being publicly recognized and being found worthy of the same concern given to anyone else in the polity. It insists on a reciprocal authenticity, both of the individual and of the community, meaning that disavowed or suppressed aspects of self can be brought into awareness, articulated, acknowledged, and synthesized with more conscious experiences of self before a concerned public. It would be a mistake to regard prioritizing this way of resuscitating subjectivity in community as an arbitrary invocation of anarchist principles. Rather, it actualizes the foundational moment of recognition within a democratic community (Honneth, 1996).

The Occupy movement has been criticized for its failure to make this encounter a part of a process culminating in a set of specific, focused demands (Hoffman, 2011). But Occupy's hesitancy to define issues reflects the understanding that potential participants had become alienated from a suppressive compromise-oriented political theater offering preordained policy options consistent with elite interests: interests that are particularly indifferent to precarity in all its dimensions. Participants needed to recover their power of speech and a confidence in their significance to the community of their representation of their world and their plight. Given their previous, long-term experience of the status quo as overwhelmingly powerful, moving too quickly to strategically anticipate confrontation could evoke a sense of cynical futility, since their recently emerged identity might seem impotent against elite power, a point one protestor implied by saying, "Demands are disempowering since they require someone else to respond" (Hoffman, 2011).

Occupy movement helps to clarify why the emphatic assertion of a counter-ideological practice, or a decolonizing of the lifeworld, is necessary. Yet, if one accepts that Occupy is not a capricious implementation of an arbitrary organizational model but instead reflects theoretically coherent praxis addressing a significant problem, and a powerful case of prefigurative politics, one is still left with the question of how this recovered self-in-democratic-community can be sustained.

We will sketch out the dilemmas associated with this problem by considering another model of political mobilization. Compare the approach taken by Occupy with that taken by Marxist organizers in the early 20th century. Marxism adamantly insists on a linkage between fundamental capitalist system dynamics and the immiseration of people and their communities (Sweezy, 1942). Profits motivate production, a concern for human welfare does not guide production decisions, and the uncertainties attendant to profit realization lead to recurrent crises. The thorough, counter-ideological expression of suffering would, in its search for remedies, lead to recognition of the need to supersede capitalism. Achieving this would require the formation of political parties of the oppressed, whose organizational structures would have to be adequate to the necessities of political and, in light of experience, political-military combat that would eventually realize a better society (Burawoy, 1982). Although recent scholarship has debunked the ideology that this organizational form was always proposed in highly centralized, undemocratic terms (Lih, 2008), the point is that prospective adherents could understand their subjective enhancement dialectically: they would recognize an inescapable logic binding expression of their grievances with necessary organizational affiliations and, eventually, duties in the social democratic movement. Experiences of the suppressive foreclosure of expression—for example, losing a vote and having to observe party discipline—could be tolerated in the belief that, the eventual achievement of socialism, offering a transparent harmony between individual and social needs, would justify current self-suppression.

In the current Occupy epoch, history may not have ended, as Fukuyama claimed (Antonio, 2000; Fukuyama, 1992), but one can no longer be confident where it is going. The experience of Stalinist state socialism, both its reality and the ideological distortions made of it, seems to say to the oppressed that, even as welfare capitalism reverts to something like the ruthless model Marx criticized, to participate in direct struggle with capitalism may be pointless. The Who's song, "Here comes the new boss, same as the old boss," captures this resignation, in both its truth and its degeneration to unexamined cliché. Thus stymied, what seems to be most readily available in the social imaginary are post-apocalyptic dystopias, contorted expressions of rage, dread, and stunted hope, in which other people are more likely to be predators than allies (Jameson, 2005). It thus becomes difficult to anticipate how the fruits, but also the necessary actions, attendant to resymbolization can be realized and carried out in a social organization also seeking to promote strategic power. Thus, the dialogic practice of Occupy is informed by a complex distrust: a distrust not only of actually existing democracy under capitalism, but also of the possibility of alternatives, given that socialism (as rendered in Stalinism) turned out be incapable of justifying its suppressive rationale.

The prefigurative political model that Occupy embodies reflects an anxiety regarding threats to a resymbolized self that is hard to allay with theory or historical example. In addition to the Stalinist nightmare, the very real processes of leadership cooptation and betrayal repeatedly experienced by radical movements appear all the more threatening if there appears to be no compelling social alternative that reliably ensures an ongoing solidarity in sacrifice in day-to-day organizational life (Hilgers, 2008; Michels, 1910/1996). Since they appear to lack any theoretical-practical justification, proposals to foster organizational strength appear, in a stereotype-infused way, to be nothing more than narcissistic in their aims.

However, the prefigurative option, defending against loss of recognition—all the harder to bear if it occurs in the midst of what was hoped to be liberatory practice—inevitably faces the practical limits imposed by preoccupations with enhanced subjectivity. Simply, as things grow worse, as people experience more widespread precariousness in jobs and in their social standing, and as they approach absolute immiseration through economic and environmental crises, the need will arise to shape the functioning of the social order by attaining collective strength. It seems that, unfortunately, the fashionable idea of a multitude in movement (Hardt & Negri, 2000) and preference for decentralized, nonhierarchical collectives among radicals (Graeber, 2009) do not adequately anticipate at the level of strategy. We hope that we will not be forced to recapitulate the vituperative debates worked through in the late 19th and early 20th centuries, wherein it was argued by Marxists that anarchism, with its wariness of collective organization, led into a cul-de-sac in which terrorist attacks against public officials—at that time, *terrorism* was the term chosen by its practitioners—defined the terms of political struggle (Lih, 2008).

In sum, we have shown how the concepts of ideology, resymbolization, and decolonization through dialogue are relevant to understanding any countermovement against oppression, ranging from the most everyday encounters with coercion to more organized opposition to institutionalized elite power. They serve to connect psychological and sociological levels of conceptualization and alert us to the subjective aspects of processes of mobilization that are often ignored, or treated in a facile manner, typically as part of sweeping claims about mass irrationality (Langman, 2005). We believe that the process models employed by the Occupy movement are acutely sensitive to this dimension of political mobilization, and argue that the strategic difficulties it has faced reflect its attempts to grapple with a problem that is inescapable in a genuinely liberatory movement.

NOTES

1. Object relations theory is the branch of psychoanalysis that focuses on how early family experiences are internalized in structures of affect and cognition that inform and constrain action.

2. One of the most impressive demonstrations of this observation can be found in Fonagy, Steele, Moran, Steele, and Higgitt (1993), in which they show how parents whose narrative depictions of their own parents are stereotypically fragmented tend to reflexively enact those stereotypes with their young children, strongly shaping their attachment patterns.

3. Throughout this chapter we refer to examples of ideology and ideological functioning within capitalist societies. We believe this emphasis appropriate given both their global predominance and because they are so often portrayed as the essence of free social arrangements. At its most useful, the critical concept of ideology interrogates such free choice claims while justifying itself in their name.

REFERENCES

Abend, S. (2005). Analyzing intrapsychic conflict: Compromise formation as an organizing principle. *Psychoanalytic Quarterly, 74*, 5–25.

Adorno, T. W., Frenkel-Brunswik, E., Levinson, D. J., & Sanford, R. N. (1950). *The authoritarian personality.* New York, NY: Harper & Row.

Antonio, R. (2000). After postmodernism: Reactionary tribalism. *American Journal of Sociology, 106*(1), 40–87.

Atlee, T. (2002). *The Tao of democracy.* North Charleston, SC: Imprint Books.

Burawoy, M. (1982). The resurgence of Marxism in American sociology. *American Journal of Sociology*, Supplement: Marxist Inquiries: Studies of Labor, Class, and States, *88*, S1–S30.

Earnest, W. R. (1992). Ideology criticism and life history research. In G. Rosenwald & R. Ochberg (Eds.), *Storied lives: The cultural politics of self-understanding* (pp. 250–264). New Haven, CT: Yale University Press.

Engels, Friedrich. (1893/1968). Letter to Franz Mehring. *Marx and Engels Correspondence.* New York, NY: International Publishers.

Fonagy, P., Steele, M., Moran, G., Steele, H., & Higgitt, A. (1993). Measuring the ghost in the nursery: An empirical study of the relation between parents' mental representations of childhood experiences and their infants' security of attachment. *Journal of the American Psychoanalytic Association, 41*, 957–989.

Freud, S. (1921). Group psychology and the analysis of the ego. *The standard edition of the complete psychological works of Sigmund Freud, Volume XVIII (1920–1922): Beyond the pleasure principle, group psychology and other Works*, 65–144.

Fromm, E. (1978). The method and function of an analytic social psychology. In A. Arato & E. Gebhardt (Eds.), *The essential Frankfurt School reader* (pp. 477–496). New York, NY: Urizen.

Fukuyama, F. (1992). *The end of history and the last man.* New York, NY: Free Press.

Geuss, R. (2008). *Philosophy and real politics.* Princeton, NJ: Princeton University Press.

Graeber, D. (2009). *Direct action: An ethnography.* Oakland, CA: AK Press.

Gramsci, Antonio. (1971). *Selections from the prison notebooks.* New York, NY: International Publishers.

Greenson, R. R. (1965). The working alliance and the transference neurosis. *Psychoanalytic. Quarterly, 34*, 155–181.

Habermas, J. (1975). *Legitimation crisis.* Boston, MA: Beacon.

Habermas, J. (1987). *Theory of communicative action. Vol. 2.* Boston, MA: Beacon.

Hardt, M., & Negri, A. (2000). *Empire.* Boston, MA: Harvard.

Held, D. (1980). *Introduction to critical theory: Horkheimer to Habermas.* Berkeley: University of California Press.

Hilgers, T. (2008). Causes and consequences of political clientelism: Mexico's PRD in comparative perspective. *Latin American Politics and Society, 50*(4), 123–153.

Hobbes, Thomas. (1660/2012). *Leviathan.* London: Oxford University Press.

Hoffman, M. (2011, October 16). Protesters debate what demands, if any, to make. *New York Times*, p. A19.

Honneth, A. (1996). The *struggle for recognition: The moral grammar of social conflicts.* Cambridge, MA: MIT Press.

Jameson, F. (2002). *A singular modernity.* New York, NY: Verso.

Jameson, F. (2005). *Archaeologies of the future.* New York, NY: Verso.

Kauppinen, A. (2002). Reason, recognition, and internal critique. *Inquiry: An Interdisciplinary Journal of Philosophy, 45*(4), 2002.

Kernberg, O. (1988). Object relations theory in clinical practice. *Psychoanalytic Quarterly, 57,* 481–504.

Kernberg, O. (2011). Limitations to the capacity to love. *International Journal of Psycho-Analysis, 92,* 1501–1515.

Langman, L. (2005). From virtual public spheres to global justice: A critical theory of internetworked social movements. *Sociological Theory, 23*(1), 42–74.

Lih, L. (2008). *Lenin rediscovered: What is to be done? in context.* Chicago, IL: Haymarket.

Lorenzer, A. (1970). *Sprachzerstorung und Rekonstruktion.* Frankfurt, Germany: Suhrkamp.

Lukács, G. (1919–23/1971). *History and class consciousness: Studies in Marxist dialectics.* Cambridge, MA: MIT press.

Luke, S. (2004). *Power: A radical view.* New York, NY: Palgrave Macmillan.

Mannheim, K. (1968). *Ideology and utopia.* New York, NY: Harcourt, Brace & World.

Marcuse, H (1964). *One-dimensional man: Studies in the ideology of advanced industrial society.* Boston, MA: Beacon.

McDougall, J. (1991). *Theaters of the mind: Illusion and truth on the psychoanalytic stage.* New York, NY: Brunner/Mazell.

Michels, R. (1910/1996). *Political parties.* New York, NY: Free Press.

Ogden, T. (1985). On potential space. *International Journal of Psychoanalysis, 66,* 129–141.

Padavic, I., & Earnest, W. R. (1994). Paternalism as a component of managerial strategy. *The Social Science Journal, 31*(4), 389–405.

Parker, I. (2007). *The revolution in psychology: Alienation to emancipation.* London, UK: Pluto.

Pollin, R. (2005). *Contours of descent: U.S. economic fractures and the landscape of global austerity.* New York, NY: Verso.

Prilleltensky, I. (1994). *The morals and politics of psychology.* Albany, NY: SUNY Press.

Rothstein, A. (2005). Compromise formation theory: An intersubjective dimension. *Psychoanalytic Dialogues, 15,* 415–431.

Shevrin, H., Bond, J, Brakel, L., Hertel, R., & William, W. (1996). *Conscious and unconscious processes: Psychodynamic, cognitive, and neuropsychologial convergences.* New York, NY: Guilford.

Sloan, T. (1996). *Damaged life: The crisis of the modern psyche.* New York, NY: Routledge.

Sweezy, P. (1942). *The theory of capitalist development: Principles of Marxian political economy.* New York, NY: Monthly Review.

Wallerstein, I. (2004). *World systems analysis: An introduction.* Chapel Hill, NC: Duke University Press.

Weeks, K. (2011). *The problem with work: Feminism, Marxism, antiwork politics, and postwork imaginaries.* Durham, NC: Duke University Press.

Williams, R. (1973). Base and superstructure in Marxist cultural theory. *New Left Review, 82,* 3–16.

Chapter 6

False Consciousness and the Maintenance of Injustice

Krystal M. Perkins and William E. Cross Jr.

> Beat and cuff your slave, keep him hungry and spiritless, and he will follow the chain of his master like a dog.
>
> —Frederick Douglass, 1855, p. 263

> When you control a man's thinking you do not have to worry about his actions. You do not have to tell him not to stand here or go yonder. He will find his "proper place" and will stay in it. You do not need to send him to the back door. He will go without being told. In fact, if there is no back door, he will cut one for his special benefit. His education makes it necessary.
>
> —Carter G. Woodson, 1933, p. 21

The fundamental "success" of oppression is when those who are oppressed actively participate in their own oppression. It is within these instances that oppression is no longer a physical policing, but a psychological one, as captured in the epigraphs that open this chapter. This is the central theme of this chapter. In particular, this chapter has been written within the intellectual spirit of Morton

Deutsch, who devoted his career in psychology to theorizing the conditions under which victims of and perpetrators of oppression *see* justice and injustice (Deutsch, 1974, 1985). These themes undergird many classical and contemporary theories in social psychology that attempt to tackle one of the more intriguing trends in modern political history—the tendency for many people to go against their economic and political interest. Although a holistic analysis of social justice and injustice would take into consideration the perceptions of perpetrators and victims alike, our focus is why so many of the disadvantaged often accept, support, and actively sustain their own unequal status. We aim to illuminate in our review the psychological conditions of, using Kinder and Sears (1985) words, "not the occasional protest, but of pervasive tranquility." Before turning to this, we provide a context to this phenomenon by first tracing its intellectual origins (topically) and its major theoretical influences within psychology.

It will be useful first to clarify up front our use of terminology. Throughout this chapter we will be using the words *low-status*, *devalued*, *disadvantaged*, *marginalized*, and *subordinate individuals/groups* interchangeably. In our view, these terms refer generally to a subgroup of the population that differs from higher-status groups and specifically to any group that is subjected to oppression and discrimination by individuals or groups in more powerful social positions. Examples of such groups include African Americans, Native Americans, Latinos, Asians, immigrants, and marginalized groups in other countries, among others.

INTELLECTUAL ORIGINS: THE CONSEQUENCES OF DOMINATION

The consequences of domination (e.g., oppression, marginalization, colonization, subjugation, etc.) on those who are dominated have a long-standing history within political and sociological theory (Fanon, 1952; Gramsci, 1971; Habermas, 1975; Marx & Engels, 1846; Woodson, 1933). In particular, Engels (Marx & Engels, 1846) invoked the concept of *false consciousness* to explain how the working classes in capitalist societies accept their working-class positions. These political theorists believed that the working classes failed to recognize their own economic and political interests by internalizing the values of their oppressors. Through institutional control over economic systems, according to Marx and Engels (1846), dominant groups in society spread ideas that served to justify and normalize their status and power. Antonio Gramsci's (1971) central concept of hegemony, outlined in his seminal book *Prison Notebooks*, explains a similar process undergirding the stability of ideological domination. Through coercive repression and control by the ideological structures of education, religion, media, and culture, consent of uneven distributions of power is produced.

Writing in the 1930s and addressing distorted and negative attitudes many African Americans held about Black history and Black culture, the historian Carter G. Woodson coined the term *miseducation*. In his classic text, *The Miseducation of the Negro*, Woodson (1933) explained that when a dominant group that is openly hostile to the interests of a minority has control over of the curriculum and schools meant to educate the marginal group, the result will be an education designed to deracinate the low-status group. Such an education will result in varying degrees of miseducation, a preoccupation with becoming assimilated and, at worst, self-hatred.

Extending Marxism, Franz Fanon (1952) developed a similar image in his analysis of the impact of colonialism on the psychology of Blacks.[1] Fanon highlighted the process of colonization and the central ideology that emerged from it, that is, White's imposition of White supremacy. Specifically, he theorized how the relationship between the colonizer and the colonized becomes normalized into one's internal psychological landscape. Fanon's theoretical work was rooted in Africa, in the context of the French colonial occupation of Algeria and the consequent war for liberation. As a trained psychiatrist working in an Algerian hospital, Fanon encountered patients who were subjected to severe racist abuse and torture; he reached the conclusion that the source, rather than the symptoms of the patients' problems, was colonial society. These colonial conditions, according to Fanon, create a "massive psychoexistential complex" from the moment of conquest (1952, p. 12). Specifically, Fanon argued that racism from White colonizers imposed an existentially false and degrading image upon Blacks that demanded their conformity to White values. This process generated harmful psychological constructs that both blinded Blacks to their subjugation of the universalized White norm and alienated their consciousness. Thus, according to Fanon, the Black man acquires a *white mask* where "the outcome of a double process is primarily economic; subsequently, the internalization—or, better the epidermalisation—of this inferiority" (1952, p. 11).

FALSE CONSCIOUSNESS AS A PSYCHOLOGICAL CONSTRUCT

> If a system that distributes outcomes unequally among its members is to survive, then its members must view the inequalities as justified and legitimate. Thus, perceived legitimacy must come not only from those who benefit from it, but also from those who are disadvantaged by the system.
>
> —Olson and Hafer, 2001, p. 157

The phenomenon of false consciousness has been imported in social psychological theorizing, resulting in several distinct but related conceptualizations such as the belief in a just world (Hafer & Olson, 1989, 1993; Janoff-Bulman, 1992; Lerner, 1980; Rubin & Peplau, 1975, illusion of control (Taylor & Brown, 1988), social identity theory (Tajfel & Turner, 1986), the depressed entitlement effect (Bem & Bem, 1970; Crosby, 1982; Crosby, Putfall, Snyder, O'Connel, & Whalen, 1989; Jost, 1997; Major, 1994; Pelham & Hetts, 2001), tolerance of injustice (Jost, 1995), paradoxical contentment (Major, 1994), outgroup favoritism (Clark & Clark, 1947; Fine & Bowers, 1984), racial colorblindness (Neville, Coleman, Falconer, & Holmes, 2005), system justification theory (Jost & Banaji, 1994), and social dominance theory (Levin & Sidanius, 1999; Levin, Federico, Sidanius, & Rabinowitz, 2002; Overbeck, Jost, Mosso, & Flisik, 2004; Sidanius, 1993; Sidanius, Levin, & Pratto, 1996; Sidanius & Pratto, 1993). A common theme among these theories is that members of some low-status groups accept, maintain, and in some instances, perpetuate their inferior position in society.

The research paradigms that support the empirical development of the body of theoretical work discussed in this chapter reflect certain dominant research traditions and epistemologies in psychology, most notably standard lab experiments and survey methods conducted both in the lab and in the field, and which rely on quantitative data. This makes the task of generalizing from these studies to the complexities of the real world challenging. However, where we can, we will attempt to articulate real-world insights from these research studies.

System Justification Theory

For nearly two decades, John Jost and his collaborators have provided extensive empirical evidence of false consciousness through the development of system justification theory (Jost & Banaji, 1994). System justification is defined as the "process by which existing social arrangements are legitimized even at the expense of personal and group interests" (Jost & Banaji, 1994, p. 2). System justification theory posits a motive to invest in and rationalize the status quo, and this motive is even present among members of disadvantaged groups. That is, a critical assumption of the system justification perspective is that even members of disadvantaged or powerless groups tend to perceive social events in such a way that hierarchical arrangements (gender, race, class) are perceived as fair and just, perhaps even natural and inevitable.

Over the years, much research has supported this phenomenon (Haines & Jost, 2000; Henry & Saul, 2006; Jost, 2004; Jost & Hunyady, 2002; Jost, Pelham, & Carvallo, 2002; Jost, Pelham, Sheldon, & Sullivan, 2003; Scott, 1990). Haines and Jost (2000), for example, found that powerless groups rationalized the status quo by accepting and bolstering weak justifications for their own inequality. They found that powerless groups attributed greater intelligence and responsibility to an outgroup when the outgroup was in a position of high power rather than equal power, and these effects were enhanced when explanations of power differences were provided.

Across five studies examining social and political attitudes, Jost and his colleagues (2003) found substantial evidence of system justification among various low-status groups. Low-status individuals (in wealth and education) and African Americans were more likely than high-income participants and Whites to express a willingness to limit criticisms of the government in the press and to limit the right of people to speak out against the government. Similarly, low-income Latinos were more likely than high-income Latinos to trust the U.S. government and to believe that the government benefits all people. Poorer participants were also more likely than wealthy participants to believe that large differences in income were necessary to motivate people to work hard. Finally, people from the South, the poor, and Southern African Americans were more likely to endorse meritocratic beliefs systems than were Northerners, the wealthy, and Northern African Americans.

Racial Colorblindness

The concept of racial colorblindness has been theorized to reflect psychological false consciousness among racial minorities (Bonilla-Silva, 2010; Ferber, 2012; Neville, 2009; Neville et al., 2005). Racial colorblindness refers to the denial, distortion, and/or minimization of race and racism. It is the belief that racism is a thing of the past and that race and racism do not play an important role in current social and economic realities (Neville et al., 2005). Theorists maintain that colorblindness is a dominant racially based framework that individuals, groups, and systems consciously or unconsciously use to justify the racial status quo or to explain racial inequalities. Racial colorblindness reinforces and reproduces contemporary systemic racial inequality by denying its reality. According to Bonilla-Silva (2010), colorblindness consists of four key frames that organize one's understanding of racial inequality: abstract liberalism, naturalization, cultural racism, and minimization of racism.

One of the contributions to this literature has been the development of a scale to assess colorblindness, the Color-Blind Racial Attitudes Scale (CoBRAS) (Neville, Lilly, Duran, Lee, & Douglass, 2000). In studies using the CoBRAS, colorblind racial attitudes were found to be associated with racist beliefs, intolerance of multiculturalism, and greater endorsement of beliefs in a just world and the presence of a level-playing field (Neville & Lilly, 2000). Among African Americans, Latinos, and Asians, beliefs in racial colorblindness were related to increased political conservatism such as voting for George W. Bush, a conservative Republican U.S. presidential candidate, less involvement in antiracism activities, and blaming racial minorities themselves for economic and social disparities.

In a later study of colorblind racial beliefs among African Americans (Neville et al., 2005) individuals who were more likely to adopt racial colorblindness attributed greater levels of social injustice to the victims of racism, adopted higher levels of anti-egalitarian beliefs to justify social inequalities (social dominance orientation), internalized more racist messages about Black Americans, preferred to associate with White American friends in comparison to other Black American friends, and had greater internalization of the racial ideology of White superiority-Black inferiority.

Taken together, acquiescent responses by low-status groups to injustice have been widely observed. Members of low-status groups have been shown to accept and even actively support hierarchical systems (gender, race, religion, class) that place them at a disadvantage (Jost & Banajii, 1994). In the next section, we turn to the central focus of this chapter and consider in greater detail what is known about why some (and not other) low-status groups would legitimize, accept, and perpetuate the sources of their inequality.

False Consciousness and Group/Personal Identity and Identification

Some theorists have proposed that people's responses to injustice are contingent on the specific identity categorization that is salient and relevant within a given context. In particular, self-categorization theory posits that self-perceptions can be conceived as a continuum ranging from perception of self as an individual to perception of self as a group member (Turner, Hogg, Oakes, Reicher, & Wetherwell, 1987). Which specific self-categorization becomes relevant to a person depends on the salience of personal versus group identity in a social situation. Salience of personal identity leads to an accentuation of differences between oneself and the ingroup such that when personal identity is salient, a person acts as an individual. Salience of one's group, in contrast, leads to an accentuation of similarities between oneself and the ingroup and differences between the ingroup and an outgroup. When group identity is made salient, an individual acts and thinks as a group member.

Recognizing oneself as a member of a group or as an individual has been found to have considerable impact on how people understand and respond to justice issues. Low-status groups show differences in beliefs about inequality and support for corrective measures when the context leads them to define themselves in terms of their group identity rather than their personal identity (Postmes, Branscombe, Spears, & Young, 1999). Kawakami and Dion's (1993) early work also found stronger feelings of deprivation and a greater likelihood of collective action intentions when group, as compared to personal, identities were made salient.

Other theorists have considered individuals' feelings toward the groups to which they belong as relevant (Ellemers, Spears, & Doosje, 1997). Social identity theory (Tajfel & Turner 1986), for example, argues that members of low-status groups may accept their alleged inferiority, but only under certain conditions. That is, they are expected to engage in outgroup favoritism when ingroup identification is low. Considerable empirical evidence supports social identity theory's claim (Levin, Sidanius, Rabinowitz, & Federico, 1998; O'Brien & Major 2005; Operario & Fiske, 2001; Sinclair, Sidanius, & Levin, 1998; Tropp & Wright, 1999). Operario and Fiske (2001), for example, found that high-identified minorities reported more vulnerability to discrimination and showed stronger reactions to prejudice than less-identified minorities who tended to overlook subtle prejudice.

False Consciousness and Social Identity Awareness Models

The 1960s and 1970s were a period of political-cultural consciousness raising that culminated in social movements for a number of historically marginalized social groups in the United States, such as gays and lesbians (Cass, 1979), people of color (Hardiman & Jackson, 1997), Latinos (Torres, 2003), and African Americans (Cross, 1991). Observers of the participants of these social movements constructed identity awareness models that mapped the multiple stages movement-participants traversed as they shifted from a social identity grounded in false consciousness toward a social identity wherein the interest of the self became more congruent with that of the social group. For gays and lesbians, it was termed the coming-out process, for women it became the embracement of feminism, and for Blacks it represented psychology of nigrescence or "becoming Black" and Afrocentric (Cross, 1991).

Such stage-models of social identity development present a nuanced depiction of identity transformation that is beyond the scope of this work. What is important to stress is that for almost every model, the starting point is the depiction of a person (stage one) whose social identity and political perspective is riddled with false consciousness or internalized oppression. Thus, women aspire to and accept as normal otherwise sexist attitudes about themselves and women in general; gays and lesbians are depicted as internalizing heterosexual norms that, in the worst-case scenario, can lead to internalized homophobia; Stage One Blacks are depicted as operating with a distorted perspective of Black history and Black culture that the late historian Carter G. Woodson (1933) captured in the phrase "the miseducation of the negro" previously discussed.

The French term *deracialization* is an existential rather than biological construct meaning to erase from a marginalized group's collective consciousness the true facts of the group's social history and replace it with one slanted toward the history and culture as written by those who have conquered, subjugated, or stigmatized the group. All of the identity models in consideration describe the process for correcting miseducation; consequently, the identity dynamics associated with advanced awareness are grounded in an in-depth knowledge of one's social, cultural, and economic history. Partly in reaction to the pejorative perspective that dominated mainstream academics, but more so as a move to fill the void of miseducation, silence, and invisibility, a handful of the social movements noted earlier catalyzed the creation of undergraduate majors and graduate studies in Africana studies, LGBT studies, women's studies, Asian American studies, disabilities studies, and Latina-Latino studies.

Empirical studies are associated with all the models noted earlier but due to space limitations we will focus on research generated by Black identity awareness models. In a review of the literature on Black identity change, Cross (1991) summarizes the research showing that in stage one (false consciousness) Blacks evidenced negative attitudes toward other Blacks, a blame the victim ideology (i.e., Blacks are their own worst enemy), the tendency to idealize White beauty and a Eurocentric aesthetic, a sense of estrangement toward other Blacks, or in the absence of outright negative attitudes, a sense of a lack of importance toward racial affairs (low salience). In the same review, Cross notes that by comparison advanced awareness has been linked to greater cultural knowledge, a sense of closeness to other Blacks, membership in organizations stressing a progressive stance toward Black issues and causes, and placing considerable emphasis on being aware and informed about Black issues (high salience).

More recent analyses have examined the process of African Americans internalizing White stereotypes about Blacks (positive and negative), called internalized racialism (e.g., an African American who believes Blacks are more prone to criminality than Whites or who believes that Blacks naturally run faster than Whites). Cokley (2002) found that stage one attitudes of miseducation and self-hatred were positively related to internalized racialism. Specifically, miseducation and self-hatred attitudes were significantly and positively related to beliefs in the mental and genetic deficiencies of Blacks. Perkins' (2010) recent analysis also found that stage one attitudes were positively associated with both system justification and racial colorblindness.

False Consciousness and Individual/National/Political Ideology

Other lines of research suggest that the mechanism through which low-status groups endorse false consciousness (or not) is ideological (Bonilla-Silva, 2010; Feagan, 2001; Ferber 2012; Hartigan, 2010). Ideology is a central feature of culture that, according to Bonilla-Silva, "consists of broad mental frameworks that social groups use to make sense of the world, to decide what is right and wrong, true or false, important or unimportant" (2010, p. 62). Some early research highlights this point in understanding the role that ideologies play in the tendency to deny or act against one's own disadvantage (Abeles, 1976; Dion, 1986; Taylor & Dube, 1986). Abeles (1976), for example, examined what factors contributed to militancy in Black college students. In his analysis, militancy was defined as a cluster of attitudes centering on a rejection of the traditional, passive, and subordinate Black role (e.g., equal treatment as human beings, equitable share in the nation's prosperity, political influence), a rejection of the racial status quo, and an acceptance of reforms or revolutionary changes in the social system. Across two studies, the best predictor of militancy was the perception that Black people in general are unfairly treated.

Some empirical studies point to the role national and political ideologies play in support of the status quo (Guimond & Dube-Simard, 1983). Guimond and Dube-Simard (1983), for example, examined feelings of group discontent and perceptions of inequality among Francophone Canadians. They found that feelings of discontent and perceptions of inequality were strongly related to a strong nationalist ideology with regard to desire for greater political autonomy for Quebec and favoring measures to protect and enhance the status of the French language and culture in Quebec. More recent analyses have found that tendencies to accept inequality in terms of outgroup favoritism (Jost & Hunyady, 2002), reduced sensitivity to discrimination (Major et al., 2002), ambivalent attitudes toward the ingroup (Jost & Burgess, 2000), ingroup blame (Major, Kaiser, O'Brien, & McCoy, 2007), and well-being (Foster & Tsarfati, 2005) were related to political ideologies.

A recent study by Cheung and Hardin (2008) experimentally examined whether conservative members of low-status groups are more likely to accept inequality. In an examination of pay expectations among foreign domestic workers in Hong Kong and among Asian and Hispanics in the United States, these workers devalued their work (paid themselves less), to the extent that they defined themselves as conservative. Endorsement of a meritocratic ideology has also been shown by several researchers to be associated with low-status groups' tolerance of their own social inequality (Foster & Tsarfati, 2005; Major et al., 2007).

Other research has emphasized the larger sociocultural messages that are embedded in both high- and low-status groups' ideology construction. This line of research argues that ones' subjectivity is not merely isolated cognitive processing, but is a compilation of one's engagement within the cultural and ideological resources available (Augustinos, 1999; Deutsch, 1974). The ideologies individuals develop are shaped by the existing materials and power relations within a society and outlines for individuals what they can legitimately expect (Deutsch, 1974). These messages often limit or enhance one's views regarding what one is entitled to. Sociocultural variables such as beliefs about upward mobility, permeability of the social system, and legitimacy have consistently been shown to play an important role in acquiescent responses among low-status groups (Overbeck et al., 2004).

System justification theory has attempted to account for the sociocultural milieu shaping ideology by hypothesizing that "system justification levels will be higher in societies in which social and economic inequality is more extreme than less extreme" (Jost, Banaji, & Nosek, 2004, p. 910). Recent applications of social identity theory also suggest that the maintenance of inequality by lower-status group members would be more prevalent in societies in which group-based status differences are seen as highly legitimate and stable (Henry & Saul, 2006). However, much of the research testing these ideas has been conducted in the relatively non-extreme and advantaged continents of North America and Europe. When research has gone outside this context, it has often involved work with college students, who are presumably coming from a position of some advantage (Uhlmann, Dasgupta, Elgueta, Greenwald, & Swanson, 2002). An exception is a recent analysis by Henry and Saul (2006), who examined system justification beliefs in severely impoverished areas in Bolivia. They examined attitudes toward the Bolivian government comparing three groups of Bolivians: indigenous members of Bolivia, the Hispanic group, and Mestizos. Low-status indigenous participants believed, more than did their Hispanic counterparts, that political dissent should be suppressed and that the Bolivian government responds to the needs of the people. The indigenous participants also felt less alienated by the government in comparison to other groups.

False Consciousness and Social Comparisons

People judge their status and outcomes according to the situation of relevant others (Crosby, 1976; see Smith, Pettigrew, Pippen, & Bialosiewicz, 2012). That is, feelings of deprivation develop on the basis of social comparisons with specific others and feelings of deprivation are a relative experience rather than an absolute one. As such, comparisons with others serve to define whether and how much deprivation and disadvantage an individual feels and experiences. For example, an individual who lacks something will be less angry if the people with whom he or she compares also lack the same thing, but will feel relatively deprived if comparable others do possess the object.

Research has theorized that characteristics of the comparison target, such as their relative advantage or disadvantage, can influence the extent to which disadvantaged individuals feel deprived (Kawakami & Dion, 1993; Tropp & Wright, 1999; Walker & Pettigrew, 1984). Early research by Stouffer, Suchman, DeVinney, Star, and William (1949) examined, among other things, why military police who were given slow promotions were more satisfied than air corpsmen who were given quick promotions. They concluded post hoc that the military police did not compare themselves with air corpsmen and therefore did not feel deprived. Kawakami and Dion (1993) also found experimentally that the magnitude of social inequalities affected feelings of satisfaction, perceived justice, and action intentions. Tropp and Wright (1999) examined comparisons of relatively advantaged outgroup (Whites) targets and targets from other disadvantaged outgroups (minorities). Consistent with theorizations on relative deprivation, Latinos and African Americans reported more deprivation in comparison with Whites than with other minorities or with their own group. Zagefka and Brown (2005) also found that interest in comparing with ingroup members negatively predicted group deprivations within a German minority sample, a London minority sample, and a longitudinal study among ethnic minorities. Consistent with previous relative deprivation research, endorsement of racial colorblindness was negatively associated with comparisons with Whites (Perkins, 2010). Moreover, the better off they felt about their situation compared to Whites, the stronger their beliefs in system justification and racial colorblindness.

THE GLOBALIZED NATURE OF FALSE CONSCIOUSNESS

The processes outlined earlier are particularly important to consider within the context of globalization, as this is a dynamic society where localized events now have global significance. In the context of the vast sweeps of global change, the individual is a distillation and manifestation of these global forces. We consider this reality as part of the backdrop within which individuals, groups, and societies think about justice and injustice. The intimate connection between the local and the global, we believe, alters the landscape under which the disadvantaged perceive their lot. In the next sections, we articulate several extensions to the question of false consciousness and intergroup relations that encompass the unique dynamics of the globalized world.

Before turning to this, our discussion of globalization draws primarily upon Scholte's (2000) delineation of globalization as comprising aspects of Westernization or Americanization. Globalization as Westernization is a dynamic process whereby social structures and modern/Western ideologies of progress (e.g., capitalism) spread throughout the world, oftentimes resulting in the destruction and subordination of the local (Scholte, 2000).

First, the present context of globalization as Americanization/Westernization mirrors the early intellectual and theoretical roots of false consciousness (Marx & Engels, 1846; Gramsci, 1971; Fanon, 1952, 1986; Habermas, 1975). The process of globalization as Americanization/Westernization appears to emulate extant systems of colonization and hegemony with very similar consequences. Specifically, the systems of power that produced domination have now reformulated and are reproducing similar types inequities with similar types of psychological consequences (false consciousness), a point we will turn to later. That is, for some researchers, globalization is something that is being imposed or driven by a few nations that define what is progress and decides who gets exploited in the implementation of that progress (Marsella, 2005, 2012). Marsella (2005, 2012), for example, argues that globalization is the hegemonic imposition of values associated with Western and American culture. Further, the push of globalization as Americanization/Westernization also highlights Fanon's (1952) original colonial critique as we believe race and privilege are the fundamental organizing principles that define what progress is and who gets exploited.

Ikenberry and Kupchan (1990) and more recently Noori (2013) also expand upon Woodson's analysis of the miseducation of African Americans to the miseducation of marginalized groups throughout the developing world as a consequence of globalization as Westernization/Americanization. They assert that Western values and ideas are being systematically exported into the educational curriculum of developing countries with an implicit mission to occupy the hearts and minds of the marginalized. Specifically, Noori (2013) describes American-style higher education in the Middle East as a form of cultural imperialism by explicitly and implicitly (through language instruction, the type of textbook used, and the curriculum) encouraging Middle Eastern students to see and value the world from an American point of view.

In addition to extending the early theoretical origins of false consciousness, the push toward globalization further elucidates the role that ideology plays in low-status groups' legitimization of their inequality. Some theorists argue that the push of globalization is creating distinct kinds of ideologies of legitimization (McQuail, 2010; Moghaddam, 2010). The widening gap between the rich and the poor, through ideologies like meritocracy, as Moghaddam (2010) points out, creates an illusion that progress made by some individuals in the status hierarchy is a result of their own hard work and talent. Further, Moghaddam (2010) asserts that the push of globalization is paradoxically shaping a unique kind of meritocratic ideology based on the belief in "The American Dream." The American dream ideology is a story that is being inculcated into the cultural zeitgeist of the third and developing world. For Moghaddam (2010), this narrative shapes how low-status groups in the developing world see and understand their disadvantaged status. The belief that society is open and that anyone can make it if they have the talent and motivation, Moghaddam (2010) asserts, may be why some of the marginalized in the developing world do not question or threaten the status quo. Thus, belief in the American dream is being advertised as a global dream/commodity that is shaping how people in the developing world see their lot. They are being cultivated to see their lot as a consequence of their own behavior.

Finally, globalization extends the current theoretical perspectives on intergroup comparisons. Relative deprivation theory and social comparison theory in general underscore the psychological significance of the social comparison process. Comparison choices have been shown to determine whether people perceive existing discrimination, whether they feel deprived, and whether they are satisfied with their own or their group's outcomes (Kawakami & Dion, 1993; Major & Konar, 1984; Walker & Pettigrew, 1984; Tropp & Wright, 1999; Zagefka & Brown, 2005). Comparison choices have also been shown to affect perceptions of injustice and entitlement, and might raise or lower people's aspirations and expectations for change. Thus, whom one compares to is central to one's evaluations and perceptions of the world.

Globalization shifts the backdrop against and within which social comparisons are made and the implications associated with those comparisons with regard to false consciousness. A more open world means that millions of people move from one country to another. Information about others is now reaching the farthest corners of the globe. Consequently, globalization has resulted in increased contact with more groups of people. However, as Shiva (2000) asserts, globalization is asymmetrical rather than uniform such that the Global South is embedded in this process to a differing degree than the Global North. For example, the global reach of the American/Western lifestyle through the media is powerful. Because of the American monopoly over the media, some theorists view the mass media as a channel of Westernization aimed at controlling, invading, and undermining the developing world (McQuail, 2010). Other theorists argue that the flow of media from the rich countries to the poorer countries may aggravate the already existing power gap (Marsella, 2012). Moghaddam (2010) also argues that the rapid movement of people across borders, in combination with the imposition of Western cultural forces via the Internet, leads to those with the least wealth either unconsciously or consciously to view themselves as least valuable.

The implications of the social comparison process appear more nuanced when considering globalization as Westernization/Americanization. In particular, comparisons with higher-status groups (e.g., the Western world) have several implications: further marginalization, as suggested by many theorists, or collective action, as evidenced by the recent Arab and African Spring movements. Social identity theory (1978) speaks to these nuances proposing that under some circumstances people might elect to compare with more advantaged targets in order to challenge the existing social hierarchy. As such, people might make comparisons with more advantaged outgroups if "equity" concerns are strong. Across several studies with minority groups, Zagefka and Brown (2006) found that motives affect comparison choices and that different comparison choices are chosen to fulfill different motives. Their data show that temporal, intragroup, and downward comparisons satisfied "enhancement" motives; and comparisons with outgroups were often motivated by equity concerns. Similarly, social identity theory also suggests that certain socio-structural conditions might render previously incomparable groups comparable (Tajfel, 1978). For example, in situations in which the social climate appears illegitimate and unstable, like the Arab and African Spring movements, people might start comparing with dissimilar more advantaged outgroups.

CONCLUSION

In this overview, we draw attention to an enduring and fundamental question of psychology. This review presented the major work that has addressed the psychological conditions under which low-status groups accept and justify their inequality. Further, we have attempted to explicate how globalization expands upon and is implicated in this process. In particular, we have offered new lenses of analysis of the current theoretical perspectives that draw out the impact of macro-systemic processes on the phenomenon of false consciousness. The evidence reviewed shows there are various personal, ideological, situational, and structural conditions that play a role and often interact with one another, affecting the likelihood that low-status groups will accept their unequal status in society. It is important to note that reactions to injustice among low-status groups encompass a large array of responses, ranging from acceptance to collective action. Social change does happen and continues to happen. Our intention in writing this chapter is not to dismiss this. Rather our intention is to document and understand more fully a ubiquitous, yet paradoxical reality that, we believe, dampens the potential for change and empowerment.

NOTE

1. We use the racial identity descriptor used by the theorist/researcher throughout the chapter.

REFERENCES

Abeles, R. P. (1976). Relative deprivation, rising expectations, and Black militancy. *Journal of Social Issues, 32,*115–133. doi: 10.1111/j.1540-4560.1976.tb02498.x

Augustinos, M. (1999). Ideology, false consciousness, and psychology. *Theory and Psychology, 9,* 295–312. doi: 10.1177/0959354399093002x

Bem, S. L., & Bem, D. J. (1970). Case study of a nonconscious ideology: Training the woman to know her place. In D. J. Bem (Ed.), *Beliefs, attitudes, and human affairs* (pp. 89–99). Belmont, CA: Brooks/Cole.

Bonilla-Silva, E. (2010). *Racism without racists: Color-blind racism and the persistence of racial inequality in America.* Lanham, MD: Rowman & Littlefield.

Cass, V. (1979). Homosexual identity development. *Journal of Homosexuality, 4,* 219–235. doi: 10.1300/J082v04n03_01

Cheung, M. H., & Hardin, C. D. Costs of conservatism: Stereotype consistent self-derogation in dollars and cents. Unpublished manuscript. Brooklyn College, New York, New York.

Clark, J. B., & Clark, M. B. (1947). Racial identification and preference for Negro children. In E. E. Maccoby, T. M. Newcomb, & E. L. Hartley (Eds.), *Readings in social psychology* (pp. 602–611). New York, NY: Holt, Rinehart, and Winston.

Cokley, K. O. (2002). Testing Cross's revised racial identity model: An examination of the relationship between racial identity and internalized racialism. *Journal of Counseling Psychology, 49,* 476–483. doi: 10.1037/0022-0167.49.4.476

Crosby, F. J. (1976). A model of egoistical relative deprivation. *Psychological Review, 83,* 85–113. doi: 10.1037/0033-295X.83.2.85

Crosby, F. J., Putfall, A., Snyder, R. C., O'Connell, M., & Whaien, P. (1989). The denial of personal disadvantage among you, me, and all the other ostriches. In M. Crawford & M. Gentry (Eds.), *Gender and thought: Psychological perspectives* (pp. 79–99). New York, NY: Springer Verlag.

Cross, W. E., Jr. (1991). *Shades of Black.* Philadelphia, PA: Temple University Press.

Dion, K. L. (1986). Responses to perceived discrimination and relative deprivation. In J. M. Olson, C. P. Herman, & M. F. Zana (Eds.), *Relative deprivation and social comparison: The Ontario Symposium* (pp. 159–179). Elkkale, NJ: Erlbaum.

Deutsch, M. (1974). Awakening the sense of injustice. In M. Lerner & M. Ross (Eds.), *The quest for justice: Myth, reality, ideal.* Montreal, QC: Holt, Rinehart & Winston.

Deutsch, M. (1985). *Distributive justice: A social psychological perspective.* New Haven, CT: Yale University Press.

Douglass, F. (1855). *My bondage and my freedom.* Modern Library.

Ellemers, N., Spears, R., & Doise, B. (1997). Sticking together or falling apart: Ingroup identification as a psychological determinant of group commitment versus individual mobility. *Journal of Personality and Social Psychology, 72,* 617–626. doi: 10.1037/0022-3514.72.3.617

Fanon, F. (1952). *Black skin, White mask.* Paris, France: Editions Du Seuil.

Fanon, F. (1986). *The wretched of the earth.* New York, NY: Grove Press.

Feagan, J. R. (2001). *Racist America: Roots, current realities, future reparations.* New York, NY: Routledge.

Ferber, A. L. (2012). The culture of privilege: Color-blindness, postfeminism, and Christonormativity. *Journal of Social Issues, 68*(1), 63–77. doi: 10.1111/j.1540-4560.2011.01736.x

Fine, M., & Bowers, C. (1984). Racial self-identification: The effects of social history and gender. *Journal of Applied Social Psychology, 14,* 136–146. doi: 10.1111/j.1559-1816.1984.tb02226.x

Foster, M. D., & Tsarfati, E. M. (2005). The effects of meritocracy beliefs on women's well-being after first-time gender discrimination. *Personality and Social Psychology Bulletin, 31*(12), 1730–1738. doi: 10.1177/0146167205278709

Gramsci, A. (1971). *The prison notebooks.* New York, NY: Columbia University Press.

Guimond, S., & Dube-Simard, L. (1983). Relative deprivation theory and the Quebec nationalist movement: The cognition-emotion distinction and the personal-group deprivation issue. *Journal of Personality and Social Psychology, 44,* 526–535. doi: 10.1037/0022-3514.44.3.526

Habermas, J. (1975). *Legitimation crisis.* (T. McCarthy, Tran.). Boston, MA: Beacon Press.

Hafer, C. L., & Olson, J. M. (1989). Beliefs in a just world and reactions to personal deprivation. *Journal of Personality, 57,* 799–823. doi: 10.1111/j.1467-6494.1989.tb00495.x

Hafer, C. L., & Olson, J. M. (1993). Beliefs in a just world, discontent, and assertive actions by working women. *Personality and Social Psychology Bulletin, 19,* 30–38. doi: 10.1177/0146167293191004

Haines, E. L., & Jost, J. T. (2000). Placating the powerless: Effects of legitimate and illegitimate explanation on affect, memory, and stereotyping. *Social Justice Research, 13,* 219–236. doi: 10.1023/A:1026481205719

Hardiman, R., & Jackson, B. W. (1997). Conceptual foundations for social justice courses. In M. Adams, L. A. Bell, & P. Griffin (Eds.), *Teaching for diversity and social justice* (pp. 23–29). New York, NY: Routledge.

Hartigan, J. Jr., (2010). *What can you say?: America's national conversation on race.* Palo Alto, CA: Stanford University Press.

Henry, P. J., & Saul., A. (2006). The development of system justification in the developing world. *Social Justice Research, 19*(3), 365–378. doi: 10.1007/s11211-006-0012-x

Ikenberry, G. J., & Kupchan, C. A. (1990). Socialization and hegemonic power. *International Organization, 44*(3), 283. doi: 10.1017/S002081830003530X

Janoff-Bulman, R. (1992). *Shattered assumptions: Toward a new psychology of trauma.* New York, NY: Free Press.

Jost, J. T. (1995). Negative illusions: Conceptual clarification and psychological evidence concerning false consciousness. *Political Psychology, 16,* 397–424. doi: 10.2307/3791837

Jost, J. T. (1997). An experimental replication of the depressed entitlement effect among women. *Psychology Women Quarterly, 21,* 387–393. doi: 10.1111/j.1471-6402.1997.tb00120.x

Jost, J. T., & Banaji, M. R. (1994). The role of stereotyping in system justification and the production of false consciousness. *British Journal of Social Psychology, 33,* 1–27. doi: 10.1111/j.2044-8309.1994.tb01008.x

Jost, J. T., Banaji, M. R., & Nosek, B. A. (2004). A decade of system justification theory: Accumulated evidence of conscious and unconscious bolstering of the status quo. *Political Psychology, 25*(6), 881–919. doi: 10.1111/j.1467-9221.2004.00402.x

Jost, J. T., & Burgess, D. (2000). Attitudinal ambivalence and the conflict between group and system justification motives in low status groups. *Personality and Social Psychology Bulletin, 26*(3), 293–305. doi: 10.1177/0146167200265003

Jost, J. T., & Hunyady, O. (2002). The psychology of system justification and the palliative function of ideology. *European Review of Social Psychology, 13,* 111–153. doi: 10.1080/10463280240000046

Jost, J. T., Pelham, B. W., & Carvallo, M. (2002). Non-conscious forms of system justification: Cognitive, affective, and behavioral preferences for higher status groups. *European Journal of Social Psychology, 33,* 13–36. doi: 10.1016/S0022-1031(02)00505-X

Jost, J. T., Pelham, B. W., Sheldon, O., & Sullivan, B. N. (2003). Social inequality and the reduction of ideological dissonance on behalf of the system: Evidence of enhanced system justification among the disadvantaged. *European Journal of Social Psychology, 33,* 13–36. doi: 10.1002/ejsp.127

Kinder, D., & Sears, D. O. (1985). Public opinion and political action. In G. Lindzey & E. Aronson (Eds.), *Handbook of social psychology* (3rd ed., pp. 659–741). New York, NY: Random House.

Kawakami, K., & Dion, K. L. (1993). The impact of salient self-identities on relative deprivation and action intention. *European Journal of Social Psychology, 23*(5), 525–540. doi: 10.1002/ejsp.2420230509

Lerner, M. J. (1980). *The belief in a just world: A fundamental delusion.* New York, NY: Plenum Press.

Levin, S., Federico, M., Sidanius, J., & Rabinowitz, J. (2002). Social dominance orientation and intergroup bias: The legitimization of favoritism for high-status. *Personality and Social Psychology Bulletin, 28,* 144–157. doi: 10.1177/0146167202282002

Levin, S., & Sidanius, J. (1999). Social dominance and social identity in the United States and Israel: Ingroup favoritism or outgroup degradation? *Political Psychology, 20,* 99–125. doi: 10.1111/0162-895X.00138

Levin, S., Sidanius, J., Rabinowitz, J., & Federico, C. (1998). Ethnic identity, legitimizing ideologies, and social status: A matter of ideological asymmetry. *Political Psychology, 19,* 373–404. doi: 10.1111/0162-895X.00109

Major, B. (1994). From social inequality to personal entitlement: The role of social comparisons, legitimacy appraisals, and group membership. *Journal of Experimental Social Psychology, 38,* 405–413. doi: 10.1037/0022-3514.68.5.826

Major, B., Gramzow, R. H. McCoy, S., Levin, S., Schmader, T., & Sidanius, J. (2002). Perceiving personal discrimination: The role of group status and legitimizing ideology. *Journal of Personality and Social Psychology, 82,* 269–282. doi: 10.1037/0022-3514.82.3.269

Major, B., Kaiser, C. R., O'Brien, L. T., & McCoy, S. K. (2007). Perceived discrimination as worldview threat or worldview confirmation: Implications for self-esteem. *Journal of Personality and Social Psychology, 92,* 1068–1086. doi: 10.1037/0022-3514.92.6.1068

Marsella, A. J. (2005). "Hegemonic" globalization and cultural diversity: The risks of global monoculturalism. *Australian Mosaic,* 12, 15–19.

Marsella, A. J. (2012). Psychology and globalization: Understanding a complex relationship. *Journal of Social Issues, 68*(3), 454–472. doi: 10.1111/j.1540-4560.2012.01758.x

Marx, K., & Engels, F. (1846/1970). *The German ideology.* (Ed. C. J. Arther). New York, NY: International Publishers.

McQuail, D. (2010). *McQuail's mass communication theory.* London: Sage Publications.

Moghaddam, F. M. (2010). *The new global insecurity: How terrorism, environmental collapse, economic inequalities, and resource shortages are changing our world.* Santa Barbara, CA: Praeger Publishers.

Neville, H. A. (2009). Rationalizing the racial order: Racial color-blindness as a legitimizing ideology. In T. Koditschek, S. K. Cha-Jua, & H. A. Neville (Eds.), *Race struggles* (pp. 115–133). Champaign, IL: University of Illinois Press.

Neville, H. A., Coleman, M. N. Falconer, J. M., & Holmes, D. (2005). Color-blind racial ideology and psychological false consciousness among African Americans. *Journal of Black Psychology, 31,* 27–45. doi: 10.1177/0095798404268287

Neville, H. A., & Lilly, R. L. (2000). The relationship between racial identity cluster profiles and psychological distress among African American college students. *Journal of Multicultural Counseling & Development, 28,* 194–207. doi: 10.1002/j.2161-1912.2000.tb00615.x

Neville, H. A., Lilly, R. L., Duran, G., Lee, R. M., & Douglas, L. (2000). Construction of the initial validation of the Color-Blind Racial Attitudes Scale (CoBRAS). *Journal of Counseling Psychology, 47,* 59–70. doi: 10.1037//0022-0167.47.1.59

Noori, N. (in press) The politics of American-style education in the Middle East. In E. Lundy & E. Lundy (Eds.), *American studies in the Middle East: A comparative encounter*. Austin, TX: Under review, University of Texas Press.

O'Brien, L. T., & Major, B. (2005). System-justifying beliefs and psychological well-being: The roles of group status and identity. *Personality and Social Psychology Bulletin, 31,* 1718–1729. doi: 10.1177/0146167205278261

Olson, J. M., & Hafer, C. L. (2001).Tolerance of personal deprivation. In J. T. Jost & B. Major (Eds.), *The psychology of legitimacy: Emerging perspectives on ideology, justice, and intergroup relations* (pp. 157–204). Cambridge, UK: Cambridge University Press.

Operario, D., & Fiske, S. T. (2001). Ethnic identity moderates perceptions of prejudice: Judgments of personal versus group discrimination and subtle versus blatant bias. *Personality and Social Psychology Bulletin, 27,* 550–561. doi: 10.1177/0146167201275004

Overbeck, J. R., Jost, J. T., Moss, C. O., & Flizik, A. (2004). Resistant versus acquiescent responses to ingroup inferiority as a function of social dominance orientation in the USA and Italy. *Group Processes & Intergroup Relations, 7,* 35–54. doi: 10.1177/1368430204039972

Pelham, B. W., & Hetts, J. J. (2001). Underworked and overpaid: Elevated entitlement in men's self-pay. *Journal of Experimental Social Psychology,* 37, 93–103. doi: 10.1006/jesp.2000.1429

Perkins, K. (2010). The acceptance of injustice among African Americans as a function of ideology and social comparison processes. New York, NY. Unpublished Doctoral Dissertation. Graduate Center of the City University of New York.

Postmes, T., Branscombe, N. R., Spears, R., & Young, H. (1999). Comparative processes in personal and group judgements: Resolving the discrepancy. *Journal of Personality and Social Psychology, 76,* 320–338. doi: 10.1037/0022-3514.76.2.320

Rubin, Z., & Peplau, L. A. (1975). Who believes in a just world? *Journal of Social Issues, 31,* 65–89. doi: 10.1111/j.1540-4560.1975.tb00997.x

Scholte, J. A. (2000). *Globalization: A critical introduction*. New York, NY: Palgrave Macmillan.

Scott, J. (1990). *Domination and the arts of resistance*. New Haven, CT: Yale University Press.

Shiva, V. (2000). *Stolen harvest: The hijacking of the global food supply*. London: Zed Books.

Sidanius, J. (1993). The psychology of group conflict and dynamics of oppression: A social dominance perspective. In S. Iyengar & W. McGuire (Eds.), *Explorations in political psychology* (pp. 183–219). Durham, NC: Duke University Press.

Sidanius, J., Levin, S., Federico, C., & Pratto, F. (2001). Legitimizing ideologies: The social dominance approach. In J. T. Jost & B. Major (Eds.), *The psychology of legitimacy: Emerging perspectives on ideology, justice and intergroup relations* (pp. 363–388). New York, NY: Cambridge University Press.

Sidanius, J., & Pratto, F. (1993). The inevitability of oppression and the dynamics of social dominance. In P. Sniderman & P. Tetlock (Eds.), *Prejudice, politics, and the American dilemma* (pp. 173–211). Stanford, CA: Stanford University Press.

Sinclair, S., Sidanius, J., & Levin, S. (1998). The interface between ethnic and social system attachment: The differential effects of hierarchy-enhancing and hierarchy-attenuating environments. *Journal of Social Issues,* 54, 741–757. doi: 10.1111/j.1540-4560.1998.tb01246.x

Smith, H. J., Pettigrew, T. F., Piplin, G. M., & Bialosiewicz, S. (2012). Relative deprivation: A theoretical and meta-analytic review. *Personality and Social Psychology Review, 16,* 203–232. doi: 10.1177/1088868311430825

Stouffer, S. A., Suchman, E. A., DeVinney, L. C., Star, S. A., & Williams, R. M. (1949). *The American soldier: Adjustment during army life* (Vol. 1). Princeton, NJ: Princeton University Press.

Tajfel, H. (1978). Social categorisation, social identity, and social comparison. In H. Tajfel (Ed.), *Differentiation between social groups: Studies in the social psychology of intergroup relations.* London: Academic Press.

Tajfel, H., & Turner, J. C. (1986). The social identity theory of intergroup behavior. In S. Worchel & W. G. Austin (Eds.), *The psychology of intergroup relations* (pp. 7–24). Chicago, IL: Nelson-Hall.

Taylor, D. M., & Dube, L. (1986). Two faces of identity: The "I" and "we." *Journal of Social Issues, 42,* 81–98. doi: 10.1111/j.1540-4560.1986.tb00226.x

Taylor, S. E., & Brown, J. D. (1988). Illusion of well-being: A social psychological perspective on mental health. *Psychological Bulletin, 103,* 191–210. doi: 193-210 0033-2909/88/$00.75

Torres, V. (2003). Validation of a bicultural orientation model for Hispanic college students. *Journal of College Student Development, 40,* 285–298.

Tropp, R. L., & Wright, C. S. (1999). Ingroup identification and relative deprivation: An examination across multiple social comparisons. *European Journal of Social Psychology, 29,* 707–724. doi: 10.1002/(SICI)1099-0992(199908/09)29:5/6<707::AID-EJSP968>3.0.CO;2-Y

Turner, J. C., Hogg, M. A., Oakes, P. J., Reicher, S., & Wetherwell, M. S. (1987). *Rediscovering the social group: A self categorization theory.* Oxford, UK: Blackwell.

Uhlmann, E., Dasgupta, N., Elgueta, A., Greenwald, A. G., & Swanson, J. (2002). Subgroup prejudice based on skin color among Hispanics in the United States and Latin America. *Social Cognition, 20*(3), 198-226. doi: 10.1521/soco.20.3.198.21104

Walker, I., & Pettigrew, T. F. (1984). Relative deprivation theory: An overview and conceptual critique. *British Journal of Social Psychology, 23,* 301–310. doi: 10.1111/j.2044-8309.1984.tb00645.x

Woodson, C. G. (1933). *The mis-education of the Negro.* Washington, DC: Associated Publishers.

Zagefka, H., & Brown, R. (2005). Comparisons and perceived deprivation in ethnic minority settings. *Personality and Social Psychology Bulletin, 31,* 467–481. doi: 10.1177/0146167204271711

Zagefka, H., & Brown, R. (2006). Predicting comparison choices in intergroup settings: A new look. In S. Guimond (Ed.), *Social comparisons and social psychology: Understanding cognition, intergroup relations and culture* (pp. 99–125). Cambridge, MA: University Press.

Chapter 7

Liberation Psychology, Feminism, and Social Justice Psychology

Geraldine Moane

Psychological theory, research, and practice may seek to advance well-being and social justice, yet many critics of psychology have questioned the degree to which psychology achieves these aims, and in some case have suggested that psychology may undermine well-being and perpetrate social oppression (Bulhan, 1985; Fine, 2006, Nelson & Prilleltensky, 2010). Critiques have arisen particularly where psychology has been applied to groups outside its original White middle-class Euro/American context (Bulhan, 1985; Dudgeon, Garvey, & Pickett, 2000). Since the 1970s, for example, feminists have criticized approaches in psychology that were based on White, male, middle-class samples, questioning their applicability to women, people of color, or those living in poverty (Norsworthy & Buranajakoernkij, 2011; Wilkinson, 1986). Historically, as applications of psychology extended to ethnic groups, critiques of racism and of insensitivity to ethnic and cultural differences emerged (Bulhan, 1985). Lesbians and gay men found that psychology could pathologize and undermine the problems that they experience by locating pathology within the interior world of the individual rather than in the relationship between the individual and oppressive social structures (Kitzinger & Perkins, 1993). Those from working class and deprived backgrounds found psychologists could be insensitive to their particular needs and social conditions (Lott, 1993).

As feminists and other groups intensified their critiques of psychology, it became clear that the discipline would need fundamental reappraisal of its knowledge production, research methods, and practices, many of which were based on the medical-scientific model. Many studies in the psychology of women, for example, that aimed to include or add women into existing theories and research identified an intrinsic deficit model of women in established psychological theories (Tavris, 1992). Feminists argued that a whole new psychology was needed.

Wilkinson (1991) expressed this view in her editorial for the first issues of *Feminism & Psychology*: "Feminist psychology is committed to developing a psychology which properly represents women's concerns in all their diversity and to the deployment of such a psychology to address a range of social inequalities including for example, race and class, as well as gender" (p. 5). Since then feminist psychologists have developed multicultural and postmodern approaches with a comprehensive analysis of intersectionality and a series of emancipatory practices in psychotherapy, counseling, research, education, and community psychology (Landrine & Russo, 2009; Lykes & Moane, 2009b; Norsworthy & Buranajakoenkij, 2011; Rutherford, Capdevila, Undurti, & Palmary, 2011).

Minority and oppressed groups came to parallel conclusions, namely that it was not enough to modify psychology to include minority perspectives, and that the discipline needed fundamental restructuring. Working with impoverished African Americans, for example, convinced Bulhan that psychology was fundamentally flawed and that its individualistic focus could perpetrate the oppressions that he witnessed. Bulhan (1985) argued that "underlying much of prevailing psychology theory and practice are the ethic of individualism, the ideal of individual autonomy, a particular conception of basic human needs, as well as an excessive emphasis on individual change which together represent cultural as well as class biases" (p. 256). Bulhan called for a psychology of liberation that would aim to transform society, thus removing many of the factors that cause or exacerbate mental illness.

In several contexts efforts to develop new psychological approaches used phrases such as psychology of liberation (Bulhan, 1985; Montero & Sonn, 2009), liberation psychology (Martín-Baró, 1994), social liberation psychology (Kagan, Burton, Duckett, Lawthom, & Siddiquee, 2011), community psychology of liberation (Nelson & Prilleltensky, 2010; Watts & Serrano-Garcia, 2003), feminist liberation psychology (Lykes & Moane, 2009b; Moane, 2011), and psychologies of liberation (Watkins & Shulman, 2008). Liberation psychologies have expanded to combine perspectives from around the globe from contexts that include poverty, violence, armed conflict, psychosocial trauma, ethnic conflict, migration, and homelessness—conditions that are linked with global injustices. Many of these contexts involve intersectionalities of race, ethnicity, class, sexual orientation, and other dimensions of oppression, a theme that has been very well developed in feminist psychology (Landrine & Russo, 2009).

Psychologies of liberation share an explicit analysis of oppression and of resistance to oppression, and an emphasis on activism and intervention. The most sustained development of such a psychology has been in Latin America, where the phrase "liberation psychology" was coined by Martín-Baró (1994) and has been developed since particularly by Montero and colleagues (Montero & Sonn, 2009). This context was characterized by totalitarian military regimes and large-scale poverty where Freire (1970), Martín-Baró (1994), and others were developing radical approaches to education as well as examining the role of psychology both as an instrument of oppression (wherein, e.g., psychologists are involved in torture and psychiatric abuse) and as an aid in liberation (wherein, e.g., psychologists are involved in empowering local communities). Martín-Baró expressed the need for a new psychology that would be less concerned with its scientific status and more oriented toward social transformation. Both Freire and Martín-Baró were the target of state oppression for their work—Freire was imprisoned in 1964 for his work on literacy, whereas Martín-Baró was assassinated in 1989.

A related approach that offers a fundamental critique of psychology and a call for new approach is that of postcolonial psychology. Postcolonial psychology was developed through the work of Fanon (1967) and Memmi (1967), both of whom described psychological patterns associated with the colonizer-colonized dynamic. Postcolonial psychology aims to challenge this duality and move from polarized binaries to more fluid multiple perspectives, which again poses a challenge to traditional psychology theory (Hook, 2012; Norsworthy & Buranajakoenkij, 2011; Reyes Cruz & Sonn, 2011). Postcolonial psychology is critical of the established fields of psychology that have been developed by dominant groups in European and American contexts and transferred to contexts and groups who have been or continue to be colonized. Often this involved the marginalization or destruction of modes of knowledge and practice that were indigenous to the colonized context, itself a form of cultural colonization (Dudgeon et al., 2000).

Clearly feminist, liberation, and postcolonial approaches provide critiques of psychology that are grounded in lived experiences of oppression, marginalization, and exclusion. Additionally, they share a common aim of developing psychological theories and practices that would aid in personal and social transformation. Such new practices often appear at odds with established theory and practice. A fundamental concern for all three approaches is that of power—power in relation to knowledge production and in relation to practice. How can those with more power and privilege work in a way that does not reproduce oppression? How can the voices and concerns of the silenced and oppressed be heard and incorporated into practice? The development of participatory approaches became central, yet also challenged many of the assumptions of psychological practice.

LATIN AMERICAN LIBERATION PSYCHOLOGY

Martín-Baró, like others in Latin American countries, was particularly aware of the conditions of warfare, poverty, class domination, and totalitarian regimes that created enormously oppressive conditions for the majority of people (the oppressed majority). Whereas these structures of oppression were seen as the root cause of oppression, and required a structural analysis, Freire (1970), Martín-Baró (1994), and others aimed to work with the oppressed majority through developing new approaches in education (pedagogy of the oppressed) and psychology (liberation psychology) that would enable the oppressed to recognize these structures. Developing a structural analysis is one of the key concepts in Latin American liberation psychology that are discussed here; they are listed in Table 7.1, along with parallel concepts from feminist psychology. Liberation psychology, as Latin American writers assert, aims to work for and with the people. Such a psychology involves working in a bottom-up or grassroots manner, with psychologists, researchers, artists, activists, and community participants engaging in the co-creation of knowledge, strategies, and interventions in specific contexts (Montero & Sonn, 2009). Martín-Baró argued that truth or knowledge is to be generated from the viewpoint and experience of the oppressed rather than through top-down scientific research. He stressed transformative goals, aiming "to create a new psychological practice in order to transform both people and societies, acknowledging their denied potential" (Martín-Baró, 1994, p. 22).

Drawing on Freire (1970), Martín-Baró referred to specific situations of oppression as *limit situations*, that is, situations where violence and poverty place limits on opportunities and on consciousness itself. People's limit situations shape psychological patterns and reactions, including consciousness. The development of critical consciousness or *conscientization* is thus central to liberation

Table 7.1
Key Concepts in Latin American Liberation Psychology and in Feminist Psychology

Liberation Psychology	Feminist Psychology
Structural analysis	Structural analysis (patriarch)
Bottom up (participatory)	Participatory
Truth from voices and experiences of the people	Experiential knowledge
Aim to develop potential/bring about change	Transformative
Limit situation	(No comparable concept)
Conscientization	Consciousness-raising/critical consciousness
Problematization	Question-posing
De-ideologization	Demystification
Historical memory	(No comparable concept)
Virtues of the people	Strengths from resistance
(No comparable concept)	Intersectionality

psychology (Freire, 1970; Martín-Baró, 1994; Montero, 2009). Freire (1970) highlights the manner in which conscientization is a process that develops over time, as oppressed groups reflect on or problematize their specific or limit-situation; take some action in relation to that; reflect on this process, and thereby further develop their analysis and their capacity for action. There is thus a developmental, cyclical, or capacity-building component to conscientization; people must start at their own level of consciousness and abilities to take action, and ultimately aim to develop their own potential and to achieve social justice. This process is not one that is imposed on people but rather is developed by them through their own agency, a position that challenges the very role of the psychologist.

Conscientization thus involves a cycle of action and reflection (praxis), that is, a process of efforts to bring about change and reflection on what these efforts reveal about power structures. It may involve problematization or de-ideologization, which is a process of posing questions that uncover or expose the ideologies that obscure power structures and inequalities. Conscientization involves making links between the personal and the political. Martín-Baró also emphasized the role of recovery of historical memory, or developing an understanding of specific conditions or limit situations as historically created and therefore as changing: "Only in so far as people and groups become aware of their historical roots, especially those events and conditions which have shaped their situations, can they gain the perspective they need to take the measure of their own identity" (1994, p. 218).

Conscientization, or awareness and transformative action, occurs through participatory practices in community contexts that acknowledge that people must be agents of their own liberation. Participatory practices are often referred to as bottom up (as opposed to top down), that is, originating from the people themselves and involving their participation. Furthermore, liberation psychology recognizes what Martín Baró called "virtues of the people," or the strengths, resources, and resilience that people develop in contexts of oppression (Martín-Baró, 1994).

As Montero (2009, p. 122) writes, "participation is a basis for liberaton." Montero (2009) explores participatory action research (PAR) as a particular example of participation. PAR places power within the hands of the groups involved, who are in control of what or how knowledge is created. It works with the resources of the group themselves, drawing on existing relationships, networks, and community resources in order "to transform their living conditions, their immediate environment and the power relations established with other groups or institutions in their society" (Montero, 2009, p. 134). Participatory action research has developed as an important emancipatory research practice in many areas of psychology and in other disciplines. Brydon-Miller (1997) argues for its ability to involve psychology in social change. Applications include Fine and colleague's use of PAR with women in prison (Fine & Torre, 2006) and with youth in education contexts (Cammarota & Fine, 2008) and Kidd and Kral's (2005) applications in counseling psychology. An example combining liberation and feminist psychology is that of Lykes, Coquillon, and Rabenstein (2009) in Guatemala (see the next paragraph).

Several examples from Latin American countries provide reviews of theory, and also detailed examples of the practices and challenges of applying of liberation psychology (Montero & Sonn, 2009). Llorens (2009) describes the difficulties and tensions of participatory research with street children in Caracas, supporting the children in their search for resources while negotiating policies with various agencies, showing that children make connections from their immediate situation to the sociopolitical situation. Hernández (2009) sets out the need for a psychology of liberation in Panama that can promote community participation and coexistence in contexts of conflict, suggesting that psychology can at least play a role in the generation of new meanings that disrupt traditional lines of conflict. Shrader McMillan and Burton (2008) describe workshops with parents in childrearing in post-war Guatemala, where again links are made between personal family contexts and the wider societal context in which violence has become normalized.

The praxis of accompaniment is described in one of the first papers on liberation psychology published in the international peer-reviewed literature (Comaz-Diaz, Lykes, & Alarcon, 1998). *Accompaniment* involves psychologists entering the lives of participants, listening to and recording their stories, and offering supportive company during contacts, including those involving community services. In Peru, Chauca-Sabroso and Fuentes-Polar (2009) describe the collection of testimonies from survivors of war and armed conflict in a process that involves becoming part of the community through providing one day workshops and emotional and psychosocial accompaniment. They chart a healing process of recovery of historical memory in which testimonies are recorded and returned to participants who are supported to participate in group mobilization.

LIBERATION PSYCHOLOGY AND FEMINISM

Latin American liberation psychology has drawn on several philosophical, theoretical, and practical traditions (Osorio, 2009), including feminism. Many practical examples of Latin American liberation psychology draw on participatory methods and are undertaken by women (and men) often working with women's groups (Luque-Ribelles, Garcia-Ramirez, & Portillo, 2009; Shrader McMillan & Burton, 2008). Conversely, there are several examples of feminist projects that draw explicitly on the Latin American liberation psychology concepts reviewed earlier—such as limit situation, conscientization, and historical memory. Additionally, well-developed feminist understandings of intersectionality, fluidity, and reflexivity are particularly relevant to liberation psychologies (Landrine & Russo, 2009). Table 7.1 provides a link between key concepts in liberation and feminist psychology; these concepts developed in very different contexts, with rich and specific meanings that overlap and enhance each other.

Feminist and participatory action research methods that enable participants to record and share experiences, provide witness and testimony, accompany and support each other, develop skills and implement strategies for transformation have developed. Participatory action research in particular involves, as Lykes et al. (2009) noted, firstly a "recognition of and collaboration with communities' local or indigenous resources" and secondly "emphasis on bringing forward the voice of participants in both the research endeavors and in broader struggles for social change" (p. 261). Collaboration, participation, diversity of methods, and a focus on change are thus key elements of feminist and liberation psychology approaches that aim for transformative rather than ameliorative interventions (Nelson & Prilleltensky, 2010). Working with individuals and groups in marginalized and oppressed contexts also highlights the power and privilege that many psychologists have access to, requiring critical self-reflection (Fine, 2006).

Feminist approaches also make links to structural inequalities, recognizing that individual and group contexts are embedded in the larger macro system, which in turn manifests in the specific situation through the particular intersections of class, gender, ethnicity, and other dimensions of inequality. In common with other emancipatory approaches, many feminist approaches (e.g., Goodman et al., 2004; Lykes & Moane, 2009) adopt a multi-leveled approach that can be linked to Bronfenbrenner's ecological model. Bronfenbrenner (1979) viewed the ecology as involving nested levels—the micro or immediate level, the meso or community level, and the macro and exo levels of structures and ideologies of society.

The development of critical consciousness, that is, the awareness of the links between individual and group experiences and social patterns of oppression, is itself seen as central to liberation. Critical consciousness, with its roots in consciousness raising, clearly a parallel concept to conscientization, develops through dialogue, in group and community contexts, and has transformative action as its goal. Several feminist writers have written of critical consciousness and of multiple consciousness (Mustakova-Possardt, 2003; Zerbe-Ens & Byars Winston, 2009). An important example is Gloria Anzeldua (1987), who challenges the binaries of colonizer/colonized and fixed ethnic categories, arguing for multiple and fluid consciousness that contains elements of both—and more. She calls for the creation of in-between spaces where the fluidity of identities can be expressed, and for working with the conflicts and ambiguities to create a new consciousness: "A *mestiza* consciousness both houses and transforms conflict and ambivalence" (Torre & Ayala, 2009, p. 388). Torre and Ayala (2009) explore this in detail, seeking the development of a space in which the binaries of "we" and "other" are challenged. This requires spaces and group processes characterized by fluidity in which new understandings can emerge through listening, and through specific methods such as opening up to uncertainty and engaging with conflict.

The special issue of *Feminism & Psychology* offers several examples of approaches that combine liberation psychology and feminism (Lykes & Moane, 2009a). Contributions combine a variety of methods and perspectives, including PAR and participatory pedagogy, and also present critical and innovative perspectives on the praxis of feminist liberation psychology. Contributions share a focus on the role that psychology can play in detailing the specificities of social context while acknowledging the impact of structural inequalities, as well as understanding and where possible, contributing to the exercise of agency. A theme that recurs throughout several of the contributions is the need to develop methodologies that can encompass class, ethnicity, privilege and, multiple dimensions of difference. They demonstrate participatory practices in action, and illustrate the challenges posed by oppressive contexts to concepts of agency and social justice (Lykes & Moane, 2009a).

Crosby's (2009) contribution describes further work with Lykes and colleagues (Lykes et al., 2009) in developing the praxis of accompaniment. Aiming to take the further step of facilitating transformative action with accompaniers, Lykes, Crosby, and colleagues brought together psychologists, lawyers, researchers, and activists from Peru, Guatemala, and Colombia who were working with and accompanying women survivors of sexual assault. Drawing on participatory action research methods, Crosby (2009) describes the challenges of accompaniment in a context where rape had been used as a weapon of war and where perpetrators have had impunity. Using creative methodologies that included mask making and theatre, Crosby and colleagues created a dialogical space in which accompaniers could consider their shared experiences of witnessing and testimony, and of their own experiences of threat and assault linked to their participation in bringing experiences of rape and sexual assault into the public domain. A particular feature of this article is its description of the attempts to build solidarity across national boundaries often fraught with historical and contemporary conflict.

Madrigal and Tejeda (2009) describe another strategy to address sexual assault and violence in El Salvador, namely a participatory education and awareness program for men that examines masculinity itself as a risk factor for perpetrating gender-based violence (GBV). They combine liberation psychology concepts, including de-ideologization, with feminist analyses of gender and of gender-based violence, to create a workshop-based dialogical space where men can work together to prevent GBV. As men share their personal experiences and consider the impact of men's violence on their own lives and communities, they develop awareness of their own capacity for violence and develop strategies for how they can act together to prevent GBV.

In another example of the use of a workshop format using participatory action research, this time in the United States, Billies, Johnson, Murungi, and Pugh (2009) describe the formation of the Welfare Warriors Research Collaborative of low-income lesbian, gay bisexual transgendered, and gender nonconforming individuals who are involved in a variety of ways with a homeless shelter in New York City. They set out to document experiences of structural and everyday violence linked to poverty, gender, and sexual orientation, and also of homeless shelter staff abuse and neglect. Using collaborative methods that include videotaping group discussions, interviews, and a survey, the group provided a context for individuals to describe and record their experiences and develop strategies for enabling homeless LGBTs to exercise agency and influence in the homeless shelter through, for example, aiding each other in asserting their rights.

An example of research interviews drawing on ethnography is offered by Chaudhry and Bertram (2009), who provide a rich and detailed description of the specific contexts and strategies of Mohajir or migrant women in Karachi, Pakistan. Combining themes from transnational feminisms and from liberation psychology, Chaudhry and Bertram document the ways in which women exercise agency despite the limits imposed by the intersections or configurations of class, ethnicity, and gender. These configurations are linked to structural inequalities that manifest in everyday violence and deprivation. Chaudhry and Bertram describe the strategies that women use to survive assaults on themselves and their family members, and provide material resources and support for their family and community.

White and Rostagi (2009) also document the strategies of women who are targets of physical and sexual assault, again at the intersections of class, ethnicity, and gender in Banda in India. In this context the breakdown of police, community, and family systems of security and retribution leaves women exposed to sexual assault and violence, grabbing of land and resources, and demands for sex in return for welfare and other resources. Through interviews and documentary material, White and Rostagi describe a group of women who form a vigilante group in response to this violence, exploring the rationale and activities of the vigilante group in terms of feminist discussion of retributive and restorative justice. White and Rostagi argue that vigilante groups can be a form of agency exercised under constraint, motivated partly by the need for retaliatory actions to prevent violence, but also by values of fairness and justice, contributing to their community through provision of food, jobs, shelter, and other resources.

Two research studies using in-depth interviews aim to record and document experiences of discrimination and oppression. Shalhoub-Kevorkian (2009) reports on focus group discussions with children who have suffered house demolitions in Palestine, giving voice to the pain and confusion of children under conditions of ongoing military assault, and also showing their resilience and hope for the future. Lorasdagi (2009) uses one-on-one interviews to allow Muslim women in Amsterdam to explore and express the meanings associated with wearing a headscarf. Their words convey complex and context-specific understandings that both acknowledge the limits of wearing a headscarf and also the emancipatory opportunities that it can offer, especially when framed in relation to their own religious and geographic location.

A great deal of feminist analysis has been applied in the context of psychotherapy and counseling, with several attempts from the early days of the women's movement to link therapy and counseling with consciousness-raising. Goodman and colleagues make this connection, defining consciousness-raising as "helping clients understand the extent to which individual and private problems are rooted in larger historical social and political forces" (Goodman et al., 2004, p. 804). Afuaepe (2011) describes her application of liberation psychology in therapy with women survivors of trauma. She uses recovery of historical memory to place trauma in historical and political context, de-ideologization to uncover sources of oppression, and utilization of the people's virtues to develop community connections and solidarity.

VOICES OF PARTICIPANTS: PARTICIPATORY PEDAGOGY IN A COMMUNITY CONTEXT

An opportunity to apply concepts from liberation and feminist psychology arose from 1999 to the present, during my involvement with the Women's Studies program in University College Dublin (UCD) in developing a community-based Certificate in Women's Studies in partnership with women's centers located in disadvantaged areas in Dublin. Later, in 2003, the program developed a Certificate in Lesbian and Queer Culture, again in partnership with LGBT community centers. The programs adopted feminist pedagogical practices that place the learner at the center of the knowledge process.

Stake and Hoffman (2000) point out that descriptions of feminist pedagogy have been "remarkably consistent" in identifying four key elements. These are firstly that learning should be participatory, and secondly that personal experience should be a valid source of knowledge and that this validation increases self-confidence. Thirdly, there is agreement that pedagogy should facilitate the development of political and social understanding and, with that, an understanding of and interest in social change. Finally, pedagogy should encourage critical thinking and capacities for independence. These themes articulate with themes in other approaches to pedagogy that emphasize participatory, emancipatory, and transformative possibilities (Burke & Jackson, 2007; Freire, 1970; Fetherston & Kelly, 2007).

The pedagogical ethos supported through the Women's Studies Outreach Programme posits that learners bring to the education process an existing knowledge base that is directly linked to their lived experiences, from which they can build and extend their intellectual capacities and critical thinking skills. Unsurprisingly, therefore, experience and reflexivity represent two central tenets of the pedagogical underpinning of the certificates. Embracing experience within both curricular and learning processes is not unproblematic, as experiences must be contextualized and critically reflected upon. Barr, for example, states: "We must devise a pedagogy and research methodology that encourages learning which is related to people's lived experiences and feelings and which develops critical thinking-so that new thoughts and new ideas can be generated" (Barr, 1999, p. 91).

Participants expressed a strong interest in a module in psychology, and in designing such a module I aimed to incorporate key insights from liberation and feminist psychology discussed earlier (Table 7.1), and to use participatory practices to facilitate the development and understanding of these concepts. Table 7.2 provides a summary of the structure of the modules (Column 1), and of the methodologies used in the modules, involving problematization (Column 2), and participatory methods (Column 3), with examples generated from these methods (Column 4).

I structured the modules by a three-component model incorporating concepts from liberation and feminist psychology that formed the curriculum for the modules and workshops. The theoretical and practical aspects of this model have been described in detail (Moane, 2003, 2010, 2011). The components are: (1) a social

Table 7.2
Participatory Pedagogy Based on Liberation and Feminist Psychology: The Three-Component Model

Component	Guiding Question	Methodology	Examples
Structural Analysis			
Society as a pyramid	Is society a pyramid? Who is at the top? How is it maintained?	Open discussion Small-group discussion	Mostly White Male, able Heterosexual
Six modes of control Violence	Provide examples from your life.	Discussion and feedback to group	Sexual assault
Political exclusion			% of women elected
Economic exclusion			Wages unpaid Labor in the home
Control of culture			Media images
Control of sexuality			Abortion Sex trade/industry
Fragmentation			Migration
Cycle of Oppression			
Vulnerabilities	How would you (or others) react to this mode of control?	Brainstorm Small-group discussion Image theatre Strike a pose	No self-worth Helplessness Depression Anger conflict Isolation Dependency
Strengths	What kind of strengths do you (or people) develop?		Humor courage Solidarity Perseverance Hope
Cycle of Liberation			
Understanding change	How does change come about?	Open discussion	System view Ripple effects
Personal	What changes can you make at the personal level?	Energy exercises Meditation Slide show	Build self-confidence Speak out
Interpersonal	What changes can you make at interpersonal level?	Small-group discussion Role play	Join a group Contribute to community
Political	What changes can you make at system level?	Personal examples	Voting Support women candidates

analysis that would facilitate a macro and structural understanding, (2) a psychological analysis that would link the personal and the political, (3) an understanding of change from the bottom up (Table 7.2).

The purpose of the social analysis is to provide a structural analysis—a clear focus and framework for the social conditions associated with oppression, and on the systemic or structural nature of oppression. Viewing society as a pyramid provides a model for exploring issues of power and control, and this part of the module draws on the Irish historical experience of colonization. More specific understanding is developed by exemplifying six patterns, which I have labeled "modes of control" (Moane, 2011, p. 35). A number of writers on oppression have described social structures or patterns associated with oppression (Moane, 2011). Four of these are violence, political exclusion, economic exploitation, and cultural control. In the context of my work with heterosexual and lesbian women, I have added control of sexuality to draw specific attention to this area of oppression. The sixth mode, fragmentation, provides further insights into the ways in which women and minorities are divided from each other. In classes and workshops, participants work in groups and draw on their personal experiences to identify examples of each of these patterns that are specific to their context or limit situation.

In the psychological analysis links are made between the political and the personal by exploring personal reactions to oppression. Reactions to oppression that recur in the literature include negative patterns such as anger, fear, helplessness, sense of inferiority, and also positive patterns or strengths that can include courage, resilience, perseverance, and generosity. These strengths, of course, can be a resource for activism and change. In courses and workshops, participants provide examples of psychological reactions based on their own experiences (Table 7.2), thus building a picture of how their psychological experiences are linked to social conditions.

Critical consciousness, conscientization, and focus on transformative action are themes throughout the modules, but are a particular focus of the third component. The analysis of transformation focuses on building strengths and on participants' own capacity for taking action for change. It provides space for a bottom-up understanding of social change through reflection and considering possibilities for action. It attends to three levels or areas of change that have been commonly identified in many different fields namely the personal level of the individual, the interpersonal level of relationships and community, and the political level of systems and structures. The phrase "cycle of liberation" is used to suggest that getting involved in change may be a developmental process whereby change at the personal and interpersonal levels facilitates change at the political level. Changes at each level can be interconnected to changes at other levels to form a cycle of liberation. Participants explore examples of involvement in change from micro acts such as confronting sexism to coalition building and lobbying. This can lead to a system view of social change that encompasses actions at every level that may accumulate to bring about change.

As noted, throughout the modules, participatory methods are used, and include (Table 7.2): open-group discussion (questions are posed to the group as a whole and responses are recorded in a flipchart); small-group discussion with or without feedback; brainstorm (one-word responses to a questions are recorded on a flipchart); role play (participants role-play an empowering action with the support of the group); image theatre (participants strike a pose that reflects their feelings or experience and then make a change); meditation and energy exercises (short exercises or visualizations that energize the group). The modules drew on participants' own personal experiences and knowledge, contextualized within the framework of feminist and liberation psychology.

Between 2000 and 2005, modules titled "Liberation Psychology for Women" were delivered as part of the Certificate in Women's Studies to four groups in four locations ranging in size from 9 to 20 and in age from 35 to 56. Modules titled "Liberation Psychology: Lesbian and Queer Perspectives" were delivered as part of the Certificate in Lesbian and Queer Studies to three groups ranging in size from 10 to 23 and in age from 21 to 61, two as modules over 12 weeks and one as a weekend module; it was also delivered in one independent workshop in a community settings to one group of 15 ranging in age from early 20s to mid-50s. Both certificates were delivered in community contexts in partnership with community centers.

Several forms of feedback were obtained from participants, one of which was open-ended questions that participants completed at the end of the modules (Moane, 2010). It was clear that all participants found the overall framework and approach accessible and helpful. It drew on their knowledge and experience of oppression, of psychological patterns, and of support and solidarity, and provided a framework for critical analysis and development of insight and understanding. The social analysis provided a clear understanding of society as a system of domination and made explicit what participants already knew. Feedback indicated that participants found this helpful rather than overwhelming, with participants using phrases in written feedback such as: "found it helpful," "very clear," "gave a language to analyze oppression," "put things in perspective," "helped to make connections with other groups," and "helped me understand personal experiences." Participants also indicated that the course made connections between the personal and the political and that this: "helped me to understand the past," "I could see what some conflicts were about," "see what was causing anxiety," "saw how society impacted," "stopped self blame," and "increased confidence." Participants saw possibilities for making changes at the personal level: "increase confidence," "hope for a better future," "enriching," "able to make changes," "not accepting the norm," "see others in different ways," and "sense of possibility." They also expressed more interest in groups and communities: "helped to reconnect," "saw the value of a group," "can be part of change," "look for and give more support," and "play a more active role." Although there was a clear sense of valuing community groups and resources, there were often reservations about getting involved in more politically oriented groups: "might at some point," "will think about it," and "if I had more time, yes."

The workshops with LGBT participants provide a very different context for applying feminist liberation psychology (Moane, 2008). Whether over a day or a weekend, workshops deliver a more intense and focused experience in which there is more sharing of personal experiences, values, and perspectives, and also greater opportunities for spontaneity, fun, support, and solidarity. The workshops involved group work methods that foster inclusion and equality of participation. There was an emphasis on safety, on confidentiality, and on creating a supportive environment. There was an expectation that the workshop would be an enjoyable as well as useful experience. As with other courses and workshops, discussions were recorded on flipcharts, and I also distributed questionnaires to participants that included questions about the social analysis, the connections between the personal and the political, and their involvement in change.

The structure of the three-component model was used for the LGBT workshops, although it obviously generated different content as it focused on LGBT experiences of oppression and liberation. The approach to the three components had to be adapted for a workshop format, as, unlike a course, which is dispersed over 10 or 12 weeks, all three components are condensed into one or two days, or even into one or two hours. In a short (2–3-hour) workshop the three components are addressed through open questions in a brainstorm format. First, questions in relation to homophobia (the social analysis) include: What is it? Where does it come from? What are the sources or origins of homophobia? Secondly, questions regarding the impact (cycle of oppression) include: What is the impact of homophobia? How does it make people feel? What are the reactions to homophobia? Thirdly, the analysis of change (cycle of liberation) can include questions such as: What needs to change? How can things change? How can participants be involved in change? Longer workshops obviously allow more detailed analysis using a variety of methodologies to allow more process and participation.

Responses to feedback questionnaires for workshops indicated several benefits were gained. Participants indicated that they found the social analysis very clear and helpful, writing that it was: "a very clear analysis," "an eye-opener," "strengthened my understanding of oppression," "was a very powerful way to show things," "equipped me to see our society more clearly," and "it was great to see the bigger picture." The course also enabled the participants to see the connection between their own personal patterns and the social pattern discussed in the social analysis: "I learnt about myself and about domination," "more aware of how I can be determined by society," and "how my surroundings affect me." Several wrote of being relieved of self-blame: "I feel a lot of relief that there is nothing wrong with me," "I stopped beating myself over the head, blaming myself," and "I wasn't so hard on myself." Finally, a sense of solidarity with others was expressed: "a sense that we all run up against the same hurdles" and "helped me to understand the connections, how we react the same."

The majority of participants indicated that they could see changes that they could make in their lives at a personal level, and that this provided them with hope and inspiration: "it lifted my heart and gave me hope for a better future," 'I found it inspiring," "it gives me a sense of possibility," "aware that I'm in a position to change things," and "I can see small changes and big changes." They felt increased confidence and strength: "I feel stronger and better equipped" and "I feel able to start to make changes." Some participants wrote of a sense of understanding and connecting better with others: "yes we all count," "see myself and others in a different way," and "it will make me more supportive." There was awareness that being visible and speaking out were important areas of change: "I want to reveal myself in a more open way" and "I want to speak out and be more forthright, challenge people."

At the political level, those participants who were already involved in groups, organizations, and communities oriented toward social change felt reenergized by the workshop experience: "It renews my commitment to community involvement," "the course validated my work in the community, I feel re-energized," and "I can see myself in further community roles." Others expressed a strong interest in or saw the value of involvement in change: "it has reinforced my commitment and belief in activism," "I can see the value of working with like-minded people," and "I would like to be more involved in the community." However, some were more ambivalent about more involvement: "I'm coming to terms with the idea that I can be part of change" and "would look at it in the future."

CONCLUSION

The theory, research, and practices described in this chapter illustrate the possibilities for the involvement of psychology in social transformation and social justice. As liberation and feminist psychology is practiced in diverse settings, the impact of oppression on daily lives is clear. Structural inequalities, war-related violence and sexual assaults, ethnic conflicts, breakdowns in justice and security systems, and everyday poverty are found in every part of the world, and also demonstrate massive global inequalities. Histories of resistance, examples of resilience, support and solidarity, strong commitments to communities, and actions for transformation are evident. Psychologists can offer many skills and resources that can facilitate making changes in conditions of oppression, play a role in documenting and inscribing such experiences, and also make links between groups and with structures of inequality. Participatory pedagogy and participatory research methods form cornerstones for approaches in liberation and feminist psychology.

By placing oppression, marginalization, social transformation, and social justice at its centre, liberation and feminist psychology proposes new understandings and interventions. Core themes include the linking of the micro and the macro through participatory and dialogical methods that bridge the local and the global, as captured in Norsworthy and Buranajakoenkij's (2011) description of their methodology: "The methodology offers participants opportunities to reflect on and analyze their current limit situations as well as 'the system of the workshop itself' through lens of power, taking into account the multiple experiences, perspectives, identities, social locations and other positionalities as they intersect with local, national and sometimes international ecological, socio-cultural and political systems" (p. 234).

Liberation psychology and feminism combine to provide analyses and interventions that recognize global systems of oppression along with specificities of local conditions and resources. Their methods are participatory, dialogical, relational and ethical, often using diversity and conflict as tools for transformation.

They have generated new spaces and new praxis for documentation, alliances, support, solidarity, and advocacy. Together, liberation psychology and feminism undertake critical interrogations of boundaries, power, and privilege, and in doing so, they problematize both psychology and social justice.

REFERENCES

Afuape, T. (2011). *Power, resistance and liberation in therapy with survivors of trauma*. London, UK: Routledge. doi: 10.1177/0959353509105621

Anzeldua, G. (1987). *Borderlands/La Frontera: The new mestiza*. San Francisco, CA: Aunt Lute.

Barr, J. (1999). *Liberating knowledge: Research, feminism and adult education*. Leicester, UK: NIACE.

Billies, M., Johnson, J., Murungi, K., & Pugh, R. (2009). Naming our reality: Low income LGBT people documenting violence, discrimination and assertions of justice. *Feminism & Psychology, 19*(3), 375–380. doi: 10.1177/0959353509105628

Bronfenbrenner, U. (1979). *The ecology of human development*. Cambridge, MA: Harvard University Press.

Brydon-Miller, M. (1997). Participatory action research: Psychology and social change. *Journal of Social Issues, 53*(4), 657–666. doi: j.1540-4560.1997.tb02454.x

Bulhan, H. (1985). *Frantz Fanon and the psychology of oppression*. New York, NY: Plenum Press.

Burke, P. J., & Jackson, S. (2007). *Reconceptualising lifelong learning: Feminist interventions*. London, UK: Routledge.

Cammarota, J., & Fine, M. (Eds.). (2008). *Revolutionizing education: Youth participatory action research in motion*. New York, NY: Routledge.

Chauca-Sabroso, R. L., & Fuentas-Polar, S. (2009). Development of historical memory as a psychosocial recovery process. In M. Montero & C. C. Sonn (Eds.), *Psychology of liberation: Theory and applications* (pp. 205–219). New York, NY: Springer.

Chaudry, L., & Bertram, C. (2009.) Narrating trauma and reconstruction in post-conflict Karachi: Feminist liberation psychology and the contours of agency in the margins. *Feminism & Psychology, 19*(3), 298–312. doi: 10.1177/0959353509105621

Comas-Díaz, L., Lykes, M. B., & Alarcon, R. D. (1998). Ethnic conflict and the psychology of liberation in Guatemala, Peru, and Puerto Rico. *American Psychologist, 53*(7), 778–791. doi: 0003.066X/98/$2.00

Crosby, A. (2009). Anatomy of a workshop: Women's struggles for transformative participation in Latin America. *Feminism & Psychology, 19*(3), 343–353. doi: 10.1177/0959353509105625

Dudgeon, P., Garvey, D., & Picket, H. (2000). *Working with indigenous Australia: A handbook for psychologists*. Perth, Australia: Gunada Press.

Fanon, F. (1967). *The wretched of the earth*. London, UK: Penguin.

Fetherston, B., & Kelly, R. (2007). Conflict resolution and transformative pedagogy: A grounded theory research project on learning in Higher Education. *Journal of Transformative Education, 5*(3), 262–285. doi: 10.1177/1541344607308899

Fine, M. (2006). Bearing witness: Methods for researching oppression and resistance—A textbook for critical research. *Social Justice Research, 19*(1), 83–108. doi: 10.1007/s11211-006-0001-0

Fine, M., & Torre, M. E. (2006). Intimate details: Participatory action research in prison. *Action Research, 4*(3), 253–269. doi: 10.1177/14767563060166801

Freire, P. (1970). *Pedagogy of the oppressed*. London, UK: Penguin Books.

Goodman, L. A., Liang, B., Helms, J., Latta, R., Sparks, E., & Weintraub, S. (2004). Training counseling psychologists as social justice agents: Feminist and multicultural principles in action. *The Counseling Psychologist, 32,* 793–837. doi: 10.1177/0011000004268802

Hernández, E. (2009). New challenges for the psychology of liberation: Building frameworks for social coexistence. In M. Montero & C. C. Sonn (Eds.), *Psychology of liberation: Theory and applications* (pp. 259–276). New York, NY: Springer.

Hook, D. (2012). *A critical psychology of the post colonial.* London, UK: Routledge.

Kagan, C., Burton, M., Duckett, P., Lawthom, R., & Siddiquee, A. (2011). *Critical community psychology*. Chichester, UK: Wiley-Blackwell.

Kidd, S. A., & Kral, M. J. (2005). Participatory action research. *Journal of Counselling Psychology, 52,* 187–195. doi: 10.1177/1541344607308899

Kitzinger, C., & Perkins, R. (1993). *Changing our minds: Lesbian feminism and psychology.* New York, NY: New York University Press.

Landrine, H., & Russo, N. F. (Eds.). (2009). *Handbook of diversity in feminist psychology.* New York, NY: Springer.

Llorens, M. (2009). Liberation psychology on the street: Working with youngsters who have lived on the streets of Caracas. In M. Montero & C. C. Sonn (Eds.), *Psychology of liberation: Theory and applications* (pp. 237–258). New York, NY: Springer.

Lorasdagi, B. K. (2009). The headscarf and emancipation in the Netherlands. *Feminism & Psychology, 19*(3), 328–334. doi: 10.1177/0959353509105623

Lott, B. (1993). *Women's lives: Themes and variations in gender learning.* New York, NY: Brooks/Cole.

Luque-Ribelles, V., Garcia-Ramirez, M., & Portillo, N. (2009). Gendering peace and liberation: A participatory action approach to critical consciousness acquisition among women in a marginalized neighbourhood. In M. Montero & C. C. Sonn, (Eds.), *Psychology of liberation: Theory and applications.* New York, NY: Springer.

Lykes, M. B., Coquillon, E., & Rabenstein, K. L. (2009.) Theoretical and methodological challenges in participatory community-based research. In H. Landrine & N. F. Russo (Eds.), *Handbook of diversity in feminist psychology.* New York, NY: Springer.

Lykes, M. B., & Moane, G. (Eds.) (2009a). Feminist liberation psychology. Special Issue. *Feminism & Psychology, 19*(3).

Lykes, M. B. & Moane, G. (2009b). Whither feminist liberation psychology? *Feminism & Psychology, 19*(3), 283–297. doi: 10.1177/0959353509105620

Madrigal, L. J., & Tejeda, W. V. (2009). Facing gender-based violence in El Salvador: Contributions from the social psychology of Ignacio Martín-Baró. *Feminism & Psychology, 19*(3), 368–374. doi: 10.1177/0959353509105627

Martín-Baró, I. (1994). *Writings for a liberation psychology.* Essays, 1985–1989, edited by A. Aron & S. Corne. Cambridge, MA: Harvard University Press.

Memmi, A. (1967). *The colonizer and the colonized.* Boston, MA: Beacon Press.

Moane, G. (2003). Bridging the personal and the political: Practices for a liberation psychology. *American Journal of Community Psychology, 31*(1/2), 129–145. doi: 0091-0562/03/0300-0091/0

Moane, G. (2008). Building strengths through challenging homophobia: Liberation workshops with young and midlife older lesbians. *Journal of Gay and Lesbian Social Services, 20*(1/2), 129–145. doi: 10.1080/105387208621799091

Moane, G. (2010). Sociopolitical development and political activism: Synergies between feminist and liberation psychology. *Psychology of Women Quarterly, 34,* 521–529. doi: 10.1111/j.1471-6402.2010.01601.x

Moane, G. (2011). *Gender and colonialism: A psychological analysis of oppression and liberation.* Basingstoke, UK: Palgrave Macmillan.

Montero, M. (2009). Methods for liberation: Critical consciousness in action. In M. Montero & C. C. Sonn, (Eds.), *Psychology of liberation: Theory and applications* (pp. 73–91). New York, NY: Springer.

Montero, M., & Sonn, C. C. (Eds.) (2009). *Psychology of liberation, theory and applications.* New York, NY: Springer.

Mustakova-Possardt, E. (2003). *Critical consciousness: A study of morality in global historical context.* Westport, CT: Praeger.

Nelson, G., & Prilleltensky, I. (2010). *Community psychology: In pursuit of liberation and well-being.* Basingstoke, UK: Palgrave Macmillan.

Norsworthy, K. L., & Buranajakoenkij, D. N. (2011). Crossing boundaries, building bridges and swimming upstream: Feminist liberatory work within South Thailand communities in conflict. *Women & Therapy, 34,* 242–260.

Osorio, J. M. F. (2009). Praxis and liberation in the context of Latin American theory. In M. Montero & C. C. Sonn (Eds.), *Psychology of liberation: Theory and applications* (pp. 11–36). New York, NY: Springer.

Reyes Cruz, M., & Sonn, C. C. (2011). Decolonizing culture in community psychology: Reflections from critical social science. *American Journal of Community Psychology, 47*(1/2), 203–214. doi: 10.1111/j.1471-6402.2010.01601.x

Rutherford, A., Capdevila, R., Undurti, V., & Palmary, I. (Eds.). (2011). *Handbook of international feminisms: Perspectives on psychology, women, culture, and rights.* New York, NY: Springer.

Shalhoub-Kevorkian, N. (2009). The political economy of children's trauma: A case study of house demolition in Palestine. *Feminism & Psychology, 19*(3), 335–342. doi: 10.1177/0959353509105624

Shrader McMillan, A., & Burton, M. (2008). From parent education to collective action: Childrearing with love in post-war Guatemala. *Journal of Community & Applied Social Psychology, 91*(3), 198–211.

Stake, J. E., & Hoffman, F. L. (2000). Putting feminist pedagogy to the test: The experience of women's studies from student and teacher perspectives. *Psychology of Women Quarterly, 24*(1), 30–38. doi: 10.1111/j.1471-6402.2000.tb01019.x

Tavris, C. (1992). *The mismeasure of women.* New York, NY: Touchstone Books.

Torre, M. E., & Ayala, J. (2009). Envisioning participatory action research Entremundos. *Feminism & Psychology, 19*(3), 387–393. doi: 10.1177/0959353509105630

Watkins, M., & Shulman, H. (2008). *Towards psychologies of liberation.* Basinstoke, UK: Palgrave Macmillan.

Watts, R., & Serrano-Garcia, I. (Eds.) (2003). Towards a community psychology of liberation. Special Issue. *American Journal of Community Psychology, 31*(1/2).

White, A., & Rastogi, S. (2009). Justice by any means necessary: Vigilantism among Indian women. *Feminism & Psychology, 19*(3), 313–327. doi: 10.1177/0959353509105622

Wilkinson, S. (Ed.) (1986). *Feminist psychology: Developing theory and practice.* Philadelphia, PA: Open University Press.

Wilkinson, S. (1991). Editorial. *Feminism and Psychology, 1*(1), 1–7. doi: 10.1177/0959353591011001

Zerbe-Ens, C., & Byars Winston, A. M. (2009) Multicultural feminist therapy. In H. Landrine & N. F. Russo (Eds.), *Handbook of diversity in feminist psychology.* New York, NY: Springer Publishing Co.

Part 2

Special Populations

Chapter 8

Healing One Story at a Time: American Indian/Alaska Native Social Justice

Virgil Moorehead and Teresa D. LaFromboise

Every November in schools nationwide, educators teach about the first Thanksgiving. They try to provide students an idea of what may have occurred in Plymouth in 1621, and to make clear how these events fit into American history. This emblematic American holiday dates back to the time when early European settlers, known as pilgrims, settled on land belonging to the Wampanoag tribe, the "people of the dawn." Stories about this encounter have a profound significance for both populations involved.

For many European Americans, Thanksgiving is a story about pilgrims discovering a new world, a place of freedom and opportunity. In addition, this story marks an occasion of gratitude. Conversely, for many Native Americans, Thanksgiving is a reminder of the onset of societal trauma by a foreign group's effort at dismantling their vision of the world. The story of Thanksgiving is a prominent example of how history can be distorted. Not surprisingly, a number of Native Americans refer to Thanksgiving as a "day of mourning." Divergent perspectives on this historic event illustrate how stories have a powerful influence on subsequent generations and possibilities for transformative social justice.

In this chapter, we will address who American Indian/Alaska Natives are and examine some significant historical experiences that have shaped them. Our overview will be followed by a description of the historical trauma construct, including an explanation of the significance of this construct for designing historically and culturally based social justice interventions. Finally, we will argue that the telling of stories, especially resilient ones, provides valuable support toward liberation from the trauma and healing for the individual.

SELECT DEMOGRAPHICS

Despite traditional interpretations, there is great diversity among the original peoples of North America. In the United States, there are 566 federally recognized American Indian/Alaska Native tribes (U.S. Bureau of Indian Affairs, 2013) and 226 additional tribes recognized by state governments but not the federal government (Manataka American Indian Council, 2009). Each recognized and non-federally recognized tribe has its own individual history, traditions, and institutions. In 1900, at the lowest point of the American Indian/Alaska Native population due to disease, warfare, and geographic relocation, fewer than 237,000 American Indian/Alaska Native people lived in the United States (Thornton, 1987). According to the 2010 U.S. Census, the American Indian/Alaska Native population has rebounded to a total of approximately 5.2 million. Within this population estimate, 2.9 million individuals identify as American Indian/Alaska Native alone, whereas nearly half of the total American Indian/Alaska Native population reports being an American Indian or Alaska Native combined with at least one or more other races.

The number who identify as either American Indian or Alaska Native alone has increased almost twice as fast as the total population, growing 18% between 2000 and 2010. This significant demographic increase is largely attributed to changes in the U.S. Census reporting system; specifically, American Indian/Alaska Native people are now counted through self-identification (Snipp & Saraff, 2011). Gone and Trimble (2012) argue that American Indian/Alaska Native identity is complicated, and should be based on self-identification as well as recognition by other tribal people. Overall, not a single effective identification measure has yet to be developed.

DEVASTATING FEDERAL GOVERNMENTAL POLICIES

To promote social justice in Indian Country,[1] a meaningful first step is to reframe current challenges in light of longer-term struggles against damaging governmental narratives. Countless colonial events could be enumerated to demonstrate how perverse U.S. governmental policies led to the devastation of thriving American Indian/Alaska Native communities (Calloway, 2003). Forcing American Indians to give up land to accommodate illegal squatters is but one example. However, we will focus upon two relatively recent policies that have shaped American Indian/Alaska Native identity: the boarding school era and the Relocation Act of 1956, which occurred between 1880 and 1930. Both were consistent with earlier U.S. governmental legislation (e.g., the Indian Removal Act of 1830, the General Allotment Act of 1880) aimed at assimilating Native people into mainstream American society (Fixico, 1986; Wilkinson, 2005). The agenda underlying these policies harkens back to initial contact between American Indians and colonizers, and to ideas pertaining to manifest destiny.[2]

During the 19th century and into the 20th century, Native children were removed from their homes and forced to attend U.S. government–run boarding schools (Adams, 1995). Every tribe experiencing this removal has recorded incredible stories of the children's experiences in those schools. Advocates of boarding schools believed that years of isolation from families along with industrial training would lessen the effect of tribalism on a new generation of American Indians, thus furthering their "civilizing mission." Most boarding schools followed a strict policy of prohibiting children from speaking their tribal languages or engaging in their cultural traditions (Churchill, 2004; Hoxie, 2001).

The impact of the boarding school era on American Indian/Alaska Native communities has been long-lasting (Child, 1998; Evans-Campbell, Walters, Pearson, & Campbell, 2012; Robbins et al., 2006). One of the most distressing consequences was its large-scale assault on effective traditional parenting practices (Metcalf, 1976; Morrissette, 1994; Schacht, Tafoya, & Mirabia, 1989), which eroded the production and reproduction of effective family systems. For example, Christensen and Manson (2001) posited that disruptive parenting patterns from the boarding school era might be passed from one generation to another. Brasfield (2001) found a shared symptomology among survivors of Canadian residential schools for First Nations children, which he calls *residential school syndrome*. The effects of this syndrome include a sense of reliving residential experiences, occasional flashbacks, diminished interest in participating in tribal activities, and feelings of relational detachment. In many ways, these symptoms fit nicely into the psychiatric diagnosis of posttraumatic stress disorder.

Similar to the boarding school policy, the U.S. government's relocation policy of the 1950s foisted further havoc on tribal communities. Implemented by the U.S. Bureau of Indian Affairs, the Relocation Act encouraged American Indians to acquire vocational skills for job placement in cities like San Francisco, Chicago, and Los Angeles (Jaimes, 1992). Due to limited resources and high rates of poverty on reservations, more than 100,000 American Indians relocated to urban areas between 1951 and 1973 (Fixico, 2000). However, the U.S. Bureau of Indian Affairs (BIA) failed to follow through on its promise to provide transitional support, producing a chronically marginalized urban Indian population. Large numbers who participated in the relocation program did not attain economic stability, but rather found themselves homeless, unemployed, and with minimal access to a cultural base. Today, nearly 70% of American Indian/Alaska Natives live in metropolitan areas (U.S. Census Bureau, 2010) compared with 45% in 1970 and 8% in 1940. This pattern suggests that despite the increasing number of American Indian/Alaska Natives in the United States, most have migrated to urban centers and, by intent or by outcome, many of these individuals have become geographically and culturally isolated from their heritage.

Individuals living in urban environments have faced distinct challenges, such as limited funding for health and social service programs and difficulty maintaining cultural traditions (Urban Indian Health Institute, 2012). Although the relocation program officially ended, most tribes and tribal members continue to suffer from pressure to assimilate as well as significant economic and cultural threat. Furthermore, successive generations of relocated American Indian/Alaska Natives exhibit ongoing health-related disparities (Castor et al., 2006; Evans-Campbell, Lindhorst, Huang, & Walters, 2006; Urban Indian Health Institute, 2009, 2011). For example, Fieland, Walters, and Simoni (2007) report that urban Native male drug users are at greater risk for HIV infection than rural counterparts due to trading sex for money, drugs, or housing.

Shawnee, Sac and Fox, Muscogee Creek, and Seminole scholar, Donald Fixico (2000) cogently describes the urban Indian experience:

> For an Indian, feeling the individualism on a crowded sidewalk of people is like drowning in water, gasping for life, and feeling helpless. This alienation has been dissolved by an identity crisis for many urban Indians and has resulted in an Indian culture of many urban tribes called "Indian neighborhoods" or "Indian ghettoes" in cities. (p. 188)

Evolving tribal stories of psychological estrangement from home continue recitation featuring themes such as when city social workers removed Indian children from their homes, when dentists thought that Native people only felt half as much pain as other patients thus giving them only half the pain killer that was necessary, and when American "new agers" discovered Native spirituality.

HEALTH/MENTAL HEALTH DISPARITIES

Today individuals from both urban and reservation Indian communities experience an increasing number and variety of health problems. Their rate of alcohol or drug use is higher than any other race (Substance Abuse and Mental Health Association, 2007). Domestic violence rates are alarming. Thirty-nine percent of American Indian/Alaska Native women experience intimate partner violence—the highest rate in the United States (Centers for Disease Control and Prevention, 2008). American Indian/Alaska Native women are 2.5 times more likely to experience sexual assault crimes compared to all other races; and one in three report having been raped during their lifetime (U.S. Department of Justice, 2000). The life expectancy of Native women and men is 72 years, nearly 5 years shorter than the life expectancy of 76.9 years for men within the general population (Whitbeck, 2011).

Mental health researchers report disproportionate levels of psychological symptoms within this population (Duran & Duran, 1995; Walters, Simoni, & Evans-Campbell, 2002; Whitbeck, Adams, Hoyt, & Chen, 2004); rates of psychiatric illnesses are higher than any other ethnic group in the United States (Beals et al., 2005; Ogunwole, 2006; Whitbeck, 2011). American Indian/Alaska Native adolescents 15 to 24 years of age have a rate of suicide 2.5 times higher than youth of the same age group within the U.S. mainstream population (LaFromboise & Fatemi, 2011; LaFromboise & Lewis, 2008). Suicide is the second leading cause of death for Native Americans between the ages of 10 and 34 years (Centers for Disease Control and Prevention, 2012). Many tribes have declared states of emergency within their communities due to suicide epidemics (Woodward, 2012).

HISTORICAL TRAUMA RESPONSE

Since 1995 researchers have linked significant levels of psychological and social problems found in American Indian/Alaska Native communities to demeaning and dehumanizing historical experiences associated with European colonization (BraveHeart & DeBruyn, 1995; Duran & Duran, 1995; Terry, 1995). Lakota scholar Maria Brave Heart defined *historical trauma* as cumulative emotional and psychological wounding over an individual lifespan and across generations, originating from massive group trauma (Brave Heart & DeBruyn, 1998). A key aspect of historical trauma is what Brave Heart terms *historical unresolved grief*. This type of grief originates from loss of lives, loss of land, and loss of fundamental aspects of culture. This grief is not only a personal loss but also a collective one. Further, each generation experiences such losses and, by social modeling and without conscious intent, this trauma is passed on from one generation to the next.

Oftentimes historical unresolved grief is referred to as "disenfranchised grief" because most of the losses that occurred are yet to be openly acknowledged or publicly mourned. Disenfranchised grief is noted to lead to an intensification of normative emotional reactions such as anger, guilt, sadness, or helplessness. Given that many American Indian/Alaska Native people are unable to process historical unresolved grief, their subsequent generations suffer from this phenomenon (Brave Heart, 2000, 2003; Duran, 2006; Walters et al., 2011).

Evans-Campbell (2008) recently posited that the intergenerational transmission of historical trauma occurs on at least two levels: the interpersonal and the societal. At the interpersonal level, intergenerational transmission may occur directly or indirectly. Indirect transmission includes traumatic events leading to poor parental mental health or poor parenting styles, resulting in higher levels of stress experienced by children. Direct transmission refers to the manner in which children vicariously experience traumatic events via stories heard about their parents' or grandparents' encounters with challenging, often destructive, colonial practices. At a societal level, the effects of a traumatic event such as relocation from reservations to cities may include multiple losses (e.g., family dispersion, estrangement or tension between reservation and urban tribal members, and identity confusion). It is hypothesized that, over time, the trauma discreetly increases and the resiliency diminishes and internal and collective resolution becomes increasingly difficult to achieve.

RACISM, DISCRIMINATION, AND MICRO-AGGRESSIONS

The effect of racism is another important consideration in American Indian/ Alaska Native health disparities. Native people have endured greater threats to their cultural identity than any other ethnic group in the United States (Mihesuah, 2009). Unflattering images of American Indian/Alaska Natives can be seen in every medium: scholarly publications, textbooks, literature, cartoons, comic books, video games, movies, television shows, and commercial logos. Sports mascots like those representing the Washington Redskins, Cleveland Indians, or Florida State Seminoles persist despite American Indian/Alaska Native activists' vitriolic rails against them. Tulalip scholar, Stephanie Fryberg, suggested that "American Indian mascots are harmful because they remind American Indians of the limited ways others see them and, in this way, constrain how they can see themselves" (Fryberg, Markus, Oyserman, & Stone, 2008, p. 208).

Consider the impact of the gigantic sculptured heads of four U.S. presidents literally carved into Mount Rushmore in the Black Hills of South Dakota overshadow majestic land held sacred to the Great Sioux Nation. Choctaw scholar, Karina Walters (2010) has explored the impact of microaggressions stimulated by the stereotypic Indian images (Chae & Walters, 2009; Walters et al., 2011). According to Sue et al. (2007), "Racial microaggressions are brief and common place indignities, whether intentional or unintentional, that communicate hostile, derogatory, or negative racial slights and insults toward people of color" (p. 271). All too often American Indian/Alaska Natives experience microaggressions directed toward them when they hear statements such as "you don't look or act like you're Indian" or "you Indian giver." These findings support existing literature on the association between perceived discrimination and American Indian/Alaska Native psychological functioning (Whitbeck et al., 2004; Yoder, Whitebeck, Hoyt, & LaFromboise, 2006; Zimmerman, Ramierez-Valles, Wahienko, Walter, & Dyer, 1996). For example, Yoder et al. (2006) found that perceived discrimination along with enculturation emerged as culturally specific variables related to the likelihood of a Native youth's thinking about suicide.

However, ideas put forth about historical trauma and the effects of perceived discrimination on mental health have led to improvements in programs and legislation that impact tribal communities (e.g., S.47: Violence against Women Reauthorization Act of 2013; Tribal Law and Order Act of 2010). Considering the increased understanding of historical trauma in tribal communities, and the social science and health communities, a next appropriate strategy is to explore what can be done to improve therapeutic interventions to reduce and, hopefully, eliminate historical trauma responses.

CALLING FORTH TRADITIONAL HEALING PRACTICES

In the field of mental health, Tewa-Apache scholar Eduardo Duran (2006) has recommended that therapy extend beyond ideas of cultural sensitivity by identifying and validating what is called the *life-world* of the people with whom professionals are working. He exhorts mental health workers to apply a mindset of *epistemological hybridity*, that is, "to think or see the truth in more than one way" (p. 14). In order to practice epistemological hybridity, mental health professionals must appreciate the cultural perspectives of the person or community seeking help. To this end, a therapeutic professional uses healing metaphors that "take the actual life-world of the person or groups as the core truth that needs to be seen as valid" (p. 14). This perspective reflects the American Psychological Association's guidelines for providing psychotherapy in a culturally appropriate manner (American Psychological Association, 2003).

Other American Indian/Alaska Native scholars have joined Duran in not only critiquing conventional individual and group therapeutic models that fail to adequately consider the importance of historical influences on current pathology but also in calling for the resurgence of traditional healing practices that assist people in recovering from problems associated with alarmingly high rates of distress (Gone & Alcantara, 2007; Gone & Calf Looking, 2011; Robbins, Hill, & McWhirter, 2008; Thomas et al., 2009; Wendt & Gone, 2012). Even if treatment approaches are culturally sensitive, years of conflict with the U.S. government have led to an overarching mistrust of mainstream mental health institutions and professionals among American Indian/Alaska Native people (Beals et al., 2005; U.S. Department of Health and Human Services, 2001). Hence, it is increasingly evident that a healing framework using effective traditional strategies is not only necessary but also imperative (Echo-Hawk, 2011).

HEALING THROUGH STORYTELLING

The use of storytelling with American Indian/Alaska Natives is a traditional healing practice consistent with this line of reasoning. Stories hold a revered status within the oral tradition that is alive and well in Indian Country. A strong emphasis on teaching and using stories is vital to American Indian/Alaska Native people envisioning their own solutions to problems. In the remainder of this chapter, we will focus first on the importance of storytelling among American Indian/Alaska Native people; second, we will provide an overview of the use of stories and narratives in various disciplines; and third, we will argue for the creation of transformative, resilient narratives at a personal, familial, and community level for psychological healing and social justice.

All cultures engage in storytelling (Bruner, 2003). Through stories, individuals create meaning. Through discursive images and cultural narratives, individuals construct identities. In one sense, it can be said that culture itself is essentially a collection of stories about a group of people. These stories provide historical, social, cultural, and spiritual information of importance to tribal life and heritage. That is, culture is created through the formation of stories about groups, their relationships, values, and aspirations (Hammack, 2011).

Stories address basically every conceivable issue there is, including the origin of the spiritual world, people, animals, plants, land, oceans, ice, and the sun (BigFoot, 2006; Cruikshank, 1998). American Indian/Alaska Native storytelling has been a major method of cultural transmission for millennia (Momaday, 1996; Ortiz, 1999; Silko, 1989; Vizenor, 2008). Told by Native American elders to their young, stories provide life instructions, inspire, teach, enumerate possibilities, establish family lines and descendants, and shed light on all aspects of life (Atkinson, 1995). Stories help sustain traditional practices such as naming ceremonies and the giving of feasts for children's achievements (Hungry Wolf & Hungry Wolf, 1987; Momaday, 1998). They identify protective and recovery factors associated with Alaska Native sobriety (Mohatt et al., 2004). They serve as an adhesive that bonds communities together. According to Caddo scholar, Delores BigFoot (2006), Native storytellers are taught from an early age to listen and re-create the exact words of the stories they hear. They are told that stories should be shared accurately since they embody the culturally sanctioned history of a tribe.

In *The Man Made of Words*, Kiowa Pulitzer Prize–winning author N. Scott Momaday (1998) claims: "At the heart of the American Indian oral tradition is a deep and unconditional belief in the efficacy of language. Words are intrinsically powerful. They are magical. By means of word one can bring about physical change in the universe" (pp. 15–16). By putting words into stories, change occurs. Similarly, the noted Laguna Pueblo writer Leslie Marmon Silko (1996) asserts, "[T]hrough the stories we hear who we are" (p. 30).

Describing storytelling in Native American culture, Momaday also writes, "In the oral tradition stories are told not merely to entertain . . . they are told to be believed" (p. 3). This observation reveals a fundamental difference between European and American Indian ways of knowing. Many American Indian/Alaska Native people place more trust in stories than in scientific evidence. They use stories to determine the truth, to cope, and to discern how to live a moral life, yet survive.

However, due to colonization and subsequent antitribal policies, many American Indian/Alaska Native stories were silenced causing cumulative damage to Native culture (Berkhofer, 1997; Mihesuah, 2009). Today, the struggle to keep cultural practices alive, including storytelling, is vitally important. Encouraging American Indian/Alaska Native people to tell their story from their own perspectives is not only an act of cultural survival, but it is also an act of resistance against social injustice.

INNOVATIVE STORYTELLING APPROACHES

Storytelling has been used in notable, innovative, and effective American Indian/Alaska Native therapeutic modalities. The Positive Indian Parenting (PIP) curriculum developed by the National Indian Child Welfare Association, for example, emphasizes the importance of incorporating traditional parenting practices into contemporary parenting education (Northwest Indian Child Welfare Institute, 1986). Stating that every parent is a born storyteller and relying heavily on values clarification, PIP uses storytelling to impart effective American Indian/Alaska Native child rearing principles and practices.

Since 1992, the Gathering of Native Americans (GONA) training process has gained widespread popularity in Indian Country. According to GONA, storytelling offers an effective method of inculcating essential values into healing work that targets alcoholism and other forms of addiction. For example, GONA employs creation stories to teach participants about the importance of knowing their culture and other types of stories to teach lessons of interdependence and generosity (Substance Abuse and Mental Health Services Administration, n.d.).

Digital storytelling has become a readily accepted therapeutic approach used in Indian Country. A contemporary version of telling stories, digital storytelling is a curative, educational tool developed with participants from a variety of contexts (Lambert, 2009). Based on the Freirean (1970) model of using images to create dialogue, digital storytelling captures individual experience through the creation of three- to five-minute videos that synthesize images, video, text, and recordings of voice and music. By having the ability to circulate stories on the Internet, first-person digital accounts highlight the authentic experiences of people who are often left out of mainstream media. Digital stories can be shared in counseling sessions, public health trainings, community education events, social marketing, and media advocacy campaigns. They can also lead to community mobilization and assist in political activism. According to Wexler, digital stories revive storytelling among American Indian/Alaska Native youth while promoting self-efficacy and positive cultural identity (Wexler, Gubrium, Griffin, & DiFulvio, 2013). One positive aspect of digital storytelling is that an historical archive of these stories is then achieved for future generations and study.

Stories are also used for other macro-level purposes. Maori scholar Linda Smith (1999) has stated, "[T]he talk about the colonial past is embedded in our political discourses, our humor, poetry, music, storytelling, and other common sense ways of passing on both a narrative of history and an attitude about history" (p. 19). In her book, *Decolonizing Methodology*, Smith recommended deconstructing the dominant narratives told about indigenous people in order to create "decolonized" research methods. Similarly, Mohawk Scholar Taiaike Alfred and

Cherokee scholar Jeff Corntassel (2005) advocate for the "restorying" of the settler version of history by questioning the imposition of colonial histories on American Indian/Alaska Native communities. In discussing what is needed for healing within indigenous communities, Cortassel (2009) asserted, "Indigenous stories of resilience are critical to the resurgence of our communities" (p. 139). In other words, whereas storytelling in and of itself is an important component to the historical preservation of Native American knowledge and belief systems, it is important to understand that trauma, without meaning to, has become part of that heritage. And to avoid perpetuating that trauma across generations, a focus on resiliency and solution needs to be similarly encouraged and practiced. Otherwise, over time one could come to believe that trauma has been part of American Indian heritage since the beginning—a fact far from the truth.

RECLAIMING AND RECONSTRUCTING HISTORIES

Although not directly created for American Indian/Alaskan Native people, Bell (2010) offers an effective model for reclaiming histories and reconstructing stories in her book *Storytelling for Social Justice: Connecting Narratives and the Arts in Antiracist Teaching.* She features stories about race and racism to help others learn to dismantle racism. Of interest is the challenging of dominant narratives that perpetuate racial inequality. For example, the dominant American narrative that espouses meritocracy or "equal opportunities exist for all" can be contested by a story that shows discrimination in hiring practices. She delineates four types of stories that describe how people talk and think about race in the United States. These stories include stock stories, concealed stories, resistance stories, and emerging and transforming stories.

Stock stories consist of the most pervasive narratives that are widespread in public discourse and common usage. Told by the dominant group, these stories often reproduce privilege of the ruling class and, by design, racism. The stock story for achieving the American dream defuses challenges to authority and perpetuates stereotypes of minority groups, suggesting that if people would just "pull themselves up by their bootstraps," they would attain success. The United States is, after all, a land of equal opportunity and meritocracy. This narrative fails to consider structural inequalities, institutional and historical racism, and chance encounters that often hinder an individual's odds of success.

The remaining three types of stories delineated by Bell can be used to contrast stock stories and remediate perpetuated fallacies. Concealed stories uncover narratives that are hidden from mainstream American society. When exposed through a critical analysis of history and juxtaposed against stock stories, concealed stories present different versions of social relations that are rooted in daily discourse among those who live in the margins of society. An example of a concealed story is the story behind large income discrepancies between White and African Americans that seldom attributes the predominantly White American accumulation of wealth to inherited assets founded upon the forced labor of African Americans. For example, the movie *Gone with the Wind* extols the virtues of a ruling Southern class and the servitude of slaves.

Resistance stories, featuring ways that people fought against conditions described in stock stories, emerge from concealed stories. These stories of struggle often revive, mobilize, and inspire people. For example, the full story of Indian fishing rights demonstrations on the Columbia River in the Northwest is a story of careful, systemic planning that resulted in a successful outcome. This story provides valuable lessons in the ways in which well-conceptualized organizing can create effective change (Wilkinson, 2005). Resistance stories are thus the foundation upon which emerging and transforming stories can be imagined.

Emerging and transforming stories also challenge stocks stories, building on and strengthening concealed and resistance stories. They help generate active strategies for advancing racial equality. Emerging and transforming stories can be created anew in each generation, as individuals engage in the process of assessing difficulties they encounter and building upon resistance narratives from the past. This will go a long way in remediating the trauma that has been more recently linked to American Indian/Alaska Native heritage.

For American Indians/Alaska Native people, Bell's typology offers a model upon which to build transformative social justice interventions. As American Indians/Alaska Natives analyze stock stories that perpetuate themes of constant struggle, they begin to reactivate resistance stories that are abundant within their cultures. Resistance stories replace narratives that simply extend the status quo and empower communities to transform stagnant conditions. It seems useful at this point to describe more closely the stock, concealed, resistant, and emerging and transforming stories of American Indian/Alaska Native people to further assess the model's utility with this population.

REMEMBERING HISTORICAL RESISTANCE STORIES

In mainstream society, stock stories concerning American Indian/Alaska Native people include allusions to them as a people who are inferior, lazy, behind the times, difficult to deal with, and in need of modernization. The image of American Indian/Alaska Native men as warriors is still prevalent. Often depicted in movies and television using bows and arrows to fight against cowboys, American Indian men are portrayed directly or indirectly as savages prone to violence. This is frequently reflected in the penchant of non-Natives to dress up as "Indian Warriors," donning war paint and carrying bows and arrows during Halloween season. The continuation of American Indian mascots strengthens this stock story and perpetuates other pathological narratives of the people. Accordingly, American Indian/Alaska Native men who are not warriors are left out of mainstream narratives. Recent controversy has arisen with the remake of the movie about the Lone Ranger and his sidekick, Tonto—which means stupid in the Spanish language.

For many American Indians/Alaska Natives, concealed stories include the "real" history of relations with the settlers in North America. For example, history texts seldom feature accounts of treaty agreements in which tribal leaders negotiated land transfers benefitting their heirs, rather than surrendering. The dubious practice, on the part of European Americans, of giving American Indian/Alaska Natives alcohol prior to treaty negotiations is often concealed from mainstream narratives. Only recently has the story been told about the influence of the Iroquois Confederacy upon the U.S. Constitution (Mander, 1999). In fact, the U.S. Congress "acknowledged the historical debt which the United States owes to the Iroquois Confederacy and other Indian nations for their demonstration of enlightened, democratic principles of government and their example of a free association of independent Indian Nations" (Taliman, 2012, p. 1)

Hoxie (2012) argues that Native American history is a story of political activism with hard-won triumphs in courts and campaigns. His scholarship uncovered "the record of remarkable men and women who managed to survive the European invasion and participate actively in the creation of the modern world." He described American Indian/Alaska Native people who "spent far more time negotiating, lobbying, and debating than they spent tomahawking settlers or shooting at soldiers" (p. 4).

Resistance stories can be found in accounts of the pursuits of a number of American Indian/Alaska Native leaders. During the late 1960s and early 1970s, American Indian/Alaska Native activists took control of their destinies while empowering hundreds of thousands of fellow Native people. The American Indian Movement (AIM), a revolutionary organization founded by a group of Indian activists to address injustices experienced by the American Indian community in Minneapolis, gained national attention in 1971 when AIM took over the BIA national headquarters in Washington, D.C., and presented a 20-point list of demands to the federal government. In 1973, AIM activists also led a 71-day armed standoff with the federal government on the Pine Ridge Indian Reservation in Wounded Knee, South Dakota. Additionally, in the early hours of November 20, 1969, a group of American Indian activists (not representing AIM) occupied Alcatraz Island in the San Francisco Bay to gain control over the island in hopes of building a center for Native American studies, an American Indian spiritual center, and an American Indian museum (Smith & Warrior, 1996). Like the seizure of the BIA and the standoff at Wounded Knee, the Alcatraz occupation gained national attention ("What took so long?" Indian activists may be unified by slaying," 1972). As historian Charles Wilkinson (2005) states in his book *Blood Struggles*, the American Indian revival of the second half of the 20th century deserves to be recognized as a major episode in American history alongside the civil rights era.

In Canada, the Assembly of First Nations (AFN) has provided a unified voice for First Nations people. This group of First Nations leaders (chiefs), who strive to protect the rights, treaty obligations, ceremonies, and claims of First Nations in Canada, has participated in drafting the U.N. Declaration of Indigenous Rights of Indigenous People, played a key role in negotiating the Indian Residential Schools settlement, and helped in the U.S. Canada Free Trade Agreement ("Assembly of First Nations," n.d.). Recently, in Canada, the Idle No More movement has gained international popularity, igniting numerous demonstrations among indigenous communities worldwide. Idle No More is a grassroots initiative launched in opposition to Canadian Bill C-45, the Canadian government's budgetary legislation that includes changes to First Nations land management (Crazy Bull, 2013).

Among all the indigenous movements in the last half-century, few have captured worldwide attention like the Zapatista movement that originated in the jungles and canyons of the southeastern Mexican state of Chiapas. The movement gained international attention on the early hours of January 1, 1994, when thousands of armed indigenous Mexicans calling themselves Zapatistas declared war against Mexico due to oppressive imperialist policies. The cry of Ya Basta!—"Enough already"—was heard worldwide as a demand for recognition, equal protection, and autonomy for indigenous people. In the years since, the movement has not only managed to survive, but it also has remained a significant force at the national and transnational levels (Khasnabish, 2010). *The New York Times* has referred to the Zapatista movement as the first postmodern revolution. Resistance stories of this kind help transform stories of suffering into stories of survivance.[3]

HEALING THROUGH HISTORICAL RESILIENCE STORIES

Tribal leaders and educators are increasingly promoting resilience narratives that highlight how, throughout history, American Indian/Alaska Natives have overcome tremendous obstacles and continued to thrive (Garrod & Larimore, 1997; Piatote, 2011). Psychologists are beginning to recognize the importance of including alternative viewpoints to historical trauma in American Indian/Alaska Native mental health treatment. Denham (2008) suggests that trauma stories may engender vulnerability to psychological problems even though they assist in ethnic/racial socialization. She argues for rethinking historical trauma by looking more closely at American Indian/Alaska Native responses to trauma. Based on person-centered ethnographic research, Denham highlighted four generations of one American Indian family who contextualized responses to historical trauma in a positive light. The Si John family reframed their traumatic past by sharing resilience strategies to achieve a positive family outlook. For example, one Si John family member, Cliff, remarked that Native people must remember the strength of their blood, "the same blood that ran through your ancestor's veins" (p. 406). By remembering his family's traumatic narratives, Cliff believed that he had greater control over his current struggles. The practice of reframing the trauma "raises questions about alternative non-pathological outcomes of exposure to historical trauma" (p. 410). However, one caveat must be kept in mind: Denham's research examined only one family and thus may not be representative of other American Indian/Alaska Native families. Nevertheless, this approach represents a potentially viable alternative to existing approaches to resolving such trauma.

Even though the historical trauma movement has been overwhelmingly beneficial and necessary, linkage of psychological trauma to colonization history, according to Gros Ventre scholar Joseph P. Gone (in press), may unintentionally encourage a discourse that does not represent the accurate range of American Indian/Alaska Native responses to colonization. He states that by so doing, historical trauma advocates may actually contribute to the dominant narrative of American Indian/Alaska Native people as victims who are fundamentally wounded.

We believe it is time to balance the teachings about what happened to American Indian/Alaska Native people, including why they suffer, with historical resilience stories (e.g., Fuller-Thomson, 2005; Heavy Runner & Marshall, 2003). This reconstructive approach not only explains why American Indian/Alaska Natives still exist, but it also reifies what is beautifully and profoundly right about Native cultures. If more resilience stories were told, America Indian/Alaska Native people would reconnect with a sense of pride in their cultural identities and cultural practices. Just as there are many collective trauma responses, there are many collective resilient responses. Just as American Indian/Alaska Native people have suffered from one of the worst forms of colonial subjugation human beings have ever had to experience, they have survived. They are still here and many, and many are thriving.

SUMMARY

For over 500 years, American Indian/Alaska Native people have encountered countless intrusions and trauma in the name of colonization and assimilation. The distortion and loss of their histories and stories, their languages, physical displacement, and governmental policies aimed at disrupting their family systems have led to a historical trauma response pattern for the culture, as well as for individuals. The psychosocial impact of this colonial legacy is evident in disheartening statistics that describe the current state of American Indian/Alaska Native health. Whereas the population of American Indian/Alaska Natives is increasing and accounts of American Indian/Alaska Natives thriving despite adversity are emerging, the number of health problems, especially mental health problems, is disproportionately increasing. In this chapter, we presented an overview of the population, including a brief description of its diversity. We emphasized that American Indian/Alaska Native people have endured numerous deleterious experiences that shaped their identities as well as their trauma. Accordingly, we argue that American Indian/Alaska Native people not only need to tell their stories, but they also need to retell their histories from a resilient perspective to prevent further cultural proselytization and outright assimilation into mainstream American society.

Bell's 2010 model offers a valuable therapeutic tool for micro- and macro-level change in Indian Country. By uncovering hidden historical resistance stories and retelling them, American Indian/Alaska Native people can chronicle, and thus protect, their true history. The telling of strength-based versions of American Indian/Alaska Native historical events adds to the historical trauma movement and advances social justice intervention. In particular, highlighting the correct and courageous legacy of generations of American/Alaska Native people better positions them into a powerful place. In doing so, the heritage of American Indian/ Alaska Natives will be restored to one that will (and should) exist without the trauma that has plagued this group for so long.

NOTES

1. Any of the self-governing American Indian/Alaska Native communities throughout the United States.

2. Manifest destiny was the belief widely held by U.S. settlers that they would ultimately occupy all of the geographical territory between the Atlantic and Pacific oceans. This belief was used to justify expansion throughout the continent and catastrophic removal or destruction of American Indian people encountered in the pursuit of that destiny (Deloria, 1969; Stephanson, 1996).

3. *Survivance* means a sense of presence, the motion of sovereignty, and the will to resist dominance. "Survival is a response; survivance is a standpoint, a worldview, and a presence" (Vizenor & Lee, 2003, p. 93).

REFERENCES

Adams, D. W. (1995). *Education for extinction: American Indians and the boarding school experience 1875–1928.* Lawrence, KS: University Press of Kansas.

Alfred, T., & Corntassel, J. (2005). Being indigenous: Resurgences against contemporary colonialism. *Government and Opposition, 9,* 597–614.

American Psychological Association. (2003). Multicultural guidelines for education and training, research, practice, and organizational development for psychologists. *American Psychologist, 58,* 377–402.

Atkinson, R. (1995). *The gift of stories: Practical and spiritual applications of autobiography, life stories, and personal mythmaking.* Westport, CT: Bergin & Garvey.

Beals, J., Novins, D., Whitesell, N., Spicer, P., Mitchell, C., Manson, S., & American Indian Service Utilization, Psychiatric Epidemiology, Risk and Protective Factors Team. (2005). Prevalence of mental disorders and utilization of mental health services in two American Indian reservation populations: Mental health disparities in a national context. *American Journal of Psychiatry, 162,* 1723–1732.

Bell, L. A. (2010). *Storytelling for social justice: Connecting narratives and the arts in the antiracist teaching.* New York, NY: Routledge Publishing.

Berkhofer, R. F. (1997). *Killing the White man's Indian: Reinventing Native Americans at the end of the twentieth century.* New York, NY: Anchor Books.

BigFoot, D. S. (2006). Storytelling as a healing tool for American Indians. In T. Witko (Ed.), *Mental health care for urban Indians: Clinical insights from Native practitioners* (pp. 133–155). Washington, DC: American Psychological Association.

Brasfield, C. R. (2001). Residential school syndrome. *British Columbia Medical Journal, 43*(2), 78–81.

Brave Heart, M. Y. H. (2000). Wakiksuyapi: Carrying the historical trauma of the Lakota. *Tulare Studies in Social Welfare, 21*(22), 245–266.

Brave Heart, M. Y. H. (2003). The historical trauma response among Natives and its relationship with substance abuse: A Lakota illustration. *Journal of Psychoactive Drugs, 35*(1), 7–13.

Brave Heart, M. Y. H., & DeBruyn, L. (1995). So she may walk in balance: Integrating the impact of historical trauma in the treatment of Native American Indian women. In J. Adelman & G. Enguidanos (Eds.), *Racism in the lives of women: Testimony theory and guides to anti-racist practice* (pp. 345–368). New York, NY: Haworth Press.

Brave Heart, M. Y. H., & DeBruyn, L. M. (1998). The American Indian holocaust: Healing historical unresolved grief. *Journal of the National Center for American Indian and Alaska Native Mental Health Research, 8*(2), 56–78.

Bruner, J. (2003). *Making stories: Law, literature, life.* Boston, MA: Harvard University Press.

Calloway, C. G. (2003). *One vast winter count: The Native American west before Lewis and Clark.* Lincoln, NE: University of Nebraska Press.

Castor, M. L., Smyser, M. S., Taualii, M. M., Park, A. N., Lawson, S. A., & Forquera, R. A. (2006). Nationwide population-based study identifying health disparities between American Indians/Alaska Natives and the general populations living in select urban counties. *American Journal of Public Health, 96,* 1478–1484.

Centers for Disease Control and Prevention. (2008). *Adverse health conditions and health risk behaviors associated with intimate partner violence.* Retrieved from http://www.cdc.gov/mmwr/preview/mmwrhtml/mm5705a1.htm

Centers for Disease Control and Prevention, National Center for Injury Prevention and Control. (2012). *Suicide: Facts at a glance.* Retrieved from http://www.cdc.gov/ViolencePrevention/pdf/Suicide_DataSheet-a.pdf

Chae, D. H. & Walters, K. (2009). Racial discrimination and racial identity attitudes in relation to self-related health and physical pain and impairment among two-spirit American Indians/Alaska Natives. *American Journal of Public Health, 99,* 144–151.

Child, B. J. (1998). *Boarding school seasons.* Lincoln, NE: University of Nebraska Press.

Christensen, M., & Manson, S. (2001). Adult attachment as a framework for understanding mental health and American Indian families. *American Behavioral Scientist, 44,* 1447–1465.

Churchill, W. (2004). *Kill the Indian save the man: The genocidal impact of American Indian residential schools.* San Francisco, CA: City Lights Publishers.

Corntassel, J. (2009). Indigenous storytelling, truth-telling, and community approaches to reconciliation. *English Studies in Canada, 35,* 137–159. doi: 10.1353/esc.0.0163

Crazy Bull, C. (2013, March 16). Idle No More brings Native voices, tribal education to the forefront. *Indian Country Today Media Network.* Retrieved from http://indiancountrytodaymedianetwork.com//opinion/idle-no-more-brings-native-voices-tribal-education-forefront-148209

Cruikshank, J. (1998). *The social life of stories: Narrative and knowledge in the Yukon Territory.* Lincoln, NE: University of Nebraska Press.

Deloria, V. (1969). *Custer died for your sins: An Indian manifesto.* New York, NY: Macmillan.

Denham, A. R. (2008). Rethinking historical trauma: Narratives of resilience. *Transcultural Psychiatry, 45,* 391–414.

Duran, E. (2006). *Healing the soul wound: Counseling with American Indians and other Native peoples.* New York, NY: Teachers College.

Duran, E., & Duran, B. (1995). *Native American postcolonial psychology.* Albany, NY: State University of New York Press.

Echo-Hawk, H. (2011). Indigenous communities and evidence building. *Journal of Psychoactive Drugs, 43*(3), 269–275.

Evans-Campbell, T. (2008). Historical trauma in American Indian/Native Alaska communities: A multilevel framework for exploring impacts on individuals, families, and communities. *Journal of Interpersonal Violence, 23,* 316–338.

Evans-Campbell, T., Lindhorst, T., Huang, B., & Walters, K. (2006). Interpersonal violence in the lives of urban American Indian and Alaska Native women: Implications for health, mental health, and helpseeking. *American Journal of Public Health, 96,* 1416–1422.

Evans-Campbell, T., Walters, K. L., Pearson, C. R., & Campbell, C. D. (2012). Indian boarding school experience, substance use, and mental health among urban two-spirit American Indian/Alaska Natives. *The American Journal of Drug and Alcohol Abuse, 38,* 421–427.

Fieland, K. C., Walters, K. L., & Simoni, J. M. (2007). Determinants of health among two spirit American Indians and Alaska Natives. In I. H. Meyer & M. Northridge (Eds.), *The health of sexual minorities* (pp. 268–300). New York, NY: Springer Press.

Fixico, D. (1986). *Termination and relocation: Federal Indian policy, 1945–1960.* Albuquerque, NM: University of New Mexico Press.

Fixico, D. (2000). *The urban Indian experience in America.* Albuquerque, NM: New Mexico Press.

Freire, P. (1970). *Pedagogy of the oppressed.* New York, NY: Continuum.

Fryberg, S. A., Markus, H. R., Oyserman, D., & Stone, J. M. (2008). Of warrior chiefs and Indian princesses: The psychological consequences of American Indian mascots. *Basic and Applied Social Psychology, 30,* 208–218.

Fuller-Thomson, E. (2005). Canadian first Nations grandparents raising grandchildren: A portrait in resilience. *The International Journal of Aging and Human Development, 60,* 331–342.

Garrod, A., & Larimore, C. (1997). *First person, first peoples: Native American college graduates tell their life stories.* Ithaca, NY: Cornell University Press.

Gone, J. (in press). Colonial genocide and historical trauma in Native North America: Complicating contemporary attributions. In A. Woolford, J. Benvenuto, & A. L. Hinton (Eds.), *Colonial genocide and indigenous North America,* Durham, NC: Duke University Press.

Gone, J. P., & Alcantara, C. (2007). Mental health interventions for American Indians and Alaska Natives: A review of the literature. *Cultural Diversity and Ethnic Minority Psychology, 13,* 356–363.

Gone, J. P., & Calf Looking, P. E. (2011). American Indian culture as substance abuse treatment: Pursuing evidence for a local intervention. *Journal of Psychoactive Drugs, 43,* 291–296.

Gone, J. P., & Trimble, J. E. (2012). American Indian and Alaska Native mental health: Diverse perspectives on enduring disparities. *Annual Review of Clinical Psychology, 8,* 131–160.

Hammack, P. (2011). *Narrative and the politics of identity: The cultural psychology of Israeli and Palestinian youth.* New York, NY: Oxford University Press.

Heavy Runner, I. & Marshall, K. (2003). Miracle survivors: Promoting resilience in Indian students. *Tribal College Journal, 14*(4), 14–18.

Hoxie, F. (2001). *A final promise: The campaign to assimilate the Indians, 1880–1920.* Cambridge, MA: University Press.

Hoxie, F. (2012). *This Indian Country: American Indian activists and the place they made.* New York, NY: Penguin Press HC.

Hungry Wolf, A., & Hungry Wolf, B. (1987). *Children of the sun: Stories by and about Indian kids.* New York, NY: William Morrow.

Jaimes, M. (1992). *The state of Native America: Genocide, colonization, and resistance.* Cambridge, MA: South End Press.

Khasnabish, A. (2010*). Zapatistas: Rebellion from the grassroots to the global.* New York: NY. Zed Books.

LaFromboise, T. D., & Fatemi, A. (2011). American Indian Life Skills: A community-based intervention for indigenous mental health. In H. Fitzgerald (Ed.), *Child psychology and mental health: Cultural and ethno-racial perspectives* (pp. 309–336). Santa Barbara, CA: Praeger.

LaFromboise, T. D., & Lewis, H. A. (2008). The Zuni Life Skills Development Program: A school/community-based suicide prevention intervention. *Suicide and Life-Threatening Behavior, 38,* 343–353.

Lambert, J. (2009). *Digital storytelling: Capturing lives, creating community.* Berkeley, CA: Center for Digital Storytelling, Digital Diner Press.

Manataka American Indian Council. (2009). Retrieved from http://www.manataka.org/page237html

Mander, J. (1999). *In the absence of the sacred: The failure of technology and the survival of the Indian nations.* Gloucester, MA: Peter Smith.

Metcalf, A. (1976). From schoolgirl to mother: The effects of education on Navajo women. *Social Problems, 23,* 535–544.

Mihesuah, D. A. (2009). *American Indians: Stereotypes & realities.* Atlanta, GA: Clarity Press Inc.

Mohatt, G. V., Rasmus, S. M., Thomas, L., Allen, J., Hazel, K., & Hensel, C. (2004). "Tied together like a woven hat:" Protective pathways to Alaska native sobriety. *Harm Reduction Journal, 1,* 10. doi: 10.1186/1477-7517-1-10

Momaday, S. (1996). *A house made of dawn.* Tucson, AZ: University of Arizona Press.

Momaday, S. (1998). *Man made of words: Essays, stories, passages.* New York, NY: St. Martin Griffin.

Morrissette, P. (1994). The holocaust of first nation people: Residual effects on parenting and treatment implications. *Contemporary Family Therapy, 16,* 381–93.

Northwest Indian Child Welfare Institute. (1986). *Positive Indian Parenting: Honoring our children by honoring our traditions: A model Indian parent training manual.* Portland, OR: Northwest Indian Child Welfare Institute.

Ogunwole, S. (2006). *We are the people: American Indian and Alaska Natives in the United States. Census 2000. Special Reports, CENSR-28.* Washington, DC: United States Census Bureau. Retrieved from http://www.bia.gov/idc/groups/public/documents/text/idc-001819.pdf

Ortiz, S. (1999). *Men on the moon: Collected short stories.* Tucson, AZ: University of Arizona Press.

Piatote, B. H. (2011). Domestic trials: Indian rights and national belonging in works by Pauline Johnson and John M. Oskison. *American Quarterly, 63*(30), 95–116.

Robbins, R., Colmant, S., Dorton, J., Schultz, L., Colmant, Y., & Ciali, P. (2006). Colonial installations in American Indian boarding school students. *Educational Foundations, 20*(3–4), 69–88.

Robbins, R., Hill, J., & McWhirter, T. (2008). Conflicting epistemologies: A case study of traditional American Indian in therapy. *Clinical Case Studies, 7,* 449–466.

Schacht, A. J., Tafoya, N., & Mirabia, K. (1989). Home-based therapy with American Indian families. *American Indian Alaska Native Mental Health Research, 3*(2), 27–42.

Silko, L. M. (1989). *Storyteller.* New York, NY: Arcade.

Silko, L. M. (1996). *Yellow woman and a beauty of the spirit.* San Jose, CA: Simon & Schuster.

Smith, L. T. (1999). *Decolonizing methodologies: Research and Indigenous peoples.* London, UK: Zed Books.

Smith, P. C., & Warrior, R. A. (1996). *Like a hurricane: The Indian movement from Alcatraz to Wounded Knee.* New York, NY: The New Press.

Snipp, M., & Saraff, A. (2011) American Indian and Alaska Native children and families: Social and economic conditions. In M. C. Sarche, P. Spicer, P. Farrell, & H. E. Fitzgerald (Eds.), *American Indian children and mental health* (pp. 27–43). Santa Barbara, CA: ABC-CLIO.

Stephanson, A. (1996). *Manifest destiny: American expansion and the empire of right.* New York, NY: Hill and Wang.

Substance Abuse and Mental Health Services Administration, Center for Substance Abuse Prevention. (n.d). *Gathering of Native Americans training curriculum.* Retrieved from http://nace.samhsa.gov/WebImages/file/TTA-GONA/GONA%20TRAINER%20GUIDE.pdf

Substance Abuse & Mental Health Services Administration, Office of Applied Studies. (2007). *Substance use and substance use disorders among American Indians and Alaska Natives. The NSDUH Report.* Retrieved from http://www.oas.samhsa.gov/2k7/AmIndians/AmIndians.htm

Sue, D. W., Capodilupa, C. M., Torino, G. C., Bucceri, J. M., Holder, A. M. B., Nadal, K. L., & Esquilin, M. (2007). Racial microaggressions in everyday life: Implications for clinical practice. *American Psychologist,* 62, 271–286.

Taliman, V. (2012, July 4). *Iroquois confederacy is foundation of United States Constitution.* Retrieved from http://www.fnx.org/blog/iroquois-confederacy-foundation-united-states-constitution/

Terry, M. J. (1995). Kelengakutelleghpat: An Arctic community-based approach to trauma. In B. H. Stamm (Ed.), *Secondary traumatic stress: Self-care issues for clinicians, researchers, and educators* (pp. 149–178). Baltimore, MD: Sidron Press.

Thomas, L. R., Donovan, D. M., Sigo, R. L. W., Austin, L., Marlatt, G. A., & Suquamish Tribe. (2009). The community pulling together: A tribal community-university partnership project to reduce substance abuse and promote good health in a reservation tribal community. *Journal of Ethnicity in Substance Abuse,* *8*(3), 283–300.

Thornton, R. (1987). *American Indian holocaust and survival: A population history since 1492.* Norman, OK: University Oklahoma Press.

Urban Indian Health Institute, Seattle Indian Health Board. (2009). *Visibility through data: Health information for Urban American Indian and Alaska Native communities.* Seattle, WA: Author. Retrieved from http://www.uihi.org/wp-content/uploads/2009/01/health_health-influencing_behaviors_among_urban_indiansupdate-121020081.pdf

Urban Indian Health Institute, Seattle Indian Health Board. (2011). *Community health profile: National aggregate of Urban Indian Health Organization service areas.* Seattle, WA: Author. Retrieved from http://www.uihi.org/wp-content/uploads/2011/12/Combined-UIHO-CHP_Final.pdf

Urban Indian Health Institute, Seattle Indian Health Board. (2012). *Addressing Depression among American Indians and Alaska Natives.* Seattle, WA: Author. Retrieved from http://www.uihi.org/wp-content/uploads/2012/08/BH-Capacity-Report-COMBINED_22August12.pdf

U.S. Bureau of Indian Affairs. (2013). *Who we are.* Retrieved from http://www.bia.gov/WhoWeAre/index.htm

U.S. Census Bureau. (2010). *The American Indian and Alaska native population: 2010*. Retrieved from http://www.census.gov/prod/cen2010/briefs/c2010br-10.pdf

U.S. Department of Health and Human Services, Center for Mental Health Services. (2001). *Mental health: Culture, race, and ethnicity—A supplement to mental health: A report of the Surgeon General*. Rockville, MD; Washington, DC: Author.

U.S Department of Justice, Office of Justice Programs, National Institute of Justice. (2000). *Full report of the prevalence, incidence, and consequences of violence against women*. Retrieved from https://www.ncjrs.gov/pdffiles1/nij/183781.pdf

Vizenor, G. (2008). *Survivance: Narratives of Native presence*. Lincoln, NE: University of Nebraska Press.

Vizenor, G., & Lee, A. R. (2003). *Postindian conversations*. Lincoln, NE: University of Nebraska Press.

Walters, K. (2010). *From Injun Joe to Big Chief: The relation between microaggression distress and substance abuse*. [PowerPoint slides]. Retrieved from http://www.seiservices.com/NIDA/1014081/Presentations/Walters.pdf

Walters, K. L., Mohammed, S. A., Evans-Campbell, T., Beltran, R. E., Chae, D. H., & Duran, B. (2011). Bodies don't just tell stories, they tell histories: Embodiment of historical trauma among American Indians and Alaska Natives. *Du Bois Review, 8*, 179–189.

Walters, K. L., Simoni, J. M., & Evans-Campbell, T. (2002). Substance use among American Indians and Alaska Natives: Incorporating culture in an "indigenist" stress coping paradigm. *Public Health Report, 117*, 104–117.

Wendt, D. C., & Gone, J. P. (2012). Rethinking cultural competence: Insights from indigenous community treatment settings. *Transcultural Psychiatry, 49*, 206–222.

Wexler, L., Gubrium, A., Griffin, M., & DiFulvio, G. (2013). Promoting positive development and highlighting reasons for living in Northwest Alaska through digital storytelling. *Health Promotion Practice, 14*(4). doi: 10.1177/1524839912462390

What took so long?: Indian activists may be unified by slaying. (1972, November 26). *The Washington Post*.

Whitbeck, L. B. (2011). The beginnings of mental health disparities: Emergent mental disorders among Indigenous adolescents. *Nebraska Symposium on Motivation, 57*, 121–149.

Whitbeck, L. B., Adams, G., Hoyt, D., & Chen, X. (2004). Conceptualizing and measuring historical trauma among American Indian people. *American Journal of Community Psychology, 33*(3/4), 119–130.

Wilkinson, C. (2005). *Blood struggles: The rise of modern Indian nations*. New York, NY: Norton.

Woodward, S. (2012, October 10). American Indian youth in crisis: Tribes grapple with a suicide emergency. *Indian Country Today Media Network*. Retrieved from http://indiancountrytodaymedianetwork.com/article/american-indian-youth-in-crisis%3A-tribes-grapple-with-a-suicide-emergency-138794

Yoder, K., Whitbeck, L., Hoyt, D., & LaFromboise, T. (2006). Suicide ideation among American Indian youths. *Archives of Suicide Research, 10*, 177–190.

Zimmerman, M. A., Ramierex-Valles, J., Wahienko, K. M., Walter, B., & Dyer, S. (1996). Enculturation hypothesis: Exploring direct and protective factors among Native American youth. In H. I. McCubbin, A. E. Thompson, A. I. Thompson, & J. E. Fromer (Eds.), *Resiliency in ethnic minority families, Native and immigrant American families* (pp. 199–219). Madison, WI: University of Wisconsin Press.

Chapter 9

Sexual Orientation and Gender Minorities

Linda M. Woolf and Danielle MacCartney

> In Iran, we don't have homosexuals like in your country.
>
> —Iranian president Mahmoud Ahmadinejad speaking on CNN, 2007

> Oh, so you're saying we should go out and start killing them? No, I'm saying the government should. They won't, but they should.
>
> —Curtis Knapp, Kansas pastor discussing gays and lesbians in the United States (U.S.: *Huffington Post*, 2012)

Around the globe, governments, communities, organizations, and individuals routinely exhibit negative attitudes, discriminatory practices, and violence against individuals identified as lesbian, gay, bisexual, transgendered, queer, or intersex (LGBTQI). Essentially, anti-LGBTQI mind-set translates into human rights violations and social justice denied. In many cases, bias is so extreme that the everyday well-being of LGBTQI individuals is threatened—their very existence as valued members of the human community is disregarded or extinguished. Anti-LGBTQI violence and oppression spans the range from slurs to potential human rights violations, including physical assaults, torture, rape, and murder. Sadly, such violence occurs with an elevated brutality not often seen in other bias-related or hate crimes (Human Rights Council [HRC], 2011; Murphy, 2001) and is frequently state sanctioned (Franklin & Herek, 2003). Anti-LGBTQI sentiment affects individuals not only on a direct personal level but also on the structural level, with bias built into the foundation of organizations and communities. Members of the LGBTI communities may experience denial of basic human rights such as the right of assembly, and violations of rights in relation to education, health care, employment, housing, and recognized relationships. All forms of anti-LGBTQI bias negatively impact individuals and communities.

Unfortunately, discrimination and violence against LGBTQI individuals occurs in every region where humans live in communities (HRC, 2011). Simply, the perception that someone is a member of a sexual or gender minority may trigger violence against that individual. The extent and degree of violence may vary by region, but no area is currently free of bias or oppression (HRC, 2011). This bias against LGBTQI individuals is not essential to human nature but rather is a product of culture and, unfortunately, is often justified through religious belief. One only has to look to history to view cultures with greater openness to human sexual and gender diversity. For example, homosexuality was legal throughout most of Europe, and gays and lesbians were largely accepted, or at minimum, viewed with indifference until the 11th through 13th centuries (Boswell, 2005). Ancient India venerated Hindu deities representing a richness of diversity, including same-gender relations and complex-gender identities (Wilhelm, 2010). Although some countries and communities may have laws protecting LGBTQI, other nation-states are extremely oppressive—homosexuality and transgenderism are criminalized with sentences ranging from imprisonment (e.g., Malaysia) to the death penalty (e.g., Sudan). As social justice concerns for LGBTQI extend across international borders, these issues must be examined through both a local and global lens.

Individuals are at risk when their sexual orientation or gender identification falls outside the norm and when their minority status is viewed pejoratively. Hence, many individuals must choose between working to fit within the norms of their community and striving to simply be themselves. Both choices involve risk. For the former, individuals risk self-oppression and long-term gender/sexual confusion and incongruence. In the latter case, individuals risk oppression and victimization at the hands of others.

DEFINITIONS

Although the terms are sometimes used indiscriminately, sex, gender identity, and sexual orientation are distinct. Typically, *sex* refers to one's biological sex (e.g., male, female, or intersex); *gender identity* refers to one's sense of being male, female, or transgender; and *sexual orientation* refers to an individual's sexual or romantic attraction to another individual based on sex or gender identity (e.g., attraction to the same sex—gay men or lesbian women; attraction to both sexes—bisexual). Sexual orientation and gender identities are not only biologically based but also personally, socially, and culturally determined. Indeed, sexual orientation, particularly for women, may exist on a continuum and be fluid across one's lifespan (Diamond, 2007; Peplau & Garnets, 2000).

Extensive variability exists in relation to defining sexual orientation and gender identification both within the United States and internationally. For example, biological sex is often viewed as a binomial classification—one is either male or female. Yet, the diversity of biological possibilities is greater and includes those who are transgendered (male-to-female or female-to-male), intersex (varying levels of ambiguity of biological factors routinely identified as male or female), and third gendered. How these variations are defined or actualized differs by individual and culture. Individuals may identify as transgendered if they are living their lives as male-to-female or female-to-male with no alterations in biological gender, if they have undertaken hormone treatments but have no surgical alterations to gender, or if they have undertaken partial or complete surgical and hormonal gender reassignment (Baird, 2003). Although their biological sex is ambiguous, intersex individuals may self-identify as male, female, neither, or something else depending on their own personal experiences and self-schemas as well as cultural norms (Preves, 2003). In some cultures, there exists a third gender classification. The hijras of India consider themselves to be a sacred third gender with some individuals born intersex whereas other individuals are castrated. Unfortunately, many members of the hijra community are forced into prostitution as a means of survival (Nanda, 1985; Thappa, Singh, & Kaimal, 2008). Additionally, third sexes include the guevedoche or machihembra of the Dominican Republic, the kwolu-aatmwol of New Guinea, the bayot or lakin-on in the Philippines, the mahu of Tahiti, and the waria of Indonesia (Denny, 1997). In the United States, there are individuals who identify themselves as a third gender—neither male nor female but rather a unique gender (Sell, 2004). Similar variability exists in relation to sexual orientation. For example, an individual may self-identify as a heterosexual but engage in same-sex sexual relationships defying culturally proscribed labels (Savin-Williams, 2001).

Each individual and community defines terms related to sexual orientation or gender differently and hence, broad categorizations such as "gay," "straight," "male," "female," or "transgendered" are, by their very nature, limiting. Something seemingly as innocuous as a questionnaire with gender categories of "male" and "female" can be experienced as a form of bias or oppression. The ambiguity and interplay between all of the aforementioned factors and the addition of other arenas of diversity such as age, ethnicity, race, and religion make simple, nonfluid sexual orientation and gender-identification incredibly challenging.

In this chapter, we use the limited term LGBTQI to represent sexual orientation and gender minorities. Currently, there is no uniform consensus over the terms used for sexual orientation or gender minorities. Indeed, there remains much debate over which terms are considered appropriate or acceptable. Many gay men and lesbian women eschew the use of the term *homosexual* as this term has been historically associated with ideas of disease, mental illness, or "nature's mistake." Individuals born with sexually ambiguous genetic factors or biological sex often prefer the term *intersex* to that of *hermaphrodite* for similar reasons (Harper, 2007).

Today, some individuals elect to use *Queer* as a more inclusive term to replace gay and lesbian and inclusive of bisexuals and transgendered individuals (Grace, Hill, Johnson, & Lewis, 2004). Although we have elected to use the broadly inclusive term *LGBTQI*, we are cognizant of the diversity of gender and sexual minority identities and that other terms and definitions could be included.

STATUS AROUND THE GLOBE

Within and outside the United States, there remain many hidden populations due to stigma, stereotype, discrimination, and legal threat. LGBTQI represent such hidden populations, more so in some communities and nations than other regions. Thus, statistics related to hidden populations can vary significantly. For example, MacKenzie, Huntington, and Gilmour (2009) estimated that 1:1,500 to 1:2,000 live births are born intersex, Preves (2003) placed the figure closer to 2%, and Gough, Weyman, Alderson, Butler, and Stoner (2008) estimated the incidence rate as closer to 4% of all live births. Hence, statistics always should be interpreted as estimates and impacted by the degree to which LGBTQI status is hidden.

Data concerning the percentage of populations identifying as LGBTQI are limited to cultures in which sexual orientation and gender minority status has been decriminalized. According to Gates (2011), approximately 3.5% of adults, or 9 million people, in the United States identify as gay, lesbian, or bisexual, and 0.3% are transgender. In Australia, 18.6% of men and 15.1% of women reported feelings of attraction to someone of the same sex, but only 1.6% of men identified as gay and 0.8% identified as lesbian (Smith, Rissel, Richters, Grulich, & de Visser, 2003). In Canada, about 1.3% of men reported being homosexual, and 0.7% considered themselves bisexual; 0.9% of women considered themselves lesbian, and 0.9% reported being bisexual (Statistics Canada, 2004). In Denmark, 2.7% of men reported engaging in same-sex sexual behavior, and 4.1% of men and 2.6 % of women in France reported at least one occurrence of same-sex intercourse (ACSF Investigators, 1992; Melbye & Biggar, 1992). These data represent demographic examples from Western cultures.

The legal status of LGBTQI individuals and organizations varies dramatically around the globe. As of 2013, only seven countries had protections for sexual orientation and gender minorities incorporated into their national constitution: Bolivia, Ecuador, Kosovo, Portugal, South Africa, Sweden, and Switzerland (HRC, 2011). Nonetheless, regional (e.g., city, province, territory) protections exist for LGBTQI individuals and communities within countries lacking broader constitutional protections. Of course, laws against discrimination do not ensure that oppressive practices and policies are absent within families, communities, the private sector, or religious groups. Legal protections are useless if not supported by the justice system within a nation-state. In 1988, a Florida judge joked during a case involving the beating death of a gay man, "That's a crime now, to beat up a homosexual," to which the prosecutor replied, "Yes, sir. And it's also a crime to kill them."

The judge replied, "Times have really changed" (Hentoff as cited in Jenness & Broad, 2009). Unfortunately, all too often the criminal justice system has turned a blind eye to discrimination and violence against LGBTQI individuals.

Eighty countries retain laws criminalizing individuals on the basis of their sexual orientation or gender identity with India recriminalizing same-sex relationships in December of 2013. Penalties range from forced sterilization to imprisonment to death. Such laws exist in opposition to current international law. According to the United Nations (UN), the criminalization of sexual behavior is considered a violation of the basic right to privacy and nondiscrimination (HRC, 2011). The UN Special Rapporteur for health stated that "sanctioned punishment by States reinforces existing prejudices, and legitimizes community violence and police brutality directed at affected individuals" (HRC, 2011, p. 14). LGBTQI individuals have a right under international law to seek asylum from nations where their sexual orientation or gender minority status is not criminalized (HRC, 2011; UN, 1950).

The principle of nondiscrimination is at the very core of the UN Universal Declaration of Human Rights (UDHR) (UN, 1948). The UDHR states that all rights are universal, indivisible, and inalienable. The UN International Covenant on Civil and Political Rights (UN, 1966a) and the UN International Covenant on Economic, Social and Cultural Rights (UN, 1966b) further affirm these rights. Sexual orientation and gender minorities are not specifically named in these covenants. Nonetheless, the UN determined in *Toonan v. Australia* that groups not explicitly named under international law are protected under these covenants (HRC, 2011). Sexual orientation and gender minorities are classified as members of a "particular social group" (UN High Commissioner for Refugees, 2008, p. 6) and hence protected from discrimination or exclusion from basic rights.

Despite the clear mandate of international law, the operational legal status of LGBTQI individuals and communities changes yearly. The International Lesbian, Gay, Bisexual, Trans, and Intersex Association (ILGA) provides up-to-date information on laws around the globe ranging from age of consent laws to restrictions related to military service to laws prohibiting discrimination. These maps can be effectively used in advocacy work to raise educational awareness concerning the legal and human rights of sexual orientation and gender minorities internationally (International Lesbian, Gay, Bisexual, Trans and Intersex Association [ILGA], 2013).

Care should be used when viewing the maps on the ILGA webpage. At first glance, it might appear that oppression is tied to poor economic development or religion. However, such conclusions would be overly simplistic. For example, many economically poor nations do not criminalize LGBTQI behaviors and wide variability exists within geographic region (e.g., Burma—illegal; Cambodia—legal). Conversely, only in recent years have same-sex physical relations been decriminalized in the United States as a consequence of the 2003 Supreme Court *Lawrence v. Texas* decision—although discrimination in employment, housing, and so on, is still legal in many states. Moreover, there is wide variability between and within religions in relation to bias against members of the LGBTQI communities. In sum, a myriad of factors play a role in the LGBTQI laws around the globe, including economics, religion, cultural traditions, and the lasting ramifications of colonization, particularly in postcolonized nations.

SOCIAL JUSTICE ISSUES

The scale of justice for LGBTQI individuals and communities unfortunately is weighted negatively. Even under the best of circumstances, LGBTQI individuals experience discrimination in their lives or through the media. Under the worst of conditions, individuals live under a cloud of oppression and fear, as their lives are considered forfeit by governmental mandates. Such bias and discrimination comes with a cost to the psychological well-being of individuals, particularly those with multiple minority status identities. Unfortunately, many LGBTQI individuals experience depression, lowered self-esteem, health-related concerns, and internalized homophobia/transphobia, as a result of discrimination, minority stress, and social stigma (Cochran & Mays, 2000; Cochran, Sullivan, & Mays, 2003; DiPlacido, 1998; Kertzner, Meyer, Frost, & Stirratt, 2009; Mays & Cochran, 2001; Meyer, 2003a, 2003b).

Issues such as freedom from violence, access to meaningful work, safe housing, and the right to a family are all at the core of what it means to be human, and are considered fundamental human rights. Our discussion is not meant to be an exhaustive list and does not represent a review of the literature for each topic. Rather, we seek to highlight some of the major social justice concerns for LGBTQI communities and the impact of social justice denied on physical and psychological health.

Violence

Violence grounded in homophobia and transphobia represents a significant violation of human rights and occurs across all global regions (HRC, 2011). Within the United States, Potok (2010) examined 14 years of federal hate crime statistics and reported that "gay people are more than twice as likely to be attacked in a violent hate crime as Jews or blacks; more than four times as likely as Muslims; and 14 times as likely as Latinos" (para. 7). LGBTQI youth are at particular risk for violence and school bullying (Horn & Nucci, 2006; Hunter, J., 1992; McFarland & Dupuis, 2001; Murphy, 2001; Nadal & Griffin, 2011; Potok, 2010). In a study of youth visiting a social service agency, Hunter (1992) found that 41% of gay and lesbian youth had been victims of a violent attack with 46% of those assaults the result of antigay sentiment. Unfortunately, those victimized youth also expressed a high degree of suicide ideation and reported attempts (41% and 34%, females and males, respectively). The Gay British Crime Survey reported that one-third of lesbian women and one-quarter of gay men had experienced a hate crime or bias incident in the past three years (Stonewall, 2009). In Australia, Hillier et al. (2010) reported the incidence of abuse and violence against lesbian and gay youth to be

61% for verbal abuse, 18% for physical abuse, and 26% reporting "other forms of homophobia" (p. ix). Unfortunately, very few nations record or report LGBTQI hate crimes and bias incidents, which makes prevention, monitoring, and intervention very difficult.

Transgendered individuals are at particular risk for physical and sexual violence (Clements-Nolle, Marx, & Katz, 2006; Lombardi, Wilchins, Priessing, & Malouf, 2001; Testa et al., 2012). These levels parallel increased risk for suicide ideation and history of single or repeated suicide attempts (Clemets-Nolle et al., 2006; Testa et al., 2012). Surveys have found that 43–60% of transgendered respondents have been victims of physical violence (Kenagy & Bostwick, 2005; Lombardi et al., 2001; Xavier, Bobbin, Singer, & Budd, 2005) with rates of 43–46% for sexual assault (Clements-Nolle et al., 2006; Kenagy & Bostwick, 2005; Xavier et al., 2005). The effects of oppression and violence on transgendered individuals are extreme. The National Transgender Discrimination Survey reported that 41% of all respondents had attempted suicide at least once with rates over 50% for those who lost a job due to discrimination or who have been bullied in school. Rates for suicide attempts exceeded 60% for those who had experienced physical or sexual assault (Grant et al., 2011).

Rape as a form of hate crime against sexual orientation and gender minorities has been well documented (HRC, 2011; Rothman, Exner, & Baughman, 2011). LGBTQI individuals are at risk for rape by members of their families, organized street gangs and hate groups, or other individuals within their communities for defying cultural and religious norms (HRC, 2011). According to the UN Special Rapporteur for women's rights, "lesbian women face an increased risk of becoming victims of violence, especially rape, because of widely held prejudices and myths . . . for instance, that lesbian women would change their sexual orientation if they are raped by a man" (HRC, 2011, p. 10). Lesbian women in some families and communities also face the reality of forced impregnation as a tool to seemingly force a change in sexual orientation (HRC, 2011).

Murders, including so-called honor killings of sexual orientation and gender minorities, have been reported around the globe (HRC, 2011). Such murders may or may not be reported, recorded, or prosecuted, depending on the laws and norms of a nation-state. The UN, the African Commission on Human and Peoples' Rights, the Inter-American Commission on Human Rights, the European Parliament, the Council of Europe, and the Organization for Security and Cooperation in Europe (OSCE) have all expressed concern about the patterns of violence targeting sexual orientation and gender minorities (HRC, 2011). Violence against LGBTQI individuals is often quite brutal involving torture, rape, cutting, mutilation, and dismemberment of genitalia and breasts (Altschiller, 2005; HRC, 2011). Altschiller (2005) laments that the extreme brutality stems from "the absolute intent to rub out the human being because of his preference" (2005, p. 28).

Nations have a responsibility to protect individuals in state custody. However, LGBTQI individuals frequently experience harassment by police and violence within the criminal justice system (Franklin & Herek, 2003). According to the UN Committee against Torture (2006), LGBTQI internees in prison or under state control are at greater risk for violence, including torture and rape, by other prisoners and need additional protections. Unfortunately, violence against LGBTQI detainees occurs all too frequently at the hands of police and guards (HRC, 2011). Reports of violence include beatings, rape, and arbitrary solitary confinement. Moreover, transgendered individuals have reported being aggressively assaulted on the breast and genitals to cause disfigurement or the rupture of implants with concomitant release of toxins. According to the National Transgender Discrimination Survey, 16% of respondents who have been in jail reported being physically assaulted and 15% reported being sexually assaulted (Grant et al., 2011). Gay men have also been subjected to forced anal examinations as a tool to "prove" sexual orientation—a practice condemned by the UN Committee against Torture. Discrimination, harassment, and abuse at the hands of those commissioned to protect lead many LGBTQI individuals to avoid contact with police. For example, 22% of transgendered individuals report harassment by police. Such harassment is so well known that almost half of all transgendered individuals report reticence in seeking police assistance (Grant et al., 2011). Moreover, in nations where sexual orientation and gender minorities are criminalized, contact with the police may result in arbitrary detention, prosecution, or criminal sentencing.

It should be acknowledged that individuals who have been supportive of LGBTQI communities and active in such support have also been subjected to acts of violence because of their pro-LGBTQI positions or activism. Documented violence has ranged from supporters having their homes ransacked to activists being murdered for their social justice stance (HRC, 2011). The UN reports that many pro-LGBTQI groups face police raids, destruction of offices, and deregistration as nongovernmental organizations (HRC, 2011). Unfortunately, raids on LGBTQI organizations, including health care clinics, place sexual orientation and gender minorities at risk. Computer hard drives may contain personal information, and client files can be used to further discriminate against LGBTQI individuals particularly in states where gay and lesbian behavior is criminalized. In some nations (e.g., Lithuania, Nigeria, Uganda), publication of supportive LGBTQI documents is banned or heavily censored—these publications are deemed a threat to "public decency" (HRC, 2010, 2011, p. 21).

Much has been written about violence against LGBTQI individuals and communities in the United States (e.g., Garnets, Herek, & Levy, 2003; Herek & Berrill, 1992; Murphy, 2001). Additionally, there are organizations that track anti-LGBTQI violence in the United States and other regions (e.g., OSCE, www.osce.org/odihr/; National Coalition of Anti-violence Programs, www.avp.org/; FRA: http://fra.europa.eu/en/theme/lgbt). It is imperative that individual teaching about anti-LGBTQI violence or working with clients who have been victimized by such violence be cognizant of the threats and consequences of such assaults. Medical and mental health practitioners need to be informed about the special needs of LGBTQI trauma victims (Garnets et al., 2003; Hyman, 2009; Katsekas, 2001; Stermac &

Sheridan, 1993). Appropriate treatment and responses to violence can assist individuals in their path to recovery as well as facilitate growth, the development of positive coping mechanisms, and resilience (Garnets et al., 2003). Conversely, uninformed treatment may result in increased anxiety, internalized homophobia, and poor mental health outcomes (Stermac & Sheridan, 1993).

Relationships and Family

Families are generally viewed as a source of support and community for individuals throughout their lives. Unfortunately, families' rejection of their LGBTQI members may be a source of great despair and oppression. Individuals face complex challenges when "coming out" to friends and families (Whitley & Kite, 2010) and risk a range of abuses and discrimination at the hands of family for their sexual orientation or gender identity. According to the UN, this abuse and discrimination can take the form of

> being excluded from family homes, disinherited, prevented from going to school, sent to psychiatric institutions, forced to marry, forced to relinquish children, punished for activist work and subjected to attacks on personal reputation. Lesbians, bisexual women and transgender people are especially at risk owing to entrenched gender inequalities that restrict autonomy in decision-making about sexuality, reproduction and family life. (HRC, 2011, p. 21)

Lesbian women may be forced into marriage or pregnancy to "cure" their sexual orientation.

In addition to often experiencing family of origin issues, LGBTQI individuals create families. Lesbian women and gay men value and benefit from long-term committed relationships and, indeed, are quite successful at such partnerships (Peplau & Fingerhut, 2007). On a range of social and psychological aspects, there is very little difference between same-sex and heterosexual relationships, inclusive of both successful and more problematic partnerships (Kurdek, 2005; Peplau & Fingerhut, 2007). State-mandated limitations placed on such bonds, and denial of committed relationships, have a negative impact on individuals in same-sex relationships. Societal denial of relationship status is associated with increased stress and adversely affects mental health (Hatzenbuehler, McLaughlin, Keyes, & Hasin, 2010; Rostosky, Riggle, & Horne, 2009). Lack of relationship recognition extends into a host of very pragmatic arenas. For example, in the United States, denial of relationship status impacts access to death benefits, access to public housing, insurance benefits, and denial of a foreign partner entry into a country. Campaigns against same-sex marriage regrettably further stigmatize gays and lesbians and can increase cultural levels of prejudice and discrimination (Herek, 2006, 2011).

In 2011, the American Psychological Association (APA) passed the Resolution on Marriage Equality for Same-Sex Couples, which highlights the research concerning same-sex marriage. This resolution not only "calls on the federal government to extend full recognition to legally married same-sex couples, and to accord them all of the rights, benefits, and responsibilities that it provides to legally married different-sex couples," but also encourages psychologists to take the lead in fighting discrimination and promoting education about the effects of stigma (APA, 2011a). The American Psychiatric Association (2005), American Sociological Association (2010–2011), the American Anthropological Association (2005), and the Canadian Psychological Association (2006) have issued similar position statements. The ILGA website (www.ilga.org) provides up-to-date information related to international same-sex marriage and LGBTQI advocacy.

Unfortunately, the UN falls short concerning marriage rights for gays and lesbians noting that nation-states are not required under international law to legalize gay marriage (HRC, 2011). Internationally, in 2012, 11 countries recognized same-sex marriage: the Netherlands, Belgium, Spain, Canada, South Africa, Norway, Sweden, Portugal, Iceland, Argentina, and Denmark. In early 2013, only 10 U.S. states (e.g., Connecticut, Iowa, Washington, Vermont), the District of Columbia, and three Native American tribes recognized same-sex marriage. The majority of U.S. states prohibited same-sex marriage, including by constitutional amendment (Human Rights Campaign, 2012). Ironically, U.S. state constitutional amendments defining marriage as a relationship solely between one man and one woman unwittingly may have nullified many marriages that involve intersex individuals and certainly do not address the issue of transgender individuals who transition following marriage. State laws are subject to federal challenge, and in early 2013, two U.S. Supreme Court cases related to the issue of same-sex marriage were heard. Hence, the issue of same-sex marriage within the United States is in a period of challenge and change.

According to the American Community Survey, approximately 19% of same-sex couple households include children (Lofquist, 2011). This survey also reported that same-sex couples have a higher percentage of adopted children than opposite-sex couples. Unfortunately, the survey does not track the number of children living in single-parent gay men or lesbian women households. Significant stigma has historically been associated with gay and lesbian parenting, including the belief that sexual orientation minorities are both morally and psychologically unfit to be parents. However, there is no empirical support for such beliefs (Patterson, 2005). Even more importantly, there is no empirical evidence that children, including adopted children, of gay and lesbian parents differ significantly in psychosocial development from children raised by heterosexual parents (Farr, Forssell, & Patterson, 2010; Patterson, 2005; Stacey & Biblarz, 2001). APA passed the 2004 Resolution on Sexual Orientation Parents, and Children, which states that the "APA opposes any discrimination based on sexual orientation in matters of adoption, child custody and visitation, foster care, and reproductive health services" and again encourages education, advocacy, and protections of the rights of gay men, lesbian women, and their children (APA, 2004).

Education

Unfortunately, children and youth identified as LGBTQI face difficulties with admission to schools and an increased risk of expulsion (HRC, 2011). While in school, LGBTQI youth often experience discrimination, taunting, bullying, and physical violence, not just by their classmates but also by their teachers (HRC, 2011). Bullying and violence against LGBTQI youth has been connected to greater absenteeism, mental health concerns (e.g., depression, low self-esteem, increased sexual risk-taking behaviors, decreased health seeking behaviors), and suicide risk (Horn & Nucci, 2006; HRC, 2011; Hunter, 1992; McFarland & Dupuis, 2001; Murphy, 2001; Nadal & Griffin, 2011; Potok, 2010; UNESCO, 2012). Hillier et al. (2010) reported that experiences with homophobic abuse negatively impacted school performance in over half of the students studied. Transgendered individuals appear to experience the greatest level of bullying and abuse with over 78% reporting harassment and 35% and 12% reporting physical assault and sexual assault, respectively (Grant et al., 2011). When schools are places of pain, LGBTQI students are much more likely to do poorly or to drop out. This denial of education has long-term impacts on future employment and well-being.

Organizations such as Teaching Tolerance: a Project of the Southern Poverty Law Center (see www.tolerance.org/) offer teaching kits, activities, publications, curricula, and school guides aimed at ameliorating prejudice, bias, and discrimination in the school system. For example, the What's So Bad about "That's So Gay"? lesson plan is aimed at elementary school children to address bias at an early age (Teaching Tolerance, 2012.) The UNESCO Rio Statement on Homophobic Bullying and Education for All calls for the following actions:

- Safe school climates free of anti-LGBTQI bias and violence;
- Access to accurate health and sexuality information relevant to the needs of all learners, including LGBTQI people;
- Teachers and school staff prepared and willing to maintain learning environments truly accessible and productive for all; and
- Mechanisms of periodic review by which educational institutions, systems and governments consult with development partners and all education sector stakeholders in order to hold themselves accountable to these principles. (UNESCO, 2011, para. 7)

The APA also sponsors the Healthy Lesbian, Gay, and Bisexual Students Project (see www.apa.org/pi/lgbt/programs/hlgbsp/index.aspx). This project provides information about the challenges faced by LGBTQI youth in schools as well as research, information, and links aimed at building safer school environments. The school staff professional development page includes a "toolbox" with resources such as model antidiscrimination and antiharassment policies for schools.

Health Care

The International Covenant on Economic, Social, and Cultural Rights (UN, 1966b) argues that all individuals should have access to health care in order to attain the highest level of physical and mental health. Obviously, many countries fall short of this goal. Minority status, lack of transportation, lack of doctors, or limited economic means all impact health care accessibility. In regions where LGBTQI status is either highly discriminated against or criminalized, many sexual orientation or gender minority individuals avoid contact with the health care system for fear of reprisals (HRC, 2011). The entire community may be impacted by LGBTQI fear of or denial of access to the medical profession. For example, health care avoidance negatively affects efforts aimed at prevention and intervention of person-to-person transmitted diseases, including HIV/AIDS (HRC, 2011). Health care risks and lack of access to medical care in many parts of the world are particularly extreme for lesbian, intersex, and transgendered women (UN Committee on the Elimination of Discrimination against Women [CEDAW], 2011) due to the added burden of multiple minority statuses.

Abuses against LGBTQI individuals and their families have occurred within health care systems around the globe. These abuses can range from denial of LGBTQI hospital or long-term care visitation for partners and spouses of individuals in same-sex relationship to forced psychiatric hospitalizations and "reparative therapies" (APA, 2009; HRC, 2011; Woolf, 2002). The UN has denounced the all-too-common practice of using the therapeutic relationship to attempt to change an individuals' sexual orientation—sometimes referred to as "reparative therapy." The UN unequivocally criticized such approaches as "unscientific, potentially harmful and contributing to stigma" (HRC, 2011, p. 18). The APA has also argued against the use of therapies designed to change one's sexual orientation and outlined its rationale in the 2009 Resolution on Appropriate Affirmative Responses to Sexual Orientation Distress and Change Efforts noting that "same-sex sexual and romantic attractions, feelings, and behaviors are normal and positive variations of human sexuality" (para. 19). In 2012, the state of California passed a law banning such "reparative" treatments for individuals under the age of 18. However, this law is currently being appealed in federal court (Eckhorn, 2013).

Health care professionals must receive appropriate training and professional competence prior to working with sexual orientation and gender minorities. Transgendered individuals have reported the need to "teach" their health care professionals about transgender care over 50% of the time (Grant et al., 2011). Individuals may avoid health care due to the effects of marginalization, despite greater health care needs resulting from challenges associated with poverty, poor housing, and the social-psychological effects of extreme oppression. Transgendered individuals have over four times the national average for HIV infection and higher rates of smoking, alcohol and drug abuse, and a host of mental health concerns, including suicide effects (Grants et al., 2011). Health care for transgendered individuals as well as intersex individuals is often ill-informed and marginalizing. Indeed, infants born intersex are at risk from birth as often they experience gender assignment in infancy. The assumption is that their intersex "condition" is a medical problem to be addressed and corrected (Gough et al., 2008; Mackenzie et al., 2009; Reis, 2009). Intersex children are frequently exposed to unnecessary surgeries based on societal norms of gender correctness, often without the child's or the parent's informed consent (CEDAW, 2011; HRC, 2011).

Mental health treatment must be multiculturally appropriate, evidence-based, and grounded in respect for the client/patient. Resources are available for those working with LGBTQI populations on mental health issues (e.g., Bieschke, Perez, & DeBord, 2007; Singh, Boyd, & Whitman, 2010). In 2011, the APA approved the Guidelines for Psychological Practice with Lesbian, Gay, and Bisexual Clients. These guidelines provide psychologists and other mental health practitioners with practical information concerning a range of topics from education and training to family-related issues (APA, 2011b). Although the need is great, formal training programs grounded in empirically based, culturally appropriate practice for work with LGBTQI individuals, families, and groups are limited.

The resolutions and training approaches discussed earlier are significant given the history of U.S. psychiatric practice and the classification of sexual orientation and minority gender status as pathologies. The *Diagnostic and Statistical Manual of the America Psychiatric Association* (*DSM*; APA) has undergone several revisions. The *DSM-I* included homosexuality as a form of "sociopathic personality disturbance" (Bohan, 1996, p. 18). The *DSM-II* was revised to change homosexuality from a personality disturbance to a sexual orientation disturbance in 1968. During this time of social change, LGBTQI activists challenged the *DSM* classification. Members of the APA Task Force on Nomenclature and Statistics met with activists to review the research related to homosexuality and discuss options (Spitzer, 1973). Dr. John E. Fryer presented as part of the annual APA Convention as Dr. H. Anonymous, complete with baggy tuxedo, mask, wig, and voice-distorting microphone. As a gay psychiatrist he discussed the damage caused by the deviance diagnosis and the lack of research evidence to support such a biased diagnosis (Clendinen, 2003). Hence, the *DSM-III* removed homosexuality from its list of disorders. Unfortunately, the *DSM-III* included the classification of ego-dystonic homosexuality for those unhappy with their sexual orientation (Spitzer, 1973). The *DSM-III-R* removed this diagnostic classification (Bayer, 1987). The World Health Organization removed homosexuality from the *International Statistical Classification of Diseases and Related Health Problems* (*ICD*) in 1992. Transgendered individuals continue to be diagnosed as Gender Identity Disorder (GID) under the *DSM-IV TR*. The *DSM-V* removed GID but replaced it with Gender Dysphoria (gender incongruence paired with dysphoria) (APA, 2013). The *ICD-10 CM* still provides a diagnostic code for transsexualism and transvestism in the "Index to Diseases and Injuries" (World Health Organization, 1992, p. 1100). Ironically, although having normative human behavior identified as a diagnosis or disorder is a form of destructive labeling, some LGBTQI advocates argue that such labeling can have benefits in terms of providing access to insurance coverage and in combating discrimination in many arenas (e.g., the workplace) (Beredjick, 2012).

Housing and Employment

As sexual orientation and gender minority statuses are not protected categories in U.S. federal housing legislation, LGBTQI people can easily face discrimination in the housing market. However, several states include sexual orientation in their housing antidiscrimination statutes (e.g., California, Delaware, Nevada, Wisconsin; Department of Housing and Urban Development, 2012). Unfortunately, laws concerning gay men and lesbian women may not be applied equally to transgendered individuals and statutes may be selectively enforced.

According to the National Transgender Discrimination Survey, transgendered respondents reported discrimination in housing with 19% turned away from an apartment or home and 11% having experienced an eviction (Grant et al., 2011). In addition, home ownership is half that of the general population and transgendered individuals have twice the level of homelessness. Many homeless transgendered individuals face harassment in shelters or are refused access altogether when seeking assistance. Unfortunately, LGBTQI youth also make up a disproportionate percentage of the homeless youth population and are at risk for discrimination and violence in shelters (Hunter, 2008).

Discrimination in employment is a violation of the UN International Covenant on Economic, Social, and Cultural Rights (UN, 1966b). Currently, 52 countries have laws that prohibit discrimination in the workplace based on sexual orientation (Itaborahy, 2012). The United States is not listed as a nation with such protections. Rather, select cities and states, but not all, provide protections from discrimination in the workplace. As such, in many parts of the United States and around the globe, individuals can be denied employment or fired from their positions with little or no recourse. For those unemployed due to their LGBTQI identification, particularly youth, an underground economy often exists involving the sex trade (Grant et al., 2011).

Despite laws aimed at preventing workplace discrimination, many LGBTQI individuals encounter bias, both implicit and explicit, in their places of employment. According to the European Union Agency for Fundamental Rights (2010),

> LGBT persons experience discrimination and homophobia in the workplace through direct and indirect discrimination (access to employment, dismissal and lack of promotion); unequal treatment in the areas of

> appreciation, performance pressure, advancement, training, and/or earnings, and/or holiday; harassment in the form of demeaning or derogatory statements, name-calling or insults, use of abusive language by colleagues, mocking, ridicule, gossip or rumours; sexually explicit remarks; and social isolation. (p. 64)

Kjaerum (2010) asserted that awareness, diversity training, dialogue, prevention, and enforcement of antidiscrimination policies are all essential to the healthy function of markets and workplaces.

In the United States, gay men earn significantly less than heterosexual men (between 11% and 27% less), whereas lesbian women tend to earn more than heterosexual women (between 20 and 34% more) (Antecol, Jong, & Steinberger, 2008; Badgett, 1995; Baumle & Poston Jr., 2011; Black, Makar, Sanders, & Taylor, 2003). Coming out at work can pose significant problems for gay and lesbian workers, including termination, loss of promotion, and job anxiety. Being open about one's sexual orientation at work is related to higher levels of job satisfaction and lower levels of job anxiety (Griffith & Hebl, 2002). Griffith and Hebl (2002) found that gay and lesbian workers were more likely to be "out" when workers evaluated the environment as "gay-friendly," but the presence of organizational structures (e.g., nondiscrimination policies or special interest groups) was not related to increased disclosure.

In the Transgender National Discrimination Survey, transgendered individuals reported twice the level of unemployment as the general population and 90% reported experiences of discrimination, harassment, and abuse at work (Grant et al., 2011). Many transgendered individuals reported delaying transitioning during employment and endeavored to hide their gender status. Ironically, individuals who opted to transition during their time of employment cited increased productivity and work satisfaction despite an increase in harassment.

CLOSING THOUGHTS

The UN actively endeavors to address issues related to sexual orientation and gender minorities and protect all individuals regardless of identity around the globe. Organizations within the UN (e.g., Office of the United Nations High Commissioner for Human Rights; Office of the United Nations High Commissioner for Refugees; United Nations Children's Fund) not only provide educational and legal resources related to LGBTQI concerns but also provide personal support for individuals who may be seeking human rights assistance, legal redress, or asylum. Of course, individuals facing extreme oppression with limited resources may not have easy access to UN assistance. Many states within the United States also have human rights commissions that respond to cases of LGBTQI abuses domestically.

There are many resources available for individuals working with LGBTQI populations or who simply want to know more about social justice concerns related to sexual orientation and gender minorities. The Public Interest Directorate of the

APA maintains a large website with resources for psychologists concerned about or working with members of the LGBTQI communities (see www.apa.org/pi/lgbt/index.aspx). Policy statements range from the resolutions discussed previously to issues such as military service, hate crimes, and transgender, gender identity, and gender expression nondiscrimination. All told, the APA has 14 resolutions as current policy on LGBTQI issues. Each policy statement is supported by scientific research on the topic, and, hence, each resolution can be used for educational as well as advocacy purposes. The APA LGBT website also includes policy news, publications, and information about current legislative actions. Extensive web links are provided on the "Advocacy" page to various organizations working on LGBTQI issues, additional resources within the APA, and current projects.

It is imperative that psychology play a role in advocacy, education, research, public policy, and practice issues related to LGBTQI individuals, communities, and social justice. As a profession, psychology is uniquely poised to address issues such as discrimination and violence from a multicultural and empirically based perspective. Together with professionals from other disciplines such as sociology, human rights, and the law, psychologists can have an impact on the local and global levels. Without action, social justice will continue to be denied, individuals will be harmed, and, unfortunately, lives will be lost.

> When individuals are attacked, abused or imprisoned because of their sexual orientation, we must speak out. We cannot stand by. We cannot be silent. Human Rights Day commemorates the Universal Declaration of Human Rights. It is not called the partial declaration of human rights. It is not the sometimes declaration of human rights. It is the universal Declaration, guaranteeing all human beings their basic human rights—without exception.
>
> UN secretary general Ban Ki-moon (2010)

REFERENCES

ACSF Investigators. (1992). Aids and sexual behaviour in France. *Nature, 360,* 407–409.

Altschiller, D. (2005). *Hate crimes.* Santa Barbara, CA: ABC-CLIO.

American Anthropological Association. (2005). *Statement on marriage and the family.* Retrieved from http://www.aaanet.org/stmts/marriage.htm

American Psychiatric Association. (2005). *Support of legal recognition of same-sex civil marriage.* Retrieved from https://ecf.cand.uscourts.gov/cand/09cv2292/evidence/PX0886.pdf

American Psychiatric Association. (2013). *Highlights of changes from DSM-IV-TR to DSM-5.* Retrieved from www.psychiatry.org/ . . . /DSM/DSM . . . /Changes-from-DSM-IV-TR—to-DSM-5.pdf

American Psychological Association. (2004). *Sexual orientation, parents, and children.* Retrieved from http://www.apa.org/about/policy/parenting.aspx

American Psychological Association. (2009). *Resolution on appropriate affirmative responses to sexual orientation distress and change efforts.* Retrieved from http://www.apa.org/about/policy/sexual-orientation.aspx

American Psychological Association. (2011a). *Resolution on marriage equality for same-sex couples.* Retrieved from http://www.apa.org/about/policy/same-sex.aspx

American Psychological Association. (2011b). Practice guidelines for psychological practice with lesbian, gay, and bisexual clients. Retrieved from www.apa.org/pi/lgbt/resources/guidelines.aspx

American Sociological Association. (2010–2011). *ASA statement against the proposed Constitutional amendment prohibiting same-sex marriage.* Retrieved from http://www.asanet.org/about/Council_Statement_on_Gay_Marriage.cfm

Antecol, H., Jong, A., & Steinberger, M. (2008). The sexual orientation wage gap: The role of occupational sorting and human capital. *Industrial & Labor Relations Review, 61,* 518–543.

Badgett, M. V. L. (1995). The wage effects of sexual orientation discrimination. *Industrial and Labor Relations Review, 48,* 726–739.

Baird, V. (2003). Transgender identities: Like stars in the sky. In S. Plous (Ed.), *Understanding prejudice and discrimination* (pp. 415–418). New York, NY: McGraw-Hill.

Baumle, A. K., & Poston Jr., D. L. (2011). The economic cost of homosexuality: Multilevel analyses. *Social Forces, 89,* 1005–1031.

Bayer, R. (1987) *Homosexuality and American psychiatry: The politics of diagnosis.* Princeton, NJ: Princeton University.

Beredjick, C. (2012, July 23). DSM-V to rename Gender Identity Disorder "Gender Dysphoria." *Advocate.* Retrieved from http://www.advocate.com/politics/transgender/2012/07/23/dsm-replaces-gender-identity-disorder-gender-dysphoria

Bieschke, K. J., Perez, R. M., & DeBord, K. A. (Eds.) (2007). *Handbook of counseling and psychotherapy with lesbian, gay, bisexual, and transgender clients* (2nd ed.). Washington, DC: American Psychological Association.

Black, D., Makar, H. R., Sanders, S., & Taylor, L. (2003). The earnings effects of sexual orientation. *Industrial & Labor Relations Review, 56,* 449–469.

Bohan, J. S. (1996). *Psychology and sexual orientation: Coming to terms.* New York, NY: Routledge.

Boswell, J. (2005). Christianity, social tolerance, and homosexuality: Gay people in Western Europe from the beginning of the Christian era to the fourteenth century. Chicago, IL: University of Chicago Press.

Canadian Psychological Association. (2006). *Marriage of same-sex couples—2006 position statement.* Retrieved from http://www.asanet.org/about/Council_Statement_on_Gay_Marriage.cfm

Clements-Nolle, K., Marx, R., & Katz, M. (2006). Attempted suicide among transgender persons: The influence of gender-based discrimination and victimization. *Journal of Homosexuality, 51,* 53–69.

Clendinen, D. (2003, March 5). John Fryer, 65, psychiatrist who said he was gay in 1972, dies. *The New York Times.* Retrieved from http://www.nytimes.com/2003/03/05/obituaries/05FRYE.html

CNN. (2007). *Ahmadinejad speaks: Outrage and controversy follow.* Retrieved from http://www.cnn.com/2007/US/09/24/us.iran/index.html

Cochran, S. D., & Mays, V. M. (2000). Relation between psychiatric syndromes and behaviorally defined sexual orientation in a sample of the US population. *Journal of Epidemiology, 151,* 516–523.

Cochran, S. D., Sullivan, J. G., & Mays, V. M. (2003). Prevalence of mental disorders, psychological distress, and mental health service use among lesbian, gay, and bisexual adults in the United States. *Journal of Consulting and Clinical Psychology, 71,* 53–61.

Committee on the Elimination of Discrimination against Women. (2011, July 29). *Concluding observations of the Committee on the Elimination of Discrimination against Women.* Retrieved from www2.ohchr.org/english/ . . . /cedaw/docs/co/CEDAW-C-CRI-CO-5-6.pdf

Denny, D. (1997). *Current concepts in transgender identity.* New York, NY: Routledge.

Department of Housing and Urban Development. (2012). *Ending housing discrimination against lesbian, gay, bisexual and transgender individuals and their families: Enriching and strengthening our nation.* Retrieved from http://portal.hud.gov/hudportal/HUD?src=/program_offices/fair_housing_equal_opp/LGBT_Housing_Discrimination

Diamond, L. M. (2007). A dynamical systems approach to the development and expression of female same-sex sexuality. *Perspectives on Psychological Science, 2,* 142–161.

DiPlacido, J. (1998). Minority stress among lesbians, gay men, and bisexuals: A consequence of heterosexism, homophobia, and stigmatization. In G. M. Herek (Ed.), *Stigma and sexual orientation* (pp. 138–159). Thousand Oaks, CA: Sage.

Eckhorn, E. (2013, April 17). Court hears gay "conversion therapy" arguments. *The New York Times.* Retrieved from http://www.nytimes.com/2013/04/18/us/day-in-court-for-california-law-banning-conversion-therapy.html

European Union Agency for Fundamental Rights. (2010). *Homophobia and discrimination on grounds of sexual orientation and gender identity in the EU Member States, Part II: The social situation (updated version).* Retrieved from http:// fra.europa.eu/fraWebsite/ . . . /FRA_hdgso_report-part2_en.pdf

Farr, R. H., Forssell, S. L., & Patterson, C. J. (2010). Parenting and child development in adoptive families: Does parental sexual orientation matter? *Applied Developmental Science, 14,* 164–178.

Franklin, K., & Herek, G. M. (2003). Violence toward homosexuals. In S. Plous (Ed.), *Understanding prejudice and discrimination* (pp. 415–418). New York, NY: McGraw-Hill.

Garnets, L. D., Herek, G. M., & Levy, B. (2003). Violence and victimization of lesbians and gay men: Mental health consequences. In L. D. Garnets & D. C. Kimmel (Eds.), *Psychological perspectives on lesbian, gay, and bisexual experiences* (2nd ed.) (pp. 188–206). New York, NY: Columbia University.

Gates, G. (2011). *How many people are lesbian, gay, bisexual and transgender?* Retrieved from http://williamsinstitute.law.ucla.edu/wp-content/uploads/Gates-How-Many-People-LGBT-Apr-2011.pdf

Gough, B., Weyman, N., Alderson, J., Butler, G., & Stoner, M. (2008). "They did not have a word": The parental quest to locate a "true sex" for their intersex children. *Psychology and Health, 23,* 493–507.

Grace, P. A., Hill, R. J., Johnson, C. W., & Lewis, J. B. (2004). In other words: Queer voices/dissident subjectivities impelling social change. *International Journal of Qualitative Studies in Education, 17,* 301–324.

Grant, J. M., Mottet, L. A., Tanis, J., Harrison, J., Herman, J. L., & Keisling, M. (2011). *Injustice at every turn: A report of the National Transgender Discrimination Survey. Washington, DC: National Center for Transgender Equality and National Gay and Lesbian Task Force.* Retrieved from http://endtransdiscrimination.org/PDFs/NTDS_Report.pdf

Griffith, K. H., & Hebl, M. R. (2002). The disclosure dilemma for gay men and lesbians: "Coming out" at work. *Journal of Applied Psychology, 87,* 1191–1199.
Harper, C. (2007). *Intersex.* Oxford, UK: Berg.
Hatzenbuehler, M. L., McLaughlin, K. A., Keyes, K. M., & Hasin, D. S. (2010). The impact of institutional discrimination on psychiatric disorders in lesbian, gay, and bisexual populations: A prospective study. *American Journal of Public Health, 100,* 452–459.
Herek, G. M. (2006). Legal recognition of same-sex relationships in the United States: A social science perspective. *American Psychologist, 61,* 607–621.
Herek, G. M. (2011). Anti-equality marriage amendments and sexual stigma. *Journal of Social Issues, 67,* 413–426.
Herek, G. M., & Berrill, K. T. (Eds.). (1992). *Hate crimes: Confronting violence against lesbians and gay men.* Thousand Oaks, CA: Sage.
Hillier, L., Jones, T., Monagle, M., Overton, N., Gahan, L., Blackman, J., & Mitchell, A. (2010). *Writing themselves in 3, the third national study on the sexual health and well-being of same sex attracted and gender questioning young people.* Australian Research Centre in Sex, Health and Society. Retrieved from www.latrobe.edu.au/ssay/assets/downloads/wti3_web_sml.pdf
Horn, S. S., & Nucci, L. (2006). Harassment of gay and lesbian youth and school violence in America: An analysis and directions for intervention. In C. Daiute, Z. Beykont, C. Higson-Smith, & L. Nucci (Eds.), *International perspectives on youth conflict and development* (pp. 139–155). New York, NY: Oxford University.
Huffington Post. (2012). *Curtis Knapp, Kansas Pastor Who Said Government Should Kill Gays, Defends Statements.* Retrieved from http://www.huffingtonpost.com/2012/05/31/curtis-knapp-kansas-pastor-death-of-gays-defense-cnn_n_1559293.html
Human Rights Campaign. (2012). *Marriage center.* Retrieved from http://www.hrc.org/marriage-center
Human Rights Council. (2010). *Promotion and protection of all human rights, civil, political, economic, social and cultural rights, including the right to development.* Retrieved from http://www2.ohchr.org/english/bodies/hrcouncil/docs/14session/A.HRC.14.23.Add.1_AV.pdf
Human Rights Council. (2011). *Discriminatory laws and practices and acts of violence against individuals based on their sexual orientation and gender identity: Report of the United Nations High Commissioner for Human Rights.* Retrieved from http://www2.ohchr.org/english/bodies/hrcouncil/docs/19session/A.HRC.19.41_English.pdf
Hunter, E. (2008). What's good for the gays is good for the gander: Making homeless youth housing safer for lesbian, gay, bisexual, and transgender youth. *Family Court Review, 46,* 543–557.
Hunter, J. (1992). Violence against lesbians and gay male youths. In G. M. Herek & K. T. Berrill (Eds.), *Hate crimes: Confronting violence against lesbians and gay men* (pp. 76–82). Thousand Oaks, CA: Sage.
Hyman, B. (2009). Violence in the lives of lesbian women: Implications for mental health. *Social Work in Mental Health, 7,* 204–225.
International Lesbian, Gay, Bisexual, Trans and Intersex Association. (2013). Maps concerning legal and human rights of sexual orientation and gender minorities. Retrieved from www.ilga.org
Itaborahy, L. P. (2012). *State-sponsored homophobia: A world survey of laws criminalising same-sex sexual acts between consenting adults.* The International Lesbian, Gay,

Bisexual, Trans, and Intersex Association. Retrieved from http://old.ilga.org/State homophobia/ILGA_State_Sponsored_Homophobia_2012.pdf

Jenness, V., & Broad, K. (2009). *Hate crimes: New social movements and the politics of violence.* New Brunswick, NJ: Aldine Transaction.

Katsekas, B. S. (2001). Psychological violence against gay men and lesbian women: An interpersonal perspective. In D. Sandhu (Ed.), *Faces of violence: Psychological correlates, concepts, and intervention strategies* (pp. 213–227). Hauppauge, NY: Nova Science.

Kenagy, G. P., & Bostwick, W. B. (2005). Health and social service needs of transgender people in Chicago. *International Journal of Transgenderism, 8,* 57–66.

Kertzner, R. M., Meyer, I. H., Frost, D. M., & Stirratt, M. J. (2009). Social and psychological well-being in lesbians, gay men, and bisexuals: The effects of race, gender, age, and sexual identity. *American Journal of Orthopsychiatry, 79,* 500–510.

Ki-moon, B. (2010). *Secretary-General's remarks at event on ending violence and criminal sanctions based on sexual orientation and gender identity.* Retrieved from http://www.un.org/sg/statements/?nid=4992

Kjaerum, M. (2010). *Challenging heterosexual norms at the workplace: Legal and policy tools. Paper presented at the LGBT Business Leader Forum in Budapest.* Retrieved from http://fra.europa.eu/fraWebsite/attachments/MK_Speech_LGBT_Leader_Forum.pdf

Kurdek, L. A., (2005). What do we know about gay and lesbian couples? *Current Directions in Psychological Science, 14,* 251–254.

Lofquist, D. (2011). *Same-sex couple households: American Community Survey briefs.* Washington, DC: United States Census Bureau. Retrieved from www.census.gov/prod/2011pubs/acsbr10-03.pdf

Lombardi, E. L., Wilchins, R. A., Priessing, D., & Malouf, D. (2001). Gender violence: Transgender experiences with violence and discrimination. *Journal of Homosexuality, 42,* 89–101.

MacKenzie, D., Huntington, A., & Gilmour, J. A. (2009). The experiences of people with an intersex condition: A journey from silence to voice. *Journal of Clinical Nursing, 18,* 1775–1783.

Mays, V. M., & Cochran, S. D. (2001). Mental health correlates of perceived discrimination among lesbian, gay, and bisexual adults in the United States. *American Journal of Public Health, 91,* 1869–1876.

McFarland, W. P., & Dupuis, M. (2001). The legal duty to protect gay and lesbian students from violence in school. *Professional School Counseling, 4,* 171–179.

Melbye, M., & Biggar, R. J. (1992). Interactions between persons at risk for aids and the general population in Denmark. *American Journal of Epidemiology, 135,* 593–602.

Meyer, I. H. (2003a). Minority stress and mental health in gay men. In L. D. Garnets & D. C. Kimmel (Eds.), *Psychological perspectives on lesbian, gay, and bisexual experiences* (2nd ed., pp. 699–731). New York, NY: Columbia University.

Meyer, I. H. (2003b). Prejudice, social stress, and mental health in lesbian, gay, and bisexual populations: Conceptual issues and research evidence. *Psychological Bulletin, 129,* 674–697.

Murphy, B. (2001). Anti-gay/lesbian violence in the United States. In D. J. Christie, R. V. Wagner, & D. Winter (Eds.), *Peace, conflict, and violence: Peace psychology for the 21st century* (pp. 28–38). Upper Saddle River, NJ: Prentice Hall.

Nadal, K. L., & Griffin, K. E. (2011). Microaggressions: A root of bullying, violence, and victimization toward lesbian, gay, bisexual, and transgender youths. In M. Paludi (Ed.),

The psychology of teen violence and victimization, (Vols. 1 and 2): *From bullying to cyberstalking to assault and sexual violation; Prevention strategies for families and schools* (pp. 3–21). Santa Barbara, CA: Praeger/ABC-CLIO.

Nanda, S. (1985). The Hijras of India: Cultural and individual dimensions of an institutionalized third gender role. *Journal of Homosexuality, 11*(3–4), 35–54.

Patterson, C. J. (2005). Lesbian and gay parents and their children: Summary of research findings. In *Lesbian and gay parenting: A resource for psychologists.* Washington, DC: American Psychological Association. Retrieved from http://www.apa.org/pi/lgbt/resources/parenting-full.pdf

Peplau, L. A. & Fingerhut, A. W. (2007).The close relationships of lesbians and gay men. *Annual Review of Psychology, 58,* 405–424.

Peplau, L. A., & Garnets, L. D. (2000). A new paradigm for understanding women's sexuality and sexual orientation. *Journal of Social Issues, 56,* 329–350.

Potok, M. (2010, Winter). Gays remain minority most targeted by hate crimes. *Intelligence Report.* Retrieved from http://www.splcenter.org/get-informed/intelligence-report/browse-all-issues/2010/winter/under-attack-gays-remain-minority-mos

Preves, S. E. (2003). *Intersex and identity: The contested self.* New Brunswick, NJ: Rutgers University.

Reis, E. (2009). *Bodies in doubt: An American history of intersex.* Baltimore, MD: Johns Hopkins University.

Rostosky, S. S., Riggle, E. D. B., & Horne, S. G. (2009). Marriage amendments and psychological distress in lesbian, gay, and bisexual (LGB) adults. *Journal of Counseling Psychology, 56,* 56–66.

Rothman, E. F., Exner, D., & Baughman, A. L. (2011). The prevalence of sexual assault against people who identify as gay, lesbian, or bisexual in the United States: A systematic review. *Trauma, Violence, & Abuse, 12*(2), 55–66.

Savin-Williams, R. C. (2001). *Mom, Dad. I'm gay. How families negotiate coming out.* Washington, DC: American Psychological Association.

Sell, I. M. (2004). Third gender: A qualitative study of the experience of individuals who identify as being neither man nor woman. In R. B. Marchesani & E. Stern (Eds.), *Saints and rogues: Conflicts and convergence in psychotherapy* (pp. 131–145). New York, NY: Haworth Press.

Singh, A. A., Boyd, C. J., & Whitman, J. S. (2010). Counseling competency with transgender and intersex persons. In J. Cornish, B. A. Schreier, L. I. Nadkarni, L. Metzger, & E. R. Rodolfa (Eds.), *Handbook of multicultural counseling competencies* (pp. 415–441). Hoboken, NJ: John Wiley & Sons.

Smith, A. M. A., Rissel, C. E., Richters, J., Grulich, A. E., & de Visser, R. O. (2003). Sex in Australia: Sexual identity, sexual attraction and sexual experience among a representative sample of adults. *Australian and New Zealand Journal of Public Health, 27,* 138–145.

Spitzer, R. L. (1973). A proposal about homosexuality and the APA nomenclature: Homosexuality as an irregular form of sexual behavior and sexual orientation disturbance as a psychiatric disorder. *American Journal of Psychiatry, 130,* 1214–1216.

Stacey, J., & Biblarz, T. J. (2001). (How) Does sexual orientation of parents matter? *American Sociological Review, 65,* 159–183.

Statistics Canada. (2004, June 15). Canadian community health survey. *The Daily.* Retrieved from http://www.statcan.gc.ca/daily-quotidien/040615/dq040615b-eng.htm

Stermac, L. E., & Sheridan, P. M. (1993). Anti-gay/lesbian violence: Treatment issues. *Canadian Journal of Human Sexuality, 2,* 33–38.

Stonewall (2009). *Homophobic hate crime: The Gay British Crime Survey 2008*. Retrieved from http://www.stonewall.org.uk/ . . . /homophobic_hate_crime__final_report.pdf

Teaching Tolerance. (2012). What's so bad about "That's so gay." Retrieved from http://www.tolerance.org/activity/thats-so-gay

Testa, R. J., Sciacca, L. M., Wang, F., Hendricks, M. L., Goldblum, P., Bradford, J., & Bongar, B. (2012, August 13). Effects of violence on transgender people. *Professional Psychology: Research and Practice.* Advance online publication.

Thappa, D. M., Singh, N., & Kaimal, S. (2008). Homosexuality in India. *Indian Journal of Sexually Transmitted Diseases and AIDS, 29*(2), 59–62.

UNESCO. (2011). *Rio statement on homophobic bullying and education for all.* Retrieved from http://www.unesco.org/new/en/hiv-and-aids/our-priorities-in-hiv/gender-equality/anti-bullying/

UNESCO. (2012). *International consultation on homophobic bullying in educational institutions.* Retrieved from http://www.unescobkk.org/news/article/international-consultation-on-homophobic-bullying-in-educational-institutions/

United Nations. (1948) *Universal declaration of human rights.* Retrieved from http://www.un.org/en/documents/udhr/

United Nations. (1950). *Convention relating to the status of refugees.* Retrieved from http://www2.ohchr.org/english/law/refugees.htm

United Nations. (1966a). *International covenant on civil and political rights.* Retrieved from http://www2.ohchr.org/english/law/ccpr.htm

United Nations. (1966b). *International covenant on economic, social and cultural rights.* http://www2.ohchr.org/english/law/cescr.htm

United Nations Committee against Torture. (2006). *Consideration of reports submitted by states parties under article 19 of the convention: Conclusions and recommendations of the Committee against Torture, United States of America.* Retrieved from http://daccess-dds-ny.un.org/doc/UNDOC/GEN/G06/432/25/PDF/G0643225.pdf?OpenElement

United Nations High Commissioner for Refugees. (2008). *UNHCR guidance note on refugee claims relating to sexual orientation and gender identity.* Retrieved from http://www.justice.gov/eoir/vll/benchbook/resources/UNHCR_Guidelines_Sexual_Orientation.pdf

Whitley, B. E., & Kite, M. E. (2010). *The psychology of prejudice and discrimination* (2nd ed.). Belmont, CA: Wadsworth.

Wilhelm, A. D. (2010). Tritiya-Prakriti: People of the third sex: Understanding homosexuality, transgender identity, and intersex conditions through Hinduism. Bloomington, IN: XLibris.

Woolf, L. M. (2002). Gay and lesbian aging. *Siecus Report: Sexuality and Aging Revisited, 30*(2), 16–21.

World Health Organization. (1992). ICD-10-CM Index to diseases and injuries. Retrieved from ftp://ftp.cdc.gov/pub/Health_Statistics/NCHS/Publications/ICD10CM/2013/

Xavier, J., Bobbin, M., Singer, B., & Budd, E. (2005). A needs assessment of transgendered people of color living in Washington, D.C. *International Journal of Transgenderism, 8,* 31–47.

Chapter 10

Disability Activism and Psychology

Daniel Holland, Laura Sturm, Nicolas Culp, and Deidra Holland

The inclusion of a chapter on disability seldom needs to be defended in a book on social justice anymore. This positive development in the realm of justice studies, however, is relatively recent. Disability has, for much of modern history, been perceived primarily as a personal or medical problem, not a minority condition significant for its social and political implications. Of course, the perception of disability solely as "sickness" or "weakness" still persists in many forms and across many settings, and this perception is often fueled and complicated by the fact that many people with disabilities, unlike other minority positions, do indeed have medical or other conditions associated with their particular form of minority status. However, the recognition of disability as more complex than a diagnosis or a by-product of a physical or mental impairment, but as a human experience that, along with other social justice issues, involves a demand for human and civil rights, is one that has clearly dawned. This recognition is indeed critical progress that has been hard-earned from the efforts of disability rights activists over years of struggle, and it is one that is, fortunately, increasingly highlighted by the inclusion of disability issues in a discussion of social justice.

It is not an overstatement to say that disability issues represent one of the most urgent human rights concerns of our time. The World Health Organization (WHO) estimates that more than 1 billion individuals worldwide are living with a disability (WHO, 2011). This number represents approximately 15% of the global population. A disproportionate number of these people are living in poverty and are in transitioning or developing regions of the world. Unlike minority conditions such as ethnicity, race, and sexual orientation, disability constitutes a porous experience that any individual can be affected by beginning at any point in life, though it is an experience that is statistically more likely as one gets older. Indeed, it is an expanding realization that people with disabilities will be one of the most rapidly growing minority groups in the world in the coming decades as the global population ages (Holland, 2008). The awareness of disability as a human and civil rights issue will increasingly benefit every citizen of every nation, and will cross-cut many concomitant struggles for inclusion and equality. Because disability is a porous minority condition, one that any individual from any background and with any racial, ethnic, or sexual identity may begin experiencing at any point in life, it is also a human and civil rights focus that, due to its universal relevance, can serve as a shared, unifying focus across realms of political activism. (Notably, however, although disability is now well recognized as a social, political, and justice issue, and has relevance across realms of political activism, it remains a human experience that is still rarely addressed in forums or formal curricula addressing diversity; Olkin, 2002). The role of psychology as a discipline and profession in this expansive social justice issue could be significant, though evolution in the field will be necessary in order for such a role to be achieved. This chapter presents some of the issues inherent in disability as a social justice issue, offers a case example of the disability rights movement in postcommunist Central and Eastern Europe (CEE) as one reference point for understanding the developmental process of disability rights, and clarifies how professional psychology might forge a relevant role in the disability rights movement.

DISABILITY RIGHTS

The economist and Nobel Laureate, Amartya Sen (2004), has said "people with physical or mental disability are not only among the most deprived human beings in the world, they are also, frequently enough, the most neglected" (p. 1). Such recognition of disability as a basis for marginalization emphasizes its political significance: a human condition that results in a need for social and political advocacy, not solely medical or psychological care. Such a political perspective does not deny the fact that some people with disabilities require individual support or intervention. What a human rights perspective does achieve, however, is a clarification that the primary barriers to inclusion for people with disabilities are essentially social and political, not intrapersonal or medical. The barriers are wittingly and unwittingly constructed in such a way that those with certain differences in function are excluded from the main. The obligation of psychologists in the 21st century is not to defer to these barriers as reified constructions or to promote adjustment and acceptance in the minds of those who encounter them, but to identify and then challenge the social, political, and institutional practices that result in such exclusion. In order to do that, however, psychologists will need to become more familiar with the concept of human rights and the manifestation of disability through this particular lens.

HUMAN RIGHTS

Human rights refer to a relationship between each individual and the society within which he or she lives. The definition of this relationship is not always clear, and therefore it is not always agreed upon. But a fundamental aspect of human rights is that they are inherently possessed, in total, by all, not earned or meted out or subject to a partial or zero sum division. The human rights idea declares that every human being, in every political society, has "rights": recognized, legitimate claims upon his or her society to specific freedoms and other goods and benefits. They are claims "as of right," not by grace, love, charity, or compassion: claims that society is morally, politically, even legally obligated to respect, ensure, and realize. Human rights are claims not only against "bad people" or tyrannical government, but even against bona fide, benevolent, representative legislatures and democratic majorities. Human rights are not absolute and may bow to the public interest, but human rights do not bow lightly; rights may "trump" even a public interest duly determined in a democratic society (Henkin, 2000, p. 5).

Human rights, therefore, are possessed by virtue of being a person. They are considered inherent in every individual regardless of national context or government, and regardless of individual differences, including those associated with disability. However, although every person may possess such human rights in theory, it is clearly the case that such rights are not accessed equally. The more excluded one is from various forms of power, influence, and visibility, the less likely one is to benefit from such inherent rights and protections, and the more likely one is to need political and social vehicles to actualize their inherency. It is also the case that people with disabilities have historically been excluded from power, influence, and visibility everywhere on the globe, putting them at high risk of having their human rights violated and resulting in a greater need for protection and advocacy.

The nature of the risks posed to the human rights of people with disabilities has taken different forms across different societal and geopolitical contexts. In developed societies with extensive infrastructures, people with disabilities have undergone denial of freedoms in the form of forced institutionalization and chronic exclusion from the built environment, educational opportunities, and employment (e.g., Fleischer & Zames, 2011). In less-developed societies, where lack of an infrastructure may prevent such institutionalized mistreatment, people with disabilities have been subjected to other forms of social exclusion or personal danger (Holland, 2007; UNICEF, 2005). For example, in developing countries people with disabilities are significantly less likely to be educated (Filmer, 2008), and are more likely to be targeted for violence during times of ethnopolitical conflict (Groce & Peaglow,

2005). Regardless of the developmental status of any societal context, however, people with disabilities are almost uniformly the most disempowered, marginalized members within most large groups. Even among already vulnerable populations, like refugees or displaced persons or excluded ethnic minorities, those who also have disabilities will be even more severely marginalized within these larger vulnerable group contexts. It is well known, for example, that, globally, people with disabilities are overrepresented among the poorest of the poor (Yeo, 2005). At the same time, the poorest have been identified as "those whom it is permissible to reject" (Hossain cited by Hickey & Bracking, 2005, p. 855). Indeed, as a global minority, people with disabilities frequently face multiple and compounded social and political conditions that can lead to compromised human rights and therefore remain among the groups most in need of advocacy, visibility, and protection.

In fact, this need for advocacy, visibility, and protection has not gone unrecognized by some of those in the international human rights community. In 2006, the United Nations General Assembly formerly adopted the UN Convention on the Rights of Persons with Disabilities. This was the first global human rights convention of the 21st century (Quinn, 2009). Although leadership in the U.S. government initially refused to participate in the drafting or ratifying of the document, under a new administration President Obama signed the convention in 2009. The UN Convention on the Rights of Persons with Disabilities provides a critical moral compass for change, as well as a vehicle for gauging and codifying change (Quinn, 2009). The convention allows the international community to monitor the rights and status of people with disabilities in a large portion of the global community, and it facilitates the sharing and transfer of best practices in the promotion of rights for those who risk marginalization due to disability. It remains important to note, however, that Article 33 of the convention recognizes that "implementation of, and compliance with, international human rights treaties are ultimately domestic issues" (United Nations, 2006). Although this international convention promoting the rights of people with disabilities is clearly a watershed in the disability rights movement, the integrity of each nation's civil rights for citizens who have disabilities remains central to its impact.

CIVIL RIGHTS

Civil rights are distinguished from human rights in that they are specific to a country and its citizens or residents. Whereas human rights are considered inalienable qualities held by any person anywhere, civil rights are formalized by a country's laws and protections and apply only to those people who fall within the context of those national laws. Disability law in the United States, for example, is determined by a number of legal statutes, including the Americans with Disabilities Act and the Individuals with Disabilities Education Act: laws that specifically address the rights of citizens with regards to the built, educational, work, and other environments within the United States.

The fact that human and civil rights exist in some articulated form does not mean they are consistently well protected. Rights frequently need to be fought for, both in their establishment and in their continued insurance. The establishment and maintenance of disability rights, both human and civil, have been no exception. Although the long history of struggle for disability rights in North America has been well documented elsewhere (Fleischer & Zanes, 2011), recent cases in the United States, Mexico, and Canada illustrate that disability law is a realm that is often locked in a struggle not to lose ground: legislation protecting the rights of people with disabilities is often challenged, and the implementation of such legislation can be uneven or unequal, and consequences for failing to abide by established laws can be nonexistent. There is, therefore, a Sisyphean nature to the establishment and maintenance of disability rights at national and international levels, though unlike Sisyphus, the task of protecting disability rights, although continuous, is not futile.

A CASE STUDY: DISABILITY IN POSTCOMMUNIST EUROPE

One region that serves as a useful and important example of the development of disability rights is postcommunist CEE. The reason CEE is such a helpful example is that disability rights, like many other forms of human and civil rights, were often severely compromised under most communist regimes for many years. With the precipitous fall of communism in CEE beginning in 1989, the potential for civil society development, civic engagement, and democratic movements was suddenly reborn. These freedoms are essential to the existence of any disability rights movement, since they permit the organizing and advocacy so often essential to changes in citizens' rights movements. The development of disability rights in CEE since 1989, then, serves as one highly visible and accelerated example for understanding the steps and vehicles necessary in the developmental process of forging disability rights. In addition, one of the authors (Daniel Holland) has spent a significant amount of time living in CEE and working on disability rights and activist causes, providing firsthand familiarity with this region as a case study.

The political and economic transformation of Central Europe since the fall of communism in 1989 has been among the most remarkable democratic developments in modern times. As impressive as this ongoing political and economic transformation has been, however, not all citizens of the postcommunist Central European nations have benefited equally or, as some suggest, even at all (Brunwasser, 2009). People with disabilities in some nations within the CEE may represent a specific minority group for which little has improved since the fall of communism almost 25 years ago. There are numerous anecdotal and eye witness accounts suggesting that a large number of people with disabilities in some countries of the postcommunist region continue to face severe economic and political marginalization, segregation, and compromised human rights (e.g., Jenkins, Klein, & Parker, 2005). These anecdotal and eye witness accounts indicate that people with disabilities are often still institutionalized in custodial settings for long periods of time, have severely limited community-based supports available to facilitate de-institutionalization, are overwhelmingly underemployed or unemployed, and continue to have few educational options. Although it is certainly true that restriction on political freedoms negatively affected the whole of communist societies, people with disabilities were particularly disadvantaged for a number of reasons. Firstly, because they had been a marginalized group even before the onset of communism, without an established network of organizations or a cohesive minority identity, they could not build on existing independent institutions the way, for example, certain faith-based groups or occupational groups (lawyers, physicians, etc.) could. Secondly, as an economically disadvantaged group, people with disabilities were dependent upon state support for their sustenance. This support, however, was framed as charitable, rather than as a provision based on individual rights, compounding the dependency of recipients and casting them in the role of beneficiaries of the state, rather than full citizens. Finally, and perhaps most importantly, because of the imposed isolation of the communist countries, people with disabilities within these countries could not benefit from worldwide developments taking place after World War II, including civil and human rights movements that included, if only marginally at first, people with disabilities. During the 1960s and 1970s, when people with disabilities in Western Europe and North America were beginning to challenge guardianship and civil commitment laws, with de-institutionalization of large asylums being proposed, and with the movement toward rights-based models of citizenship gaining influence, their peers living in the communist countries of CEE were experiencing no such reforms. Indeed, people with disabilities in the communist countries did not even possess reliable knowledge that such reforms were occurring elsewhere (Holland, 2008).

A central feature of life for people with disabilities during the communist period, and often a defining feature of second-class citizenship in any political context, was their segregation from the mainstream of society. Many people with disabilities in many of the countries of the communist bloc were placed in facilities that still exist in high number and are still referred to as "social care homes," which were the equivalent of what the sociologist Goffman (1961) termed "total institutions." These institutions were typically large (many of them housing more than 50 to 100 persons) and located in remote and rural locations far away from concentrated residential areas. Residents of the social care institutions were classified as "voluntary" service users, but in fact could not leave without being granted permission, and so were de facto detained. Most of the residents of these institutions spent their entire lives in them, with no systematic processes of being re-integrated into the community. People, particularly children or young adults with developmental disabilities, were most likely to be placed in such institutions, but those with other disabilities like cerebral palsy or spina bifida or other complex conditions might also find themselves in such settings (Holland, 2003). It is important to note that placement in these institutions was most often driven by economic pressures upon families, more so than social pressures (Holland, 2008). A family who had a member with a disability faced few options in most of the communist countries: there were frequently no community-based support services for disability, no inclusion in the regular schools, and no realistic possibility for one parent to remain unemployed in order to provide care in the home. The result was enormous economic and practical pressure on the individual and family to rely on institutional care. The postcommunist governments of CEE have inherited these institutions and their persisting institutional inertia from their communist predecessors.

Even for those children with disabilities who were not institutionalized, segregated educational environments were imposed, resulting in another form of compromised opportunity. As noted in a fact-finding report for UNICEF conducted in 1999 by Mental Disability Rights International (MDRI):

> During [the first half of the 20th century], educational philosophy insisted on a State where as many children as possible could be brought up to standards that were predicated on "normal" development. This tradition still prevails today in Russia and much of Central and Eastern Europe. . . . Thus, instead of making schools accessible to children with disabilities, the child is excluded from school until he or she can be "corrected." In practice, some children will never conform to an inflexible "norm" and will remain in separate, segregated schools her or his entire life. (p. 10)

Many of the economic, philosophical, and infrastructural pressures that resulted in institutionalization or segregation of people with disabilities under communism are present today within the more market-driven economic systems these countries have adopted. Economic insecurity for many families in postcommunist bloc is significant, and community-based resources for people with disabilities, such as inclusive or special schools, or community mental health programs, are frequently not available. The result is that families who have a member with a disability are often left with limited options for the care, education, or support of that family member except for centralized residential options that could be far from home. The result can be the placement of someone in institutional care due to a lack of financial and community-based resources that would allow that individual to remain in his or her own community.

One crucial response to this situation, and a response that has been almost entirely due to increasing democratic freedoms in the postcommunist region, has been the development of nongovernmental organizations (NGOs) and other activist groups that have disability issues as their central cause. These NGOs and activist groups have been highly effective at forging progress along two fronts in a number of postcommunist countries. One front has to do with the development and provision of community-based services that provide necessary support to people with disabilities and their families in order to prevent or decrease the pressure for institutional care. Examples of such groups include the Kompa program in the Slovak Republic, which has been instrumental in establishing a model school program for children with disabilities (Holland, 2010). The other front in the disability rights movement in the postcommunist region involves policy and legislative activism. This front addresses the problem of existing laws, such as civil commitment and guardianship laws that fail to protect the rights and sovereignty of people with disabilities. An example of one such activist organization is the Mental Disability Advocacy Centre in Budapest, which serves a watchdog and advocacy function for the entire postcommunist region and whose lawyers have successfully brought cases of disability human rights violations in front of the European High Court for Human Rights in Strasbourg.

The central role of NGOs in securing disability rights in postcommunist Europe illustrates the critical importance that civil society has in promoting such minority rights. Because postcommunist Europe has been undergoing a rapid evolution in civil society freedoms, the degree to which such freedoms facilitate the development of disability rights can be more clearly recognized. It is the freedom exercised by regular citizens, unrestrained by the dominance of elite powers on the one hand, and unaccountable to the priorities of purely profit-driven demands on the other, who have been able to promote the interests and rights of the marginalized among them, including those with disabilities.

Indeed, the case of some nations in the postcommunist region of CEE illustrates what appears to be a consistent theme in the development of disability rights across geopolitical and cultural contexts, and throughout different eras. The evolution of such rights appears to follow a consistent process that depends upon individual activists, freely organized civil society groups, legislative process, and ongoing monitoring. The initial demand for recognition that people with disabilities are excluded or marginalized, for example, often appears to be dependent upon the efforts of a few individual activists. In CEE, as in North America and elsewhere, these early individual activists have often been those with direct experience of an urgent and even desperate need for reform: people who have disabilities themselves, or parents of children who do (see profiles of Erzsebet Szekeres and Javid Abedes in Bornstein, 2004). Following upon these few early voices has come the gradual influence of nongovernmental organizations and civil society groups, coalescing around specific issues or specific disability subtypes, where collective action has resulted in greater visibility and influence. Building upon the influence of organized civil society groups, the eventual representation of rights for people with disabilities in various realms of government policy and law takes place, though this stage in the evolution of disability rights can be slow and uneven, entailing long periods of plateau in the progress toward change. Finally, following on the establishment of legislative protections of disability rights, continued watchdog functions must be carried out at multiple levels of protection and advocacy in order to ensure that the formalized rights are respected. Following this evolutionary process in the postcommunist region has been helpful for elucidating the inter-dependence of citizen activism, civil society development, and democratic reform in government all within a relatively concentrated span of time, recognizing, too, that a good deal of development in disability rights still needs to occur.

Psychologists as Disability Activists

With the exception of a small number of intellectuals and activists (e.g., Gill, 1987, 2004; Linton, 1998; Mona, 1998; and a few others) professional psychologists have not been highly visible in the disability rights movement. This lack of involvement has probably occurred for a number of reasons. Psychologists (particularly clinical and counseling psychologists) are often educated and trained within a pathology-oriented paradigm (Holland, 2008). Such pathology-oriented approaches to disability wittingly or unwittingly place the burden of inclusion on the individual: the person with the disability is expected to make the effort necessary to transcend the condition in order to rejoin the nondisabled majority (Campbell, 2009; Holland, 2008; Linton, 1998). But such expectations ignore the social and political implications of disability, and neglect to address the fact that an inclusive social environment is still often essential for many people who have differences that are not amenable to change, even if change were sought.

A critical balance to strike in the engagement of psychologists in disability activism is the recognition that advocacy need not prohibit clinical care. The recognition that disability is a sociopolitical issue does not mean people with disabilities are removed from the same need for psychological care that people without disabilities often have, or that disability framed as a social and political issue cannot also be addressed as an individual concern. What it does mean, however, is that the sociopolitical context within which the person with a disability lives is relevant to that individual's psychological experience, and any psychological care of that individual needs to understand the social and political forces interacting with whatever personal issues that individual must confront.

The disability activist and psychologist, Linton (1998), called attention to the uncomfortable split between disability studies and disability rights on the one hand, and applied fields, such as psychology and other helping professions, on the other. Historically, this split has represented divergent approaches to disability, with applied fields viewing disability through a medical model of deficit and impairment, and disability studies and disability activism promoting a view that emphasizes a minority experience with political implications. But Linton identified the potential for ideas from disability studies and disability activism to retain independence from the medically driven and professionally oriented guilds, a position which suggests some restraint in her hopefulness. She nevertheless envisioned a possibility in which applied psychology can become more aware of the broader political meanings of disability, integrating such awareness into clinical work.

The clinical care of people with disabilities need not adhere to the biomedical paradigm of the past, a paradigm that has had an unfortunate hold over some corners of the field. In addition to symptom reduction, psychological care can involve promotion of an awareness that a broader disability community exists; a community to which one can belong and contribute, and from which one can draw politically and socially engaged sustenance. Psychotherapy is not equivalent to consciousness-raising, nor should it ever involve a form of proselytizing. Integrating a social and contextual perspective into the psychological care of people with disabilities remains essential, since there must co-exist, along with focused, evidence-based treatment, a consciousness of the ways in which broader environmental forces can contribute to the experiences of those who have disabilities in a world that is often not inclusive. This is an approach to clinical treatment that recognizes the importance of macrosystemic influences as identified in Bronfenbrenner's (1975) ecological systems theory, and approaches an understanding of the individual within a cultural and societal context, as proposed by the biopsychosocial model (Engel, 1977). An orientation to the sociopolitical context in which an individual finds himself or herself in is not a tangent or a distraction, but a critical element of effective intervention for those who, as a result of these contextual forces, are often at higher risk for needing psychological care (i.e., Gannon, 1982).

In many ways the field of psychology is already equipped to integrate a stronger social justice approach regarding disability into its mission. Professional psychology and graduate education for the field has increasingly attended to contextual factors, rather than adhering solely to a biomedical model of mental health and illness, particularly over the past two decades (e.g., Khubchandani & Williams-Nickelson, 2003). Professional psychology has long held a value for social justice issues as they impact minority concerns elsewhere. Indeed, professional psychologists who are also disability activists (e.g., Mona, 1998; Olkin & Pledger, 2003) outline specific ways that professional psychology and the more rights-oriented approach of disability studies can "join hands," emphasizing that such a hybrid model for professional psychology, uniting clinical care and social activism, is within reach. The key to such progress, however, may be for psychology to resolve its own long-standing identity confusion when it comes to its role as both a profession and a social cause, and this is a conflict that is rarely articulated or discussed.

PSYCHOLOGY'S IDENTITY CONFUSION AND ITS IMPLICATION FOR DISABILITY ACTIVISM

Professional psychology has long struggled with a dual identity that rarely gets articulated and, in fact, may at times hamper its relevance in the world at large. This dual identity concerns whether psychology, particularly clinical, counseling, and school psychology, is primarily a professional field, or, conversely, primarily a social cause. The problem with these dual identities is that they are, in some critical respects, mutually exclusive. A professional field, by definition, is exclusionary.

It exists as a realm of endeavor or practice that serves to exclude others who do not qualify in some way, cordoning off activities and reserving them only for those who gain entry through approved training, credentials, fees, or all three. A social cause, on the other hand, typically seeks to be as inclusive as possible. Often, the only criterion for membership in a social cause is a shared belief in its mission. Psychology, however, has often tried to serve both realms and, as a result, may have compromised its influence in each. Professional psychology has increasingly focused on cordoning off certain realms of practice in order to protect those realms for its constituent members. There is nothing inherently wrong with this; it is the same protective function taken by virtually all professions or guilds. A foundation based upon professional membership and credentialing, however, works in opposition to psychology's identity as a social cause, an identity increasingly embraced by the field and represented by advocacy and activist efforts by psychologists with a concern for social justice issues, including those tied directly to psychological health (del Soto, 2008; Eidelson & Eidelson, 2003). The result of this clash of priorities is an often confused and somewhat disoriented identity for the profession, one that strives to protect "turf" and economic priorities while at the same time promoting social issues that can benefit directly from what the profession has to offer.

The first step socially concerned psychologists might take in order to address the conflict between these dual identities is to relax their own professional allegiance, rather than perceive it solely as an asset. Although education and training in psychology can be valuable for understanding the complex issues facing people who are marginalized for any reason, adhering to the inherent process of exclusion that professional membership entails serves to undercut this advantage. Of course, such a path of departure from professional identity may mean forgoing the financial rewards and status of entrenched professional membership, and that may not be feasible for all of those psychologists who wish to be activists. But recognizing the contradiction embedded in the perception of psychology as both a professional guild and a social cause is essential to understanding the complications one faces when trying to simultaneously adopt the priorities of each. Only following reflection upon this contradiction can one make reasoned and constructive decisions regarding activist and professional choices (or activist *versus* professional choices) when working with marginalized groups generally and people with disabilities specifically.

CONCLUSION

As in any era, psychologists are currently in an age of many challenges for those who are dedicated to social justice issues. Those who possess an awareness of the complexities faced by people with disabilities, particularly what are often underrepresented psychological disabilities like mental illness or developmental delay, have an enormous contribution to make in the social justice realm. This involvement, however, necessitates a number of adjustments that extend beyond the typical education, training, and focus of professional psychologists. These typical emphases are on the acquisition of clinical knowledge that conceptualizes disability as a condition to be treated, with adjustment or amelioration as the goal. Such a goal is indeed worthy in many cases and is not to be flippantly devalued here. But such a goal is not the primary aim of disability activism. In order to be most effective in disability activism, one must gain an understanding of the broader social and political forces that impact those with disabilities, and recognize the vehicles or roles helpful for promoting the rights of those who are disabled. The disability activist must be prepared to identify the target of intervention, not the individual who is different, but the formal and informal patterns in the social and political environment that serve to oppress or devalue that individual because he or she is different. Such an activist mission bares an unusual challenge for the person educated and trained as a psychologist, since such professional preparation is particularly valuable for understanding the impact of oppressive forces on the person, but also tends to place the burden of change on that person. The point here, then, is that psychologists are both urgently needed in the continued global struggle for disability rights and possibly somewhat underprepared for it. Ultimately, however, the call to social justice so many psychologists seem constitutionally prone to hear will prevail in the lives of many. As more of those with a background in psychology enter into the realm of disability activism, they will recognize the need for change across multiple fronts. Much of that need for change, of course, will be in the broader political landscape, but some, as is the case with all activism, will be in their own previously learned assumptions. The result of more psychologists becoming invested in disability activism and the promotion of disability rights, however, cannot help but be a critically beneficial development for the cause.

REFERENCES

Bornstein, D. (2004). *How to change the world: Social entrepreneurs and the power of new ideas*. New York, NY: Oxford.

Bronfenbrenner, U. (1975). *Influences on human development*. New York, NY: Holt.

Brunwasser, M. (2009, January 5). Memo from Pravda: In Eastern Europe, lives languish in mental facilities. *New York Times*, A-7.

Campbell, F. (2009). Medical education and disability studies. *Journal of Medical Humanities, 30*(4), 221–235.

del Soto, A. G. (2008). Vulnerability, resiliency, and dignity: Psychosocial dimensions of the refugee experience. *Refuge: Canada's Journal on Refugees, 25*(1), 3–5.

Eidelson, R. J., & Eidelson, J. I. (2003). Dangerous ideas. *American Psychologist, 58*(3), 182–192.

Engel, G. L. (1977). The need for a new medical model: A challenge for biomedicine. *Science, 196*, 129–136.

Filmer, D. (2008). Disability, poverty, and schooling in developing countries: Results from 14 household surveys. *The World Bank Economic Review, 22*(1), 141–163.

Fleischer, D. Z., & Zames, F. (2011). *The disability rights movement: From charity to confrontation*. Philadelphia, PA: Temple University.

Gannon, L. (1982). The role of power in psychotherapy. *Women and Therapy, 1*(2), 3–11.

Gill, C. (1987). A new social perspective on disability and its implications for rehabilitation. *Occupational Therapy in Health Care, 4*(1), 49–55.

Gill, C. (2004). Depression in the context of disability and the "right to die." *Theoretical Medicine, 25,* 171–198.

Goffman, I. (1961). *Asylums: Essays on the social situation of mental patients and other inmates*. New York, NY: Anchor Books.

Groce, N. E., & Peaglow, C. (2005). *Violence against disabled children*. UN Secretary Report on Violence Against Children. New York, NY: UNICEF.

Henkin, L. (2000). Human rights: Ideology and aspiration, reality, and prospect. In S. Power, & G. Allison (Eds.), *Realizing Human Rights* (pp. 3–38). New York, NY: Palgrave Macmillan.

Hickey, S., & Bracking, S. (2005). Exploring the politics of chronic poverty: From representation to a politics of justice? *World Development, 33*(6), 851–866.

Holland, D. (2003). Grassroots promotion of community health and human rights for people with disabilities in post-communist Central Europe: A profile of the Slovak Republic. *Disability and Society, 18(2),* 133–144.

Holland, D. (2007). Disability and international human rights: Sisyphus reconsidered. In R. J. Eidelson, J. Laske, & L. Cherfas (Eds.), *Peacemaker 101: Careers confronting conflict*. Philadelphia, PA: Solomon Asch Center for Study of Ethnopolitical Conflict, University of Pennsylvania.

Holland, D. (2008). The current status of disability activism and non-governmental organizations in post-communist Europe: Preliminary findings based on reports from the field. *Disability and Society, 26*(6), 543–556.

Holland, D. (2010). Social entrepreneurs and NGOs for people with mental disabilities in post-communist Europe: Implications for international policy. *Review of Disability Studies: An International Journal, 6*(4), 7–24.

Jenkins, R., Klein, J., & Parker, C. (2005). Mental health in post-communist countries. *British Medical Journal, 331,* 173.

Khubchandani, A., & Williams-Nickelson, C. (2003). *Resource guide for psychology graduate students with disabilities*. Washington, DC: American Psychological Association.

Linton, S. (1998). *Claiming disability*. New York, NY: NYU.

Mental Disability Rights International (1999). *Children in Russia's institutions: Human rights and opportunity for reform*. Washington, DC: Author.

Mona, L. (1998). Sexuality and persons with physical disabilities: Unexplored no longer. *The Journal of Sex Research, 35*(2), 217–220.

Olkin, R. (2002). Could you hold the door for me? Including disability in diversity. *Cultural Diversity and Ethnic Minority Psychology, 8*(2), 130–137.

Olkin, R., & Pledger, C. (2003). Can disability studies and psychology join hands? *American Psychologist, 58,* 296–304.

Quinn, G. (2009). The United Nations Convention on the Rights of Persons with Disabilities: Toward a new international politics of disability. *Texas Journal on Civil Liberties and Civil Rights, 15*(1), 33–52.

Sen, A. (2004, November 30). Disability and justice. Keynote address at World Bank conference. "Disability and Inclusive Development: Sharing, Learning, and Building Alliances." Washington, DC.

UNICEF (2005). *Children and disability in transition in CEE/CIS and Baltic States*. Florence, Italy: UNICEF Innocenti Research Centre.

United Nations. (2006). Convention on the rights of persons with disabilities. New York, NY: United Nations.

World Health Organization (2011). *World report on disability*. Geneva, CH: Author.

Yeo, R. (2005). Disability, poverty, and the new development agenda. London, UK: Disability Kar Programme; UK Department for International Development.

Chapter 11

Vulnerability and Privilege among the Elderly: Social Justice Issues in Gerontology and Psychology

Monika Ardelt and Harris L. Friedman

The world is facing one of the most profound demographic shifts in the history of humankind as a dramatically increasing proportion of the globe's human population is rapidly aging (Powell, 2010; Victor, 2010). This rapid change challenges all societies, starting with the profound effects occurring in Japan (Metzler, 2012), and is increasingly affecting Western European nations and the United States—with the effects percolating throughout the rest of the world (Magnus, 2009). In fact, the United States can see into its likely future by looking at the demographics in Japan where the challenges from the aging of that society are most stark and precipitously worsening (Victor, 2010). Our chapter focuses mostly on the interface of social justice, psychology, and gerontology in the United States, mainly because a global approach would take an entire book to cover with even minimal adequacy, but the larger context of many of these issues affects everyone.

The theme we emphasize is that the elderly are both a vulnerable and a privileged group in the United States (Moody & Sasser, 2012). For example, older adults disproportionally benefit from public programs while facing reduced social status as well as diminishing health that inevitably accompanies aging. These complementary disparities are related to differential public resource allocations for younger and older age groups that have many psychological implications for social justice. Generational differences affect the psychological functioning and well-being of the elderly in complex ways that speak to both advantages and disadvantages of the aged. Although there are similar dynamics in some other countries, such as Sweden where there are both improving economic prospects for the elderly accompanied by worsening economic prospects for youth, causing an increasing generation gap (Vogel, 2002), the specific dynamics differ considerably from nation to nation (Uhlenberg, 2013; Victor, 2010). Consequently, our discussion of the United States should not be overgeneralized but, rather, serve as a case study of one particular nation's situation.

As a chapter written primarily from a psychological perspective on gerontology, various anthropological and sociological perspectives, which have long dominated the discourse on social justice in this population, are used in addition to psychological frameworks. One anthropological vantage, for example, is that modern Western cultures, such as the United States, tend to be future-oriented, which devalues the aged compared to the young, who are intimately more comfortable with the fast-paced evolution of technology. In contrast, in more traditional cultures (as defined by sociologists such as Durkheim, 1964 [1893]), the elderly are given greater value, as they carry the myths and knowledge from the past (Achenbaum, 2010; Cowgill & Holmes, 1972). There are many tales in such cultures of an older person, as the keeper of the legends, being able to resolve a problem using a solution from the past that was known only through oral history or actual lived remembrance. In the modern world, however, with data electronically archived and knowledge cumulatively progressing, the role of the aged as keepers of history is diminished. Even in more traditional cultures, much about the world that the elderly knew has changed, such as knowledge of animal migration routes important in hunting cultures that have been disrupted due to environmental alterations, diminishing the relevance of such memories, if not making them obsolete. In addition, the likelihood of someone living into old age has increased, so elders, who were formerly seen as rare cultural treasures, can now be reduced to just one of a growing cohort of useless people who are seen as taking rather than contributing to society (Peterson, 1996; Thurow, 1996). Likewise, one sociological perspective from demography suggests that the growing proportion of older people in the United States might create a burden on the rest of the population if the proportion of dependent older adults keeps growing, while the proportion of working adults declines (Moody & Sasser, 2012). One example is the many unexpected consequences of life extension through technological advances that has resulted in increased survival rates of the oldest of the ageing population but also in increasing health care costs for this fastest-growing group (Victor, 2010).

Translating these types of insights from sociology and anthropology to the interface of social justice, psychology, and gerontology in the United States requires extrapolation. Disparities that both elevate and denigrate the aged pose deep social justice dilemmas as to how resources, both material and psychological, are utilized, and that can be broadly classified under forms of distributive, procedural, and interactional justice. From a psychological vantage, we focus primarily on the individual level of analysis, but of course individuals can never be separated from their social and environmental contexts. Through this psychological lens, we examine the ways in which benefits and detriments are distributed to the elderly as well as the procedural and interactional accompaniments to this distribution.

THE GRAYING OF THE WORLD (DEMOGRAPHY AS DESTINY)

Life expectancy is steadily increasing in the world (United Nations, 2013). In the developed regions of the world, during the past 50 years, life expectancy at birth has increased from 64.8 years to 73.4 years for men and from 70.4 years to 80.4 years for women. Even in the least developed countries, life expectancy at birth has increased from 38.0 years to 57.3 years for men and from 40.0 years to 59.5 years for women. In the United States, life expectancy at birth was 75.6 years for men and 80.6 years for women for the period 2005–2010, which is somewhat lower compared to Western Europe (77.3 and 83.0 years, respectively) and Japan (79.2 and 86.0 years, respectively). Of course this change in the U.S. life expectancy has not benefited all equally, as it varies by factors such as race. In 2009, U.S. life expectancy at birth was 78.8 years for Whites but only 74.5 years for Blacks, with a 4.8-year and 6.5-year gender difference for Whites and Blacks, respectively (Federal Interagency Forum on Aging-Related Statistics, 2012). Due to a longer life expectancy and lower birth rates, the 65 and older population has increased in all regions of the world, while the proportion of the 0–14 population decreased during the same time period with the exception of the least developed countries (see Table 11.1). By 2030, it is projected that fully 20% of the population in the

Table 11.1
Population Aging by Country/Region

	Population Aged 0–14		Population Aged 65+	
Country/Region	**1950 % (million)**	**2010 % (million)**	**1950 % (million)**	**2010 % (million)**
More developed regions	27.5% (223.2)	16.4% (203.7)	7.7% (62.7)	16.1% (199.4)
Least developed countries	41.4% (80.7)	40.9% (342.7)	3.3% (6.4)	3.5% (29.0)
United States of America	27.0% (42.6)	19.8% (61.9)	8.3% (13.0)	13.1% (40.8)
Western Europe	23.4% (33.3)	15.7% (30.0)	10.1% (14.4)	18.5% (35.3)
Japan	35.4% (29.1)	13.3% (16.9)	4.9% (4.1)	23.0% (29.2)

Source: Population Division of the Department of Economic and Social Affairs of the United Nations Secretariat, *World Population Prospects: The 2012 Revision*, http://esa.un.org/unpd/wpp/index.htm

United States will be 65 or older, while a staggering 25% in Western Europe and 31% in Japan will be in this age group (United Nations, 2013). These statistics clearly set the stage for understanding coming demographic shifts and their expected impact on social justice for the aged.

GENERATIONAL EQUITY

An example of privilege that inures to the elderly is that older adults hold a disproportionate amount of wealth in the United States, and this is often the benefit from a lifetime of individual efforts, as well as from favorable social programs designed to disproportionately help the elderly (Moody & Sasser, 2012). In the United States, many believe that resources are increasingly being shifted to the aged at the expense of the shrinking proportion of the young who must bear the burden of past promises. In essence, the argument is that the elderly, as a political voting bloc, exert disproportionate power to the detriment of other vulnerable groups, such as children who cannot vote for their self-interests. The result is that education, health care, and social service dollars are siphoned away from others to pay for benefits for the elderly (Peterson, 1996; Thurow, 1996; Williamson, Watts-Roy, & Kingson, 1999). This perception results in growing resentment, known as "age rage" (Cravit, 2012).

The U.S. poverty rates for children are higher than those in every other developed country, which, again, some blame on the voting power of older adults (Moody & Sasser, 2012). In 1959, the poverty rate among U.S. children below the age of 18 was 27% and, although it decreased in 2010, it remained high at 22%. By contrast, the poverty rate among adults age 65 and above declined from 35% to 9% in the same time period (Federal Interagency Forum on Aging-Related Statistics, 2012). This presents a picture of a nation whose children are vastly impoverished compared to its elderly. However, it is hard to interpret these statistics as the poverty line for older adults is set lower than for younger individuals. For example, in 2011 the poverty line for two-person households for people under the age of 65 was $15,063, while it was $13,596 for two-person households age 65 and above (DeNavas-Walt, Proctor, & Smith, 2012). The operationalization and measurement of U.S. poverty is problematic for many reasons, as the measure does not take into account the costs of health care, housing, child care, and other expenses and, therefore, considerably underestimates poverty (Brady, 2004).

The working young also face an increasing burden to support the elderly, as their numbers diminish comparatively. With less resources produced by the shrinking percentage of working young, greater resentment toward the aged appears likely. Already the elderly are often relegated to the sidelines of life, seen as serving no useful purpose in society, and judged less favorably than the young (Kite, Stockdale, Whitley, & Johnson, 2005).

One way to interpret these demographic shifts is through understanding generational equity, namely how life burdens may be shared across and within generations with varying degrees of fairness. This is sometimes broken down into *intergenerational equity* between younger and older generations and *intragenerational equity* within a generation (rather than across generations). We start by examining the two major U.S. programs designed primarily to benefit the elderly.

Intergenerational Equity: Medicare and Social Security

Older adults in the United States are eligible for the government-sponsored health insurance program, Medicare, at the age of 65 if they or their spouse is entitled to receive Social Security payments (Kaiser Family Foundation, 2010). Older adults account for one-third of all health care expenditures in the United States, even though Medicare covered only 60% of enrollees' health care costs in 2008 (Federal Interagency Forum on Aging-Related Statistics, 2012; Moody & Sasser, 2012). In 2012, 13.5% of the federal budget was spent on Medicare to provide health care coverage to about 48 million older adults as well as to younger people with permanent disabilities (Center on Budget and Policy Priorities, 2013).

At the age of 62, many people in the United States also become eligible to receive partial Social Security benefits, which is the public retirement pension system. However, to receive full benefits, a person must be 66 years of age (born in 1943–1954) and must have worked for at least 10 years in a job where Social Security taxes were deducted. The retirement age for full benefits will increase to 67 for those born in 1960 or later (Social Security Administration, 2013). Retirement benefits are calculated based on earnings averaged over 35 years of work (indexed for inflation) with the appropriate number of zeros added for persons who worked less than 35 years (Johnson, 2011; Moody & Sasser, 2012). In 2012, 22% of the federal budget went to Social Security payments for 36.7 million retired workers and 2.9 million spouses and children of retired workers. In addition, 6.3 million children and spouses of deceased workers and 10.9 million disabled workers and their eligible dependents also received benefits (Center on Budget and Policy Priorities, 2013). So not all, but most, of these benefits go to the aged. The cost of providing these benefits is considerable and growing as people are living longer, notwithstanding that retired workers have paid contributions into the system. The large expenditures for Medicare and Social Security fuel the generational equity argument that the United States spends too much money on the older population at the expense of the young, especially to its children's detriment.

It is clear that Medicare and Social Security help the elderly. For example, without Social Security, 45% of older Americans and, more specifically, almost half of older women would have lived below the poverty line in 2008 (Van de Water & Sherman, 2010). In 2010, 65% of the 65 and over population received at least half of their total income from Social Security with 36% receiving 90% or more (Social Security Administration, 2012). Higher-income beneficiaries, by contrast, often have other resources and even have to pay taxes on their Social Security payments (Moody & Sasser, 2012). In this context, it is worth noting that public support for the preservation of Social Security remains strong, and not only among the older generations. A 2012 survey by the National Academy of Social Insurance revealed that 72% had a favorable view of Social Security. Not surprisingly, 85% of the oldest generation (those born before 1946) viewed Social Security favorably, but so did 65% of the so-called Millennium generation born in 1980 or later. People of all income levels and across all political leanings shared this favorable view of Social Security, including 79% of Democrats, 74% of Independents, and a majority (59%) of Republicans (Tucker, Reno, & Bethell, 2013).

Perhaps this favorable view stems from the fact that Social Security and Medicare do not just benefit the elderly and the disabled but also provide security for middle-aged and younger adults who are aware that they may depend on these programs for their future retirement or in case of disability. Without Social Security and Medicare, older adults might also be more dependent on their adult children to take care of them after their savings are depleted. In this way, Social Security and Medicare protect not only older adults from poverty and financial ruin but also their children from having to provide financial assistance and possibly co-residency to their impoverished older parents (Minkler, 1991; Williamson et al., 1999). This leads to the recognition that intergenerational equity is only one way to discuss the fair distribution of scarce economic resources across generations. Another possibility is to look at generational interdependence between age groups (Williamson et al., 1999). Generations are not typically independent of one another, as intergenerational family transfers flow from the older generation to the younger generation in forms of social, psychological, and financial support and inheritance (Angel & Mudrazija, 2011).

One of the most vexing concerns expressed about the Social Security and Medicare programs is that, by differentially benefitting the elderly, the aged are responsible for the high poverty rate of U.S. children by depriving them of their equitable share of resources. However, it can be equally argued that childhood poverty is more likely the result of increasing single-parent families, stagnant and declining (inflation-adjusted) low-income wages, unemployment, and a public unwillingness to provide assistance to the poor (Williamson et al., 1999). In fact, Minkler (1991) called the intergenerational equity debate "the new victim blaming," in which the elderly are scapegoated for many of U.S. society's problems, fueling the so-called age rage. The social justice implications for this controversy are clear and one can only wonder how this translates into psychological issues for older adults who might internalize this blame as an additional psychological burden to the other challenges posed by aging.

Intragenerational Equity: Cumulative Advantage and Disadvantage across the Life Course

Socioeconomic status (SES), defined as a combination of education, income, occupation, and wealth, influences to a large extent the life course of individuals and constitutes a basis for diversity among the aged. Children who are born to low SES parents tend to grow up in disadvantaged neighborhoods with higher social stress and lower social capital (e.g., intellectual stimulation and social support) (Ainsworth, 2002; Leventhal & Brooks-Gunn, 2000; Sampson, Morenoff, & Gannon-Rowley, 2002). They also often receive inadequate nutrition, which leads to health problems early in life, such as developmental delays, obesity, hypertension, and diabetes (Baker et al., 2005; Bradley & Corwyn, 2002). Low SES children are more likely to struggle in school than high SES children, whose parents can afford private (pre-)schools, tutoring, summer camps, and vacations abroad, which tend to translate into higher grades and test scores that determine admission to the most prestigious universities (Entwisle, Alexander, & Olson, 2004; Kozol, 2005). Moreover, after obtaining a university degree, high SES parents can provide social connections that help their offspring to secure a well-paying job, whereas lower SES individuals have to compete for jobs in the labor market, further widening the gap between the rich and poor (Lin, 1999). Higher SES individuals also tend to work in white-collar occupations that offer health insurance, whereas lower SES adults are more likely to experience chronic stress and have physically and psychosocially demanding jobs, often without affordable health insurance or without being offered any health insurance benefits at all (Adler & Newman, 2002; Culpepper, 1993; Warren, Hoonakker, Carayon, & Brand, 2004). As a consequence, lower SES adults who do not qualify for the government-sponsored Medicaid program for the poor or Medicare for older adults tend to avoid or delay doctor's visits, resulting in untreated or undertreated illnesses (Card, Dobkin, & Maestas, 2008; Zuvekas & Taliaferro, 2003). Even if low SES individuals see a physician, they often cannot pay for the medication to treat their illness (Klein, Turvey, & Wallace, 2004; Mojtabai & Olfson, 2003). Health behaviors, such as nutrition, exercise, smoking, drinking, and drug use, also vary by SES, due to health education and social circumstances, and exacerbate the difference in health between those with low and high SES (Adler & Newman, 2002; Bradley & Corwyn, 2002; Warren et al., 2004). The whole process leads to cumulative advantage for high SES individuals and cumulative disadvantage for low SES persons (Dannefer, 2003; O'Rand, Binstock, & George, 2006; O'Rand, Isaacs, & Roth, 2010), resulting in widening health disparities by SES across the life course and greater life expectancies for those with higher SES (Adler & Newman, 2002; Frytak, Harley, & Finch, 2004; Palloni, 2006; Willson, Shuey, & Elder, 2007). The government-sponsored Medicare program is often the first health insurance program that lower SES adults can access at age 65 (Card et al., 2008). Therefore, even though the aged poor might have some advantages over the younger poor due to their eligibility for Medicare, by the time they reach this status, they often carry a lifetime of cumulative deprivation.

The elderly are hardly homogenous in terms of financial well-being, and many are suffering deprivations. Among people 65 and older, 2010 poverty rates tended to be higher for the oldest-old (12.3% for persons 85 and older versus 8.1% for elders 65–74), women (10.7% versus 6.7% for men), elders living alone (16.8%

versus 4.2% for married couples), and minority groups (18% for both Blacks and Hispanics versus 6.8% for Whites) (Federal Interagency Forum on Aging-Related Statistics, 2012). Hence, Social Security income is particularly important for minority elders in the United States, as 49% of Blacks and 55% of Hispanics received 90% or more of their retirement income from Social Security (Social Security Administration, 2012). Overall, the statistics suggest that lower SES over the life course tends to result in cumulative disadvantage in old age (Dannefer, 2003) and that poor children are also more likely to experience poverty later in life (O'Rand et al., 2010). Without doubt, the economic conditions of the low SES elderly provide psychological challenges related to social justice as most younger adults have greater prospects and opportunities than the aged to rectify economic deprivation and overcome their poverty.

Older Workers versus Early Retirees

One approach to deal with economic issues related to the rapidly graying population of the United States is to encourage or require older people to work longer to contribute to society and to delay Social Security payments and Medicare spending. In the United States, mandatory retirement was abolished in 1986 for most workers, and in 1994 for university professors (S. P. Smith, 1991), as continuing to work adds considerable resources to ailing government programs (Johnson, 2011). Indeed, the trend toward earlier retirement for men has been reversed since the mid-90s (see Figure 11.1). In 1963, 76% of men between the age of 62 and 64 were in the labor force, which declined to 45% in 1995 and rose to 53% in 2011. This trend is even more pronounced for those aged 65–69. In 1967, 43% of this age group was in the labor force, compared to only 24–26% between the mid-1980s to the early 1990s. Yet, since the mid-1990s, labor force participation has steadily increased to 37% in 2011. Among men 70 years of age and older, 15% were working in 2011. As shown in Figure 11.2, the labor force participation of women, by contrast, was relatively steady between 1963 and the early 1990s but has increased for all age groups since the mid-1990s. In 1963, only 29% of women age 62–64, 17% of those age 65–69, and 6% of 70-year-olds and above were in the labor force, compared to 45%, 27%, and 8%, respectively, in 2011 (Federal Interagency Forum on Aging-Related Statistics, 2012).

However, many workers in the United States now expect to work into their 70s. According to the 2013 Retirement Confidence Survey conducted by the Employee Benefit Research Institute, only 2% of workers expected to delay retirement until age 66–69 and only 9% until age 70 or above in 1991 compared to 10% and 33%, respectively, in 2013 (Helman, Adams, Copeland, & VanDerhei, 2013). The major reasons workers gave to delay retirement include the poor economy (25%), a lack of faith in Social Security or the government (25%), not enough money saved to be able to retire (21%), and wanting to ensure sufficient money to retire comfortably (16%).

Figure 11.1
Labor Force Participation Rates of Men Age 55 and Over, by Age Group, Annual Averages, 1963–2011.

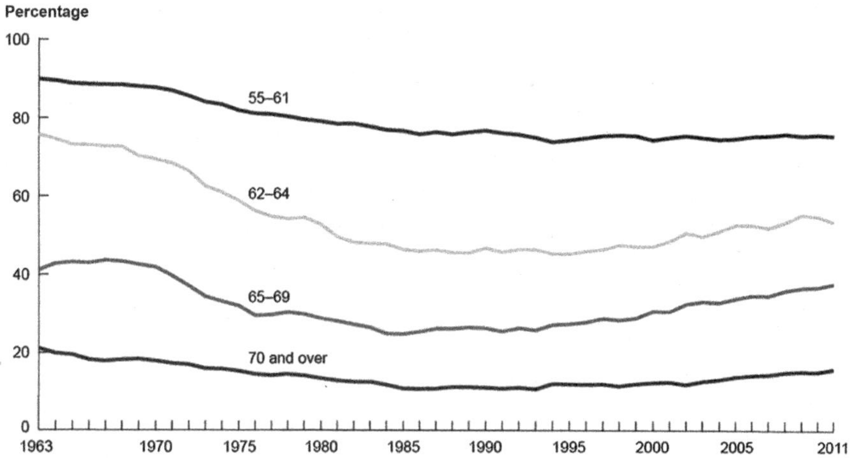

Source: Bureau of Labor Statistics, Current Population Survey. (Federal Interagency Forum on Aging-Related Statistics, 2012, p. 18)

Figure 11.2
Labor Force Participation Rates of Women Age 55 and Over, by Age Group, Annual Averages, 1963–2011.

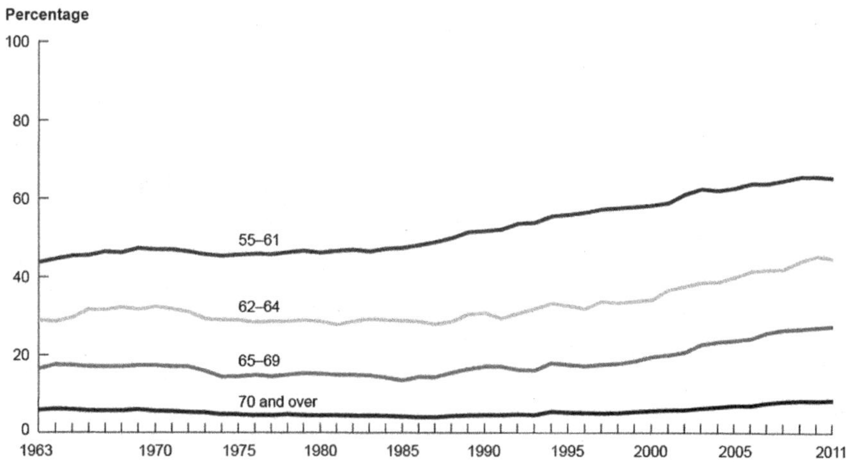

Source: Bureau of Labor Statistics, Current Population Survey. (Federal Interagency Forum on Aging-Related Statistics, 2012, p. 19)

Yet, not everyone who wants to work longer is actually able to do so. Older workers tend to be healthy, highly educated, and less likely to work in physically demanding jobs with difficult working conditions (Calvo, 2006; Johnson, Mermin, & Resseger, 2011; Juhn & McCue, 2012). By contrast, 47% of retirees in 2013 reported that they had retired earlier than planned, whereas only 6% said that their retirement came later than planned (Helman et al., 2013). The majority of retirees (55%) cited health problems or disabilities as the reason for an earlier than planned retirement, followed by downsizing, plant closures, or other work-related reasons (49%), the ability to afford an earlier retirement (32%), and caregiving responsibilities for a family member (23%). Only 7% of the survey respondents mentioned exclusively positive reasons for an earlier than planned retirement. Although older workers have lower unemployment rates than younger workers due to their seniority, when displaced they tend to need a longer time to find a new job, often at a lower salary and with fewer benefits, if they can find another job at all (Johnson & Mommaerts, 2011). In fact, many older workers decide to retire early rather than face prolonged unemployment (Moody & Sasser, 2012; Munnell & Rutledge, 2013). Extending the retirement age poses a number of social justice challenges for the elderly, especially for unskilled manual workers for whom continuing employment into their later years would be much more difficult than for white-collar and professional workers.

Understanding Some of the Macro-Level Forces Driving Retirement

Although our focus is on the interface of psychology and gerontology, there are macro-level forces driving many of the dynamics involving social justice. For example, the shift from defined benefit pension plans, which promise a specific or defined amount of pension income for the remainder of life at retirement, to defined contribution plans, whose pension income depends the amount employers and employees have contributed to the fund over the years and on how successfully it was invested, might be partially responsible for workers' desire to delay retirement (Friedberg & Webb, 2005). In 1980, almost 40% of workers in the private sector had defined benefit pension plans compared to 17% who were covered by defined contribution plans. Starting in 1989, however, the percentage of private sector workers who were covered by defined contribution plans exceeded the percentage of workers in defined benefit plans with the gap widening ever since. In 2011, only 14% of workers in the private sector had defined benefit pension plans compared to 42% with defined contribution plans (Lind, Hill, Hiltonsmith, & Freedman, 2013). In defined benefit plans, investment risks are carried primarily by the employer, whereas in defined contribution plans all the investment risks, including investment choices, market downturns, and contribution rates, are shifted to the employee. Hence, a stock market crash is much more devastating for workers with defined contribution plans than those with defined benefit plans. For example, during the Great Recession from 2007 to 2009, the value of equities in defined contribution and individual retirement accounts decreased by $2.8 trillion (Munnell & Rutledge, 2013). Although workers are encouraged through tax deductions to save for retirement, only few are able to save enough or procure the expertise to invest their retirement savings wisely. In the 2013 Retirement Confidence Survey, 57% of workers and 55% of retirees reported total savings and investments of less than $25,000, excluding the value of the primary residence and any defined benefit pension plans (Helman et al., 2013).

The excessive fees of defined contribution and individual retirement accounts drain retirement savings even more. According to calculations by Hiltonsmith (2012), account fees can add up to $155,000 over a lifetime for a median-income, two-earner family and might reduce their investment returns by almost a third. Overall, it costs about 46% more to provide the same target benefit amount in retirement in a defined contribution pension plan compared to a defined benefit plan due to higher fees, a less balanced portfolio, and no longevity and risk pooling (Almeida & Fornia, 2008). As a result, workers with a defined contribution plan retire on average almost two years later than workers with a defined benefit plan (Friedberg & Webb, 2005).

Even though older workers continue to contribute to society and to government programs, they might also add to a higher unemployment rate and occupational stagnation among the young, particularly in a recession. If older workers do not retire, the young might be unable to find jobs, and younger and middle-aged workers cannot get promoted to the positions that some older workers occupy (Caro, Bass, & Chen, 1993). One possible solution might be to offer part-time work, flexible work arrangements, and phased retirement to older workers (Uhlenberg, 2013). This would allow for their continuing contribution to society and their retirement funds, but also give them more leisure time to explore other interests, such as hobbies, self-development, volunteering, and grandchildren, and make room for the young to enter the work force and middle-aged workers to take on more responsibilities (Moody & Sasser, 2012). Yet, this might require a general change in employer policies to provide fringe benefits and retirement contributions not only to full-time but also to part-time workers, which in fact would be a boon to all part-time workers (Johnson, 2011). Clearly, decisions about retirement have major impacts on psychological concerns of the elderly, such as well-being and quality of life.

The Psychological Cost of Generational Disparities

From the perspective of many of the most privileged U.S. elderly, the so-called golden years may promise opportunities to reap the rewards of a lifetime of effort through pursuing leisure activities, such as golf within gated upscale-retirement communities where children are banned. If forced to continue to work into the older years, these rewards may never be obtained. Yet, even if obtained, this romanticized notion of retirement does not always live up to expectations. For example, the segregation of the aged often leads to isolation, as social losses (e.g., of family and peers who have been outlived) and physical losses (e.g., of mobility, vision, and hearing) mar the idealized happiness of retirement living. The high rates of suicide among U.S. men above the age of 64 perhaps reflect these dynamics, as they are consistently higher than among younger men. White older men, in particular, tend to have the highest suicide rates (Centers for Disease Control and Prevention, 2012), possibly due to the attempt to maintain a sense of control, autonomy, and independence that was available throughout their lives (Sullivan, Hedberg, & Fleming, 2000). Of course, there are many ways in which aging occurs, and these negative trajectories are not universal for all.

Unfortunately, older adults often buy into the very anti-aging myths that are promulgated in the media, such as physical beauty being the measure of worth for women (Smirnova, 2012) and various forms of potency, such as earning power, being the measure of worth for men (Culpepper, 1993). With the increased likelihood of infirmity and diminished cognitive capacity that can lead to subtle and overt discrimination from both others as well as from self-debasement, the dreams still held by many of the elderly can no longer be achieved, yet there are no viable alternatives so far for substitution in the modern world.

PHYSICAL AND MENTAL HEALTH

The older people grow, the higher the probability they will suffer from diminished physical and mental health, which might make their continuing participation in the labor force impossible. Although most hope they will live long and healthy lives, the reality is that advanced age increases the risk for chronic health conditions, functional limitations, and mental health disorder (e.g., depressive symptoms). In 2008–2010, among people 65 and older in the United States, 55.9% reported having hypertension, 51.2% arthritis, 30.4% heart disease, 24.0% cancer, and 20.5% diabetes (Federal Interagency Forum on Aging-Related Statistics, 2012). Among Blacks, the rate of hypertension was even higher with 69.2% (compared to 57.2% for Hispanics and 54.2% for Whites), possibly the result of greater lifelong stress due to racial discrimination and an increased likelihood of poverty (Baum, Garofalo, & Yali, 1999; Davis, Liu, Quarells, & Din-Dzietham, 2005; Klonoff & Landrine, 2000; Troxel, Matthews, Bromberger, & Sutton-Tyrrell, 2003; Williams & Neighbors, 2001). Moreover, functional limitations (e.g., being able to stoop/kneel, walk 2–3 city blocks, or lift 10 lbs.) and depressive symptoms increased with age, whereas self-assessed health declined (Federal Interagency Forum on Aging-Related Statistics, 2012). Among individuals age 65–74, 12.9% of men and 18.7% of women reported at least one functional limitation, and 21.2% of men and 20.7% of women rated their health as fair or poor. Those percentages increased in the age 85 and above group to 39.6% for men and 53.0% for women with respect to functional limitations and to 34.4% for men and 32.3% for women for self-assessed fair or poor health. Self-assessed health of older minorities, however, tended to be worse than that of Whites. Among adults aged 65–74, 32.8% of

Blacks and 34.5% of Hispanics reported having fair or poor health compared to only 18.1% of Whites. Even in the age 85 and above group, racial differences remained, with 45.8% of Blacks, 48.2% of Hispanics, and 30.6% of Whites reporting fair or poor health. Similarly, depressive symptoms increased from 9.7% for men and 14.5% for women age 65–69 to 18.9% for men and 17.9% for women for adults age 85 and over.

Accompanying such physical health issues are a plethora of implications, such as the disproportionate amount of health care dollars that go to serve the aged. In 2012, $472 billion was spent for Medicare and accounted for 13.5% of the federal budget (Center on Budget and Policy Priorities, 2013). Especially concerning are so-called heroic efforts that extend life by a few weeks or months but do little to improve the quality of life and yet cost outrageous amounts of money (Moody & Sasser, 2012). Although the proportion of older adults who died in acute care hospitals decreased from 32.6% in 2000 to 24.6% in 2009 and the proportion of those who died under hospice care increased from 21.6% to 42.2%, the percentage of older adults who spent some time in the intensive care unit (ICU) during their last month of life also increased from 24.3% to 29.2%. Moreover, among hospice patients in 2009, 28.4% used the service for three days or less, and 40.3% of late hospice enrollees came from hospitals that included an ICU stay (Teno et al., 2013). Those statistics suggest a trend toward more, rather than less, aggressive treatment for older adults at the end of life, with hospice care added only as an option of last resort during the dying phase instead of providing comfort care during the last stage of life (Byock, 1996; Lattanzi-Licht & Connor, 1995). The biomedicalization of aging contributes to this trend. Many medical procedures that used to be cutting-edge are now offered by physicians as routine medical care to older adults, such as angioplasty, coronary artery bypass graft surgery, heart defibrillator, kidney dialysis, and kidney transplants, which makes it difficult to reject such procedures, particularly if they are reimbursed by Medicare (Kaufman, Shim, & Russ, 2004). It also makes it difficult to view physical decline and death as a natural part of life and provides the false hope that life can be extended endlessly (Kaufman, 2005) if we are only willing to invest enough resources in medical research and health interventions (De Grey, 2007). In a society that highly values independence, autonomy, and control, becoming physically dependent, frail, and vulnerable is perceived as the ultimate failure that needs to be prevented at all costs (Holstein, 2010). Yet, because resources are inherently limited, each society needs to decide how to distribute those resources across all segments of society.

One possibility to reduce the costs of health care spending for the old is to ration health care for life-extending treatments for the very old in exchange for better long-term care and access to health care for all age groups (Callahan, 1987, 1990). Yet, such a plan would be difficult to implement for several reasons. First, chronological age by itself is not a good predictor of who might benefit from a medical procedure. Healthy older adults in their 70s or even 80s might live another 10 years or more after receiving a life-extending intervention, such as coronary artery bypass graft surgery, a heart defibrillator, or a kidney transplant, whereas chronically or terminally ill persons in their 50s or 60s might be less suitable candidates for such procedures (Schneider, 1993; Winslow, 1993). Second, some life-extending treatments, such as antibiotics, are actually quite inexpensive, whereas the average yearly costs of living in a low-technology long-term care facility was over $60,000 in 2008 (Federal Interagency Forum on Aging-Related Statistics, 2012). Third, without a universal health care system for all, there is no guarantee that the money saved through age-based health care rationing would actually be used to provide health care to younger people (Holstein, 1990). Fourth, age-based rationing would only restrict health care to those who depend on Medicare and cannot afford private health care, which would further disadvantage older adults with lower SES, perpetuating their struggle to access health care earlier in life (Schneider, 1993; Wetle & Besdine, 1990). Fifth, age-based health care rationing by itself might only save less than 1% of national annual health care expenditures (Binstock, 1994).

Age stereotypes, by contrast, might be the reason why older adults are often excluded from health promotion and disease-prevention programs, and why physicians might misdiagnose older adults' physical symptoms (Ory, Hoffman, Hawkins, Sanner, & Mockenhaupt, 2003). An example is the prevention and detection of HIV infections among older adults who comprise a growing number of AIDS-related deaths, because the disease is either discovered too late or its symptoms are mistaken for other illnesses (Adekeye, Heiman, Onyeabor, & Hyacinth, 2012). Due to stereotyping, many maladies of the aged might be dismissed as due just to aging, denying proper diagnosis, treatment, and follow-up. Again, this illustrates how both privilege and deprivation affect the elderly at the same time.

The area of mental health is even more complex. Real physical ailments are often dismissed as not just part of aging per se, but as mental illness. It is extremely common to confuse delirium, a transitory state of confusion due to metabolic disorders, infections, or medications, with dementia, a more lasting trait (Espino, Jules-Bradley, Johnston, & Mouton, 1998). For example, an elderly individual given multiple medications to treat different ills can become disoriented due to medication interactions, particularly if there is no singular provider monitoring all the medications and their interactions (Mallet, Spinewine, & Huang, 2007; Steinman et al., 2006). Then, to compound this problem, psychotropic medications, often prescribed to treat the confusion, add to the cacophony (Aparasu & Mort, 2004; Mort & Aparasu, 2000). This is a woefully common failure of the health care system. An alternative might be to implement a model of appropriate medication use that takes into account the patients' life expectancy, the time it will take to achieve the benefits of the medication, and whether the goal of care is life prolongation, treatment of an acute illness, or palliative symptom control (Holmes, Hayley, Alexander, & Sachs, 2006). Hence, older adults might be simultaneously over- and undertreated, and finding the right balance between providing needed health care and acknowledging the finitude of resources and the limits of medicine remains a challenge.

This is an area that impacts many practicing psychologists who interact professionally with the elderly. Psychologists are often called upon to play roles that are fecund with social justice implications, such as when institutions want help to manage the elderly more easily. Reasonable protests about quality of care by elderly residents of health care and long-term care facilities, for example, can be mislabeled as disruptive behavior, which psychologists might be asked to document to justify the use of pacifying medications or physical restraints that allow for less staff to be employed. In addition, practicing psychologists are often asked to render opinions about the competency of the elderly by those who might benefit from a judicial ruling of incompetence. These sorts of dilemmas are rampant in treatment settings focused on the elderly (see Pruchno & Smyer, 2007).

LONG-TERM CARE

Providing adequate health care for older adults is expensive, but the financing of long-term care for chronic diseases and disabilities is especially problematic. Contrary to a basic misconception, Medicare does not pay for long-term care but, rather, pays only for short-term rehabilitative care in a skilled nursing facility after a qualifying hospital stay of three days or more. The first 20 days in a nursing facility are fully covered, whereas days 21–100 require a co-payment. After 100 days, older adults either have to leave the nursing facility or pay out of pocket for nursing home care (http://www.medicare.gov/coverage/skilled-nursing-facility-care.html). Once their financial assets are depleted, Medicaid pays for nursing home care. A whole legal industry exists to help older adults spend down, transfer, or convert their financial assets to an exempt form, such as a trust fund, so that they can qualify for Medicaid payments for nursing home care without being actually impoverished (Budish, 1990, 1995; Moses, 1990). In 2008, Medicaid paid 52% of long-term care facility costs (Federal Interagency Forum on Aging-Related Statistics, 2012), and about two-thirds of the $346 billion in Medicaid spending in 2009 went to older adults and disabled individuals (The Kaiser Commission on Medicaid and the Uninsured, 2013). Social justice issues involve the generational equity of Medicaid paying for the long-term care needs of older adults rather than for the medical needs of poor children, and whether families should be allowed to preserve their assets while relying on Medicaid to pay for their elder relatives' nursing home costs.

From a psychological perspective, many U.S. elderly are relegated to poor qualities of life by being warehoused in nursing homes and other long-term care facilities (Ogden & Adams, 2009), which tend to deprive the aged of dignity and, when dementia is involved, heighten the loss of a sense of personhood (Holstein, 2010; Kayser-Jones, 2002). Even though only 4% of U.S. adults age 65 and above are in nursing homes at any one point in time, nearly half of this age group is predicted to spend at least some time in nursing homes or similar long-term care facility during the course of their lives (Moody & Sasser, 2012). In addition, during these times, there are often family members or court-appointed guardians who control the elderly's assets and whose motivations may not be in the best interest of the elderly they are supposed to protect. One possibility to avoid placing the aged in dehumanizing institutions is to reimburse informal family caregivers for their caregiving time (Kunkel, Applebaum, & Nelson, 2003; Simon-Rusinowitz, Mahoney, & Benjamin, 2001). This might allow older adults to remain in their homes instead of having to move to an often impersonal institutional setting where they are often forced to give up their privacy, dignity, autonomy, and sense of self (Holstein, 2010). Yet, politicians are reluctant to implement such a policy, because they are afraid of the "woodwork-effect," that is, families "coming out of the woodwork" to demand payments for services that they did not provide before or that they would have provided for free (Arling & McAuley, 1983). However, females rather than males often provide this free long-term care for older relatives in the home at the cost of their own career advancements or job prospects, and sometimes, their physical and mental health (Holstein, 2010), again demonstrating the interdependency approach to understanding generational equity. For example, in 2009 about 61.6 million family caregivers provided care to an adult with functional limitations at some point in time during the year at an estimated economic value of approximately $450 billion, which exceeded total expenditures for Medicaid and approached spending for the Medicare program (Feinberg, Reinhard, Houser, & Choula, 2011). Middle-aged women in the "sandwich generation" often take care of both children and parents (Brody, 1985, 1990), and older women tend to care for their husbands and then spend the last years of their own lives in assisted living facilities or nursing homes, where they are most likely cared for by underpaid, undervalued, and overworked female caregivers (Culpepper, 1993; Holstein, 2010). Consequently, the fairness of asking women to disproportionately bear the primary costs for long-term care needs of older adults requires examination. If family caregivers do not receive additional help in the form of respite care, community support, and paid home care, they might become overburdened and are more likely to send their older relatives to long-term care facilities whose costs ultimately tend to be paid by taxpayers through Medicaid. As Holstein (2010, p. 636) remarked, care for the elderly, "who need assistance, is not a private matter deserving only some small assistance from the state but rather it is a public matter calling for broad risk-sharing."

ELDER ABUSE AND NEGLECT

Providing long-term care for an older adult with physical or cognitive impairments is highly stressful, which increases the risk of elder abuse and neglect (Fulmer et al., 2005; Johannesen & LoGiudice, 2013). Moreover, older adults are often vulnerable victims of financial exploitation as well (Moody & Sasser, 2012).

Holding disproportionate resources, while being less able to mentally and physically defend them, invites exploitation in the form of financial abuse (Wilber & Reynolds, 1996). For example, older adults are often the victims of online fraud, unscrupulous telemarketers, and scam artists who promise riches or lucrative investments for their retirement funds with high returns, but swindle them out of their money instead (Barnard, 2010; Hines, 2002; Mouallem, 2002). Older adults who are cognitively impaired are at particular risk for financial abuse, because they have diminished decision-making capacities and might not understand the implications of their financial actions (Wilber & Reynolds, 1996). In this case, a guardian of the estate who manages the older person's financial affairs and property can be appointed (Ritter, 1995). Yet, there is a fine line between the protection of older adults from financial abuse and their right and freedom to engage in financial transactions of their choice, even if they appear foolish to others (Wilber & Reynolds, 1996). Moreover, children and other relatives who become court-appointed guardians of an older adult's estate might use the assets for their own benefits rather than those of the elderly person. Emotionally and physically dependent older adults and those who need extensive care due to physical or cognitive impairments are at higher risk for exploitation and might also be reluctant or unable to report the mistreatment and seek help if financial abuse is enforced through verbal and physical abuse or if they feel that their future well-being depends on the financially abusive caregiver (Moody & Sasser, 2012; Nerenberg, 2010; Wilber & Reynolds, 1996).

In a U.S. representative study of community-dwelling older adults between the ages of 57 and 85 years, 9% reported experiencing verbal abuse, 3.5% financial abuse, and 0.2% physical abuse by a family member (Laumann, Leitsch, & Waite, 2008). Women and physically vulnerable older adults were more likely to suffer verbal abuse, whereas African Americans and those without a partner were more likely to suffer financial abuse than Whites and respondents with marital or romantic partners. Risks for elder neglect include characteristics of the aged care recipient, such as greater physical and cognitive impairment, depressive symptoms, history of childhood physical abuse and neglect, and less social support, and characteristics of the caregiver, such as greater functional impairment and the experience of childhood neglect (Fulmer et al., 2005). The results indicate that it might be more difficult and stressful to care for older adults who are sicker, have no other social support, and are often depressed. Moreover, caregivers who are not physically well themselves might be too overwhelmed by their caregiving burden. The finding that a history of childhood neglect of the caregiver and recipient is a risk factor for experiencing neglect in old age is further evidence of the cumulative advantage and disadvantage model across the life course (Dannefer, 2003).

A meta-analysis of 49 studies on elder abuse experienced by community-dwelling older adults concluded that risk factors were related to characteristics of the older person, the perpetrator, the relationship, and the environment (Johannesen & LoGiudice, 2013). More specifically, elder abuse was more likely to occur if the older person suffered from cognitive or physical impairments, psychiatric illness or psychological problems, or past trauma and abuse, was functionally dependent on others, exhibited provocative or aggressive behavior problems, or had low income or wealth. Elder abuse was also related to caregiver burden or stress, psychological problems of the caregiver, family disharmony, a problematic relationship between caregiver and care recipient, and low social support (Johannesen & LoGiudice, 2013). This suggests that elder abuse cannot be solely blamed on the perpetrator but could be alleviated if caregivers would receive greater community and family support and advice on how to cope with the stresses of caring for an incapacitated, frail, and sometimes difficult older adult in order to reduce overall caregiver burden and stress (Anetzberger et al., 2000; Judge, Yarry, Looman, & Bass, 2013; Mittelman, Roth, Haley, & Zarit, 2004; Nerenberg, 2010; T. L. Smith & Toseland, 2006).

However, elders in long-term care settings appear to be at even greater risk of abuse. In a random survey of relatives of long-term care recipients age 60 and above, 16.2% reported observing neglect (e.g., failure to prevent bed sores, to provide adequate nutrition, hygiene, comfort, or personal safety, or to respond to requests for help), 13.0% emotional abuse (e.g. being disrespectful or prevention of contact with others), 12.7% caretaking abuse (e.g., the over- or under-administration of drugs, inappropriate use of physical restraints, or unjustified force feeding), 11.2% verbal abuse (e.g., yelling, cursing, insults, threats, intimidation, humiliation, or harassment), 9.2% material abuse (e.g., misuse or theft of money, possessions, property, or assets, sometimes by forcing or deceiving the older person into signing documents or gifting possessions), and 4.2% physical abuse (e.g., striking, hitting, beating, pushing, shoving, shaking, slapping, kicking, pinching, or burning) by formal paid caregivers (Post et al., 2010). Elders who were verbally or physically abusive themselves were, in turn, most at risk for all types of abuse by paid caregivers, except material abuse, compared to those elders with physical and cognitive impairments, suggesting a negative abuse spiral. Caretakers who were abused by their charges tended to retaliate with abuse. It also highlights the risks of "talking back" to an abusive caretaker who has the power to make the life of a dependent older person miserable. Problems related to physical functioning increased the risks for verbal and emotional abuse and neglect, whereas cognitive impairment by itself was unrelated to increased abuse (Post et al., 2010).

One way to prevent elder abuse and neglect appears to be through a strong social support network of family and friends who can look out for the older person, both in a family environment and in formal paid care situations (Luo & Waite, 2011; Shugarman, Fries, Wolf, & Morris, 2003). Moreover, support from family, friends, and the community helps to alleviate caregiver burden and stress and, hence, decreases the likelihood of elder abuse (Anetzberger et al., 2000; Lai & Thomson, 2011; Mittelman et al., 2004; Nerenberg, 2010; T. L. Smith & Toseland, 2006; Thompson, Futterman, Gallagher-Thompson, Rose, & Lovett, 1993). Therefore, reducing social isolation among older adults and caregivers might lower the risk for elder abuse and neglect, and improve older adults' well-being (Ferguson &

Goodwin, 2010; Thoits, 2011). Clearly the psychological aspects of elder abuse involve multiple concerns related to social justice.

AGING IN PRISONS

On the other side of the spectrum of abuse are older adults who have a history as perpetrators rather than as victims. Older prisoners are a special needs subgroup of the elderly highlighted in this chapter, although many other subgroups, such as those belonging to various minorities, could also be discussed in detail, but are not due to space limitations.

Prisoners tend to age more rapidly than nonprisoners, which makes them about 10 years older physiologically, on average, compared to not imprisoned same-age peers (Rikard & Rosenberg, 2007). About half a million people over the age of 50 are arrested each year in the United States (Wahidin & Aday, 2010). Due to overzealous mandatory life sentences (only in the United States can a teen receive life without parole for a crime committed as a youth), three-strikes laws and "tough on crime" policies with longer mandatory minimum sentences, reduced possibilities for early parole, the aging baby boom cohort, and a longer life expectancy, the prison population is graying (Rikard & Rosenberg, 2007). The proportion of U.S. prisoners age 50 and above increased from 4.9% in 1990 to 11.6% in 2007 (Wahidin & Aday, 2010). In 2009, 13.6% of the federal prison population was older than 50 years (Human Rights Watch, 2012). It is estimated that by 2020, 21–33% of the prison population will consist of elderly inmates (Rikard & Rosenberg, 2007).

For example, a report by the State of Florida Correctional Medical Authority (2010) described the characteristics of their oldest prisoners as follows:

> As of June 30, 2010 the oldest male inmate was 90 and was admitted to DC [Department of Corrections] at age 82 with a 15 year sentence. The oldest female inmate was 91 and was admitted at age 87 to serve a 31 year sentence. The ages of the ten oldest male inmates range from 86 to 90; the average age is 87.5 and seven of the ten are serving a sentence of 50 years or more. The shortest sentence is the 90 year old with a fifteen year sentence. The ages of the ten oldest female inmates range from 76 to 91; the average age is 79.2 and three of the ten are serving a sentence of 50 years or more. The shortest sentence for the ten oldest female inmates is a 79 year old serving a seven year sentence. For the 20 oldest inmates, the average sentence length is 34.7 years and the youngest age of admission was a 76 year old female inmate admitted at age 35. (p. 53)

Older inmates are more likely than younger prisoners to have been convicted of a violent crime that typically results in a longer sentence with a lower probability for parole (Rikard & Rosenberg, 2007). In 2009, 65% of state prisoners age 55 and older served prison time for a violent crime compared to 50% of the under age 55 inmate population. Among state prisoners over the age of 50, 21% served a life sentence in 2009 compared to 8% of inmates age 50 and younger (Human Rights Watch, 2012). Older prisoners who are often physically too weak to pose any credible threat to anyone remain incarcerated (Wahidin & Aday, 2010). These elderly inmates not only languish in prisons unnecessarily, but also inflict a major financial burden on society due to their higher medical needs in terms of health care, medical devices and equipment, prescription drugs, and housing accommodations (Rikard & Rosenberg, 2007). Older inmates are more likely to suffer from chronic health conditions and worse physical and mental health, which makes their incarceration about three times more expensive than for younger prisoners (Anno, Graham, Lawrence, & Shansky, 2004; Binswange, Krueger, & Steiner, 2009; State of Florida Correctional Medical Authority, 2010; Williams, Sudore, Greifinger, & Morrison, 2011). Ironically, older prisoners with medical needs might receive better medical care than non-incarcerated older adults under the age of 65 without health insurance (Wahidin & Aday, 2010). Hence, it might be time to return the focus of the criminal justice system from incapacitation and punishment to rehabilitation and reintegration, so that inmates can learn how to become valuable and productive members of society rather than grow old and die in prisons at an increasing cost to taxpayers (Rikard & Rosenberg, 2007). Prisoners, as well as other aged special populations, warrant greater attention, as the elderly are a diverse group and have many challenging social justice concerns.

CONCLUSION

The proportion and number of elderly in the United States is expected to dramatically increase and will have major impacts on all sectors of society. However, the experience of aging varies considerably by sex, race, and socioeconomic status, so it is difficult to discuss the interface of psychological issues with aging related to social justice in a simple way. In fact, older adults tend to be more diverse in terms of health, wealth, income, and social support than younger adults due to the process of cumulative advantage and disadvantage over the life course (Dannefer, 2003). To even speak about the elderly as a coherent class is somewhat misleading. Those with economic assets and good health can enjoy their later years of life by engaging in leisure pursuits, such as travel, whereas others struggle with poverty and ill health.

To address the many challenges, some major societal restructuring might be needed. Hence, a not so radical proposal would be to bolster Social Security for all, rather than reducing it (Geoghegan, 2011; Lind et al., 2013). This could be financed in part through increased taxes on higher-income earners and wealth accumulation (Polivka, 2010). Because defined benefit pension plans in the private sector have been largely replaced by defined contribution plans that make pension income vulnerable to individual investment success and failure and the volatility of the stock market, it might be time to replace private pension plans and retirement savings with a universal Social Security floor that everyone eligible for Social Security would receive in addition to the traditional Social Security payments (Lind et al., 2013). This would increase retirement security for all and eliminate the need for Supplemental Security Income (SSI) payments to older adults living in poverty and tax deductions for private retirement contributions that primarily favor wealthier individuals with enough money to save for retirement.

Similarly, rather than pitting poor children and young adults against older adults in terms of perceived intergenerational conflict when deciding how to reign in the costs of Medicare and Medicaid spending, it might make more sense to provide Medicare for all and to implement a public mandatory long-term care insurance program (Conyers, 2008; Miller, 2012). The United States spends more money for health care than any other industrialized nation without offering universal health insurance coverage and with demonstrably worse health outcomes (Starfield, 2000). As Seidman (2013) has argued, Medicare for all would: (1) provide universal and portable health insurance coverage that is not tied to an employer, which would eliminate the need to choose employment based on insurance coverage and free business managers and entrepreneurs from the bureaucratic burden of purchasing cost-efficient health insurance for themselves and their employees; (2) eliminate the marketing costs for private health insurance and substantially reduce administrative costs; (3) be relatively simple to implement through a bureaucratic structure that is already in place and a set of taxes earmarked for Medicare that would replace private health insurance premiums, and (4) reduce health care costs by using the bargaining power of a single-payer system. In fact, Medicare pays much less for hospital procedures than private health insurance companies and uninsured individuals because by law, the payments need to approximate the actual costs of the procedures, including salaries, equipment, and overhead (Brill, 2013). This means that Medicare has to reimburse providers for their services, but providers are not allowed to overcharge Medicare. No such provision against overcharging exists for patients with private insurance or those without insurance. Clearly, this health care dilemma is a major social justice issue, which has yet to be resolved but is on the forefront of current discourse.

Other possible ways to adjust for these concerns include increasing the retirement age for receiving full or partial Social Security payments, reducing Medicare benefits, or privatizing Social Security and Medicare. In terms of addressing issues of generational equity, however, there is considerable skepticism that the money saved by reducing or privatizing Social Security and Medicare would be used to fund needed services for children and younger adults rather than to maintain tax cuts or tax loopholes for rich individuals and corporations or the current defense budget (Minkler, 1991; Polivka, 2010). Binstock (1983) remarked that although in public discourse it is often emphasized how many workers it takes to support a retired person on Social Security and Medicare, it is not often discussed how many are needed to finance an aircraft carrier or a tax break for special interest groups.

In addition to these major issues, there are many other concerns that revolve around the interface of psychology, gerontology, and social justice. At the individual level, issues involving meaning attached to life extension, especially in those who are infirm but kept alive (such as the growing number of people afflicted with degenerative brain diseases) challenge current values (Kaufman, 2005). In contrast, new ways of envisioning the positive aspects of aging, such as taking advantages of opportunities to enhance wisdom and spirituality in ways that perhaps can be obtained only at the latter stages of life, are exciting (Ai, Wink, & Ardelt, 2010; Ardelt, 2000, 2011; Ardelt & Oh, 2010). In addition, issues of empowerment, which involve changing attitudes and stereotypes, are possible as demographics shift toward a greater number of elderly in the population (Glendenning, 1995; Woodward, 2003). It also needs to be kept in mind that, somewhat paradoxically, despite the prospects of failing health and other difficulties, the elderly seem to experience sustained or even enhanced well-being compared to other age groups (Cheng, 2004; Diener & Suh, 1998; Gana, Bailly, Saada, Joulain, & Alaphilippe, 2013; George, 2010). Psychologists and others who work with and are concerned about the elderly have much to consider due to these rapidly shifting patterns, especially as they relate to implications for social justice.

We end our chapter by addressing two cutting-edge issues as examples for the many difficult challenges, as well as exciting opportunities, that an aging world faces. The first involves housing and transportation. The modern world is built with certain assumptions, such as people can cross a street in a designated amount of time or read street signs from a distance. The elderly, as well as many other groups (e.g., the disabled), are not always able to navigate this built environment that ignores their special needs (Rosenberg, Huang, Simonovich, & Belza, 2013; Shumway-Cook et al., 2002). One solution is to warehouse such people in nursing homes or similar institutions, especially due to the breakdown of other supporting institutions (e.g., the extended family). Ostensibly, this provides some protection, but it also serves the purpose of preventing the elderly from disrupting others, such as slowing down traffic as they might take extra time for street crossings (Langlois et al., 1997). Designing housing and transportation that can facilitate quality of life for the elderly is an area related to social justice as, without these supports, opportunities for independence are denied. In this regard, it is interesting to speculate about the possible changing appearance of the built environment as it might evolve to accommodate the growing population of the aged (Cunningham & Michael, 2004).

The second is the issue of transhumanism, which changes the very constituents of what it means to be human. With the growing opportunity for life extension through cybernetic enhancement for the haves, but not for the have-nots (Hook, 2004; McNamee & Edwards, 2006; Wenning & Cruz, 2006), we can imagine a world in which the wealthy are augmented in many ways, presaged by many people now wearing innovations such as Bluetooth phones and likely soon to be wearing other devices, such as Google glasses. Future developments, such as robotic exoskeletal suits that might enable the elderly to not only be active but to excel over others athletically, appear to loom just over the horizon, as science fiction rapidly becomes science fact. Likewise, cognitive deficits might be replaced by enhancements, such as brain-implanted computer chips, that advantage the wealthy elderly who can afford them. Perhaps society might eventually develop the technology, medical breakthrough, and wealth that all can have enhancements that change the very meaning of being old, possibly even leading to a humanity where the young are rare anomalies and the majority are extraordinarily healthy people who happen to have lived many years (De Grey, 2007).

As the future becomes the present, the transition between these exciting, and also scary, possibilities contrasts with the dire circumstances of many of the elderly and the social crises that loom over the coming demographic shifts. Psychology, as a scientific discipline and praxis, has much to offer now and to what will evolve.

REFERENCES

Achenbaum, W. A. (2010). Past as prologue: Toward a global history of ageing. In D. Dannefer & C. Phillipson (Eds.), *The SAGE handbook of social gerontology* (pp. 20–32). Thousand Oaks, CA: Sage.

Adekeye, O. A., Heiman, H. J., Onyeabor, O. S., & Hyacinth, H. I. (2012). The new invincibles: HIV screening among older adults in the U.S. *PLoS ONE, 7*(8), e43618. doi: 10.1371/journal.pone.0043618

Adler, N. E., & Newman, K. (2002). Socioeconomic disparities in health: Pathways and policies. *Health Affairs, 21*(2), 60–76.

Ai, A. L., Wink, P., & Ardelt, M. (2010). Spirituality and aging: A journey for meaning through deep interconnection in humanity. In J. C. Cavanaugh & C. K. Cavanaugh (Eds.), *Aging in America* (Vol. 3: Societal Issues, pp. 222–246). Santa Barbara, CA: Praeger.

Ainsworth, J. W. (2002). Why does it take a village? The mediation of neighborhood effects on educational achievement. *Social Forces, 81*(1), 117–152. doi: 10.1353/sof.2002.0038

Almeida, B., & Fornia, W. B. (2008). *A better bang for the buck. The economic efficiencies of defined benefit pension plans.* Washington, DC: National Institute on Retirement Security.

Anetzberger, G. J., Palmisano, B. R., Sanders, M., Bass, D., Dayton, C., Eckert, S., et al. (2000). A model intervention for elder abuse and dementia. *The Gerontologist, 40*(4), 492–497. doi: 10.1093/geront/40.4.492

Angel, J. L., & Mudrazija, S. (2011). Aging, inheritance, and gift-giving. In R. H. Binstock & L. K. George (Eds.), *Handbook of aging and the social sciences* (7th ed., pp. 163–173). San Diego, CA: Elsevier.

Anno, B. J., Graham, C., Lawrence, J. E., & Shansky, R. (2004). *Correctional health care: Addressing the needs of elderly, chronically ill, and terminally ill inmates.* Washington, DC: U.S. Department of Justice, National Institute of Corrections.

Aparasu, R. R., & Mort, J. R. (2004). Prevalence, correlates, and associated outcomes of potentially inappropriate psychotropic use in the community-dwelling elderly.

American Journal of Geriatric Pharmacotherapy, 2(2), 102–111. doi: 10.1016/s1543-5946(04)90015-3

Ardelt, M. (2000). Intellectual versus wisdom-related knowledge: The case for a different kind of learning in the later years of life. *Educational Gerontology: An International Journal of Research and Practice, 26*(8), 771–789. doi: 10.1080/036012700300001421

Ardelt, M. (2011). Wisdom, age, and well-being. In K. W. Schaie & S. L. Willis (Eds.), *Handbook of the psychology of aging* (7th ed., pp. 279–291). Amsterdam, The Netherlands: Elsevier.

Ardelt, M., & Oh, H. (2010). Wisdom: Definition, assessment, and its relation to successful cognitive and emotional aging. In D. Jeste & C. Depp (Eds.), *Successful cognitive and emotional aging* (pp. 87–113). Washington, DC: American Psychiatric Publishing.

Arling, G., & McAuley, W. J. (1983). Feasibility of public payments for family caregiving. *Gerontologist, 23,* 300–306. doi: 10.1093/geront/23.3.300

Baker, S., Barlow, S., Cochran, W., Fuchs, G., Klish, W., Krebs, N., et al. (2005). Overweight children and adolescents: A clinical report of the North American Society for Pediatric Gastroenterology, Hepatology and Nutrition. *Journal of Pediatric Gastroenterology and Nutrition, 40*(5), 533–543. doi: 10.1097/01.MPG.0000161147.16590.12

Barnard, J. W. (2010). Deception, decisions, and investor education. *Elder Law Journal, 17*(2), 201–237.

Baum, A., Garofalo, J. P., & Yali, A. M. (1999). Socioeconomic status and chronic stress: Does stress account for SES effects on health? *Annals of the New York Academy of Sciences, 896*(1), 131–144. doi: 10.1111/j.1749-6632.1999.tb08111.x

Binstock, R. H. (1983). The aged as scapegoat. *Gerontologist, 23*(2), 136–143. doi: 10.1093/geront/23.2.136

Binstock, R. H. (1994). Old-age-based rationing: From rhetoric to risk? *Generations, 18*(4), 37–41.

Binswange, I. A., Krueger, P. M., & Steiner, J. F. (2009). Prevalence of chronic medical conditions among jail and prison inmates in the USA compared with the general population. *Journal of Epidemiology and Community Health, 63*(11), 912–919. doi: 10.1136/jech.2009.090662

Bradley, R. H., & Corwyn, R. F. (2002). Socioeconomic status and child development. *Annual Review of Psychology, 53*(1), 371–399. doi: 10.1146/annurev.psych.53.100901.135233

Brady, D. (2004). Reconsidering the divergence between elderly, child, and overall poverty. *Research on Aging, 26*(5), 487–510. doi: 10.1177/0164027504266587

Brill, S. (2013). Bitter pill: How outrageous pricing and egregious profits are destroying our health care. *Time, 181*(8), 16–24, 26, 28 passim.

Brody, E. M. (1985). Parent care as a normative family stress. *The Gerontologist, 25*(1), 19–29. doi: 10.1093/geront/25.1.19

Brody, E. M. (1990). *Women in the middle: Their parent-care years.* New York, NY: Springer.

Budish, A. D. (1990). Avoiding the Medicaid trap. *Retired Officer, 46*(9), 37–39.

Budish, A. D. (1995). *Avoiding the Medicaid trap: How to beat the catastrophic costs of nursing-home care.* New York, NY: H. Holt.

Byock, I. R. (1996). The nature of suffering and the nature of opportunity at the end of life. *Clinics in Geriatric Medicine, 12*(2), 237–252.

Callahan, D. (1987). *Setting limits: Medical goals in an aging society.* New York, NY: Simon & Schuster.

Callahan, D. (1990). Why we must set limits. In P. Homer & M. Holstein (Eds.), *A good old age? The paradox of setting limits* (pp. 23–36). New York, NY: Simon & Schuster.

Calvo, E. (2006). Does working longer make people healthier and happier? *Issue in Brief. Work Opportunities for Older Americans, Series 2, February 2006*. Retrieved from http://crr.bc.edu/wp-content/uploads/2006/02/wob_2.pdf

Card, D., Dobkin, C., & Maestas, N. (2008). The impact of nearly universal insurance coverage on health care utilization: Evidence from Medicare. *American Economic Review, 98*(5), 2242–2258. doi: doi 10.1257/aer.98.5.2242

Caro, F. G., Bass, S. A., & Chen, Y.-P. (1993). Introduction: Achieving a productive aging society. In S. A. Bass, F. G. Caro & Y.-P. Chen (Eds.), *Achieving a productive aging society* (pp. 3–25). Westport, CT: Auburn House.

Center on Budget and Policy Priorities. (2013, April 12, 2013). Policy basics: Where do our federal tax dollars go? Retrieved from http://www.cbpp.org/cms/?fa=view&id=1258

Centers for Disease Control and Prevention. (2012). Web-based injury statistics query and reporting system (WISQARS). Fatal injury reports. Retrieved from National Center for Injury Prevention and Control http://www.cdc.gov/injury/wisqars/index.html

Cheng, S.-T. (2004). Age and subjective well-being revisited: A discrepancy perspective. *Psychology and Aging, 19*(3), 409–415. doi: 10.1037/0882-7974.19.3.409

Conyers, J. (2008). A fresh approach to health care in the United States: Improved and expanded medicare for all. *American Journal of Public Health, 98*(Suppl 1), S58. doi: 10.2105/AJPH.98.Supplement_1.S58

Cowgill, D. O., & Holmes, L. D. (1972). *Aging and modernization*. New York, NY: Appleton-Century-Crofts.

Cravit, D. (2012). *Beyond age rage: How the boomers and seniors are solving the war of the generations*. La Vergne, TN: BPS Books.

Culpepper, E. E. (1993). Ageism, sexism, and health care: Why we need old women in power. In G. R. Winslow & J. W. Walters (Eds.), *Facing limits. Ethics and health care for the elderly* (pp. 191–209). Boulder, CO: Westview Press.

Cunningham, G. O., & Michael, Y. L. (2004). Concepts guiding the study of the impact of the built environment on physical activity for alder adults: A review of the literature. *American Journal of Health Promotion, 18*(6), 435–443. doi: 10.4278/0890-1171-18.6.435

Dannefer, D. (2003). Cumulative advantage/disadvantage and the life course: Cross-fertilizing age and social science theory. *Journals of Gerontology: Series B: Psychological Sciences and Social Sciences, 58B*(6), P327-P337. doi: 10.1093/geronb/58.6.S327

Davis, S. K., Liu, Y., Quarells, R. C., & Din-Dzietham, R. (2005). Stress-related racial discrimination and hypertension likelihood in a population-based sample of African Americans: The metro Atlanta heart disease study. *Ethnicity & Disease, 15*(4), 585–593.

De Grey, A. (2007). *Ending aging: The rejuvenation breakthroughs that could reverse human aging in our lifetime*. New York, NY: St. Martin's Press.

DeNavas-Walt, C., Proctor, B. D., & Smith, J. C. (2012). *U.S. Census Bureau, Current population reports, P60-243, Income, poverty, and health insurance coverage in the United States: 2011*. Washington, DC: U.S. Government Printing Office.

Diener, E., & Suh, M. E. (1998). Subjective well-being and age: An international analysis. In K. W. Schaie & M. P. Lawton (Eds.), *Annual review of gerontology and geriatrics* (Vol. 1717, pp. 304–324). New York, NY: Springer Publishing.

Durkheim, É. (1964 [1893]). *The division of labor in society*. New York, NY: Free Press of Glencoe.

Entwisle, D. R., Alexander, K. L., & Olson, L. S. (2004). The first-grade transition in life course perspective. In J. T. Mortimer & M. J. Shanahan (Eds.), *Handbook of the life course* (pp. 229–250). New York, NY: Springer.

Espino, D. V., Jules-Bradley, A. C., Johnston, C. L., & Mouton, C. P. (1998). Diagnostic approach to the confused elderly patient. *American Family Physician, 57*(6), 1358–1366.

Federal Interagency Forum on Aging-Related Statistics. (2012). *Older Americans 2012: Key indicators of well-being*. Washington, DC: U.S. Government Printing Office.

Feinberg, L., Reinhard, S. C., Houser, A., & Choula, R. (2011). *Valuing the invaluable: 2011 update. The growing contributions and costs of family caregiving*. Washington, DC: AARP Public Policy Institute.

Ferguson, S. J., & Goodwin, A. D. (2010). Optimism and well-being in older adults: The mediating role of social support and perceived control. *The International Journal of Aging & Human Development, 71*(1), 43–68. doi: 10.2190/AG.71.1.c

Friedberg, L., & Webb, A. (2005). Retirement and the evolution of pension structure. *Journal of Human Resources, 40*(2), 281–308.

Frytak, J. R., Harley, C. R., & Finch, M. D. (2004). Socioeconomic status and health over the life course: Capital as a unifying concept. In J. T. Mortimer & M. J. Shanahan (Eds.), *Handbook of the life course* (pp. 623–643). New York, NY: Springer.

Fulmer, T., Paveza, G., VandeWeerd, C., Fairchild, S., Guadagno, L., Bolton-Blatt, M., et al. (2005). Dyadic vulnerability and risk profiling for elder neglect. *The Gerontologist, 45*(4), 525–534. doi: 10.1093/geront/45.4.525

Gana, K., Bailly, N., Saada, Y., Joulain, M., & Alaphilippe, D. (2013). Does life satisfaction change in old age: Results from an 8-year longitudinal study. *Journals of Gerontology Series B: Psychological Sciences and Social Sciences, 68*(4), 540–552. doi: 10.1093/geronb/gbs093

Geoghegan, T. (2011, June 19). Get radical: Raise social security, *The New York Times*.

George, L. K. (2010). Still happy after all these years: Research frontiers on subjective well-being in later life. *The Journals of Gerontology: Series B: Psychological Sciences and Social Sciences, 65B*(3), 331–339. doi: 10.1093/geronb/gbq006

Glendenning, F. (1995). Education for older adults: Lifelong learning, empowerment, and social change. In J. F. Nussbaum & J. Coupland (Eds.), *The handbook of communication and aging research* (pp. 467–498). Mahwah, NJ: Lawrence Erlbaum.

Helman, R., Adams, N., Copeland, C., & VanDerhei, J. (2013). The 2013 retirement confidence survey: Perceived savings needs outpace reality for many. *EBRI Issue Brief, no. 384, March 2013*. Retrieved from www.ebri.org

Hiltonsmith, R. (2012). *The retirement savings drain: The hidden & excessive costs of 401(k)s*. New York, NY: Dēmos.

Hines, J. (2002). Impact of science and technology on the elderly: Telemarketing fraud upon the elderly: Minimizing its effects through legislation, law enforcement and education. *Albany Law Journal of Science & Technology, 12*, 839–917.

Holmes, H. M., Hayley, D. C., Alexander, G. C., & Sachs, G. A. (2006). Reconsidering medication appropriateness for patients late in life. *Archives of Internal Medicine, 166*(6), 605–609. doi: 10.1001/archinte.166.6.605

Holstein, M. (1990). Voices of the old. In P. Homer & M. Holstein (Eds.), *A good old age? The paradox of setting limits* (pp. 37–43). New York, NY: Simon & Schuster.

Holstein, M. (2010). Ethics and old age: The second generation. In D. Dannefer & C. Phillipson (Eds.), *The SAGE handbook of social gerontology* (pp. 630–640). Thousand Oaks, CA: Sage.

Hook, C. C. (2004). Transhumanism and posthumanism. In S. G. Post (Ed.), *Encyclopedia of bioethics* (3rd ed., pp. 2517–2520). New York, NY: Macmillan.

Human Rights Watch. (2012). *Old behind bars. The aging prison population in the United States*. Retrieved from http://www.hrw.org/sites/default/files/reports/usprisons 0112webwcover_0.pdf

Johannesen, M., & LoGiudice, D. (2013). Elder abuse: A systematic review of risk factors in community-dwelling elders. *Age and Ageing, 42*(3), 292–298. doi: 10.1093/ageing/afs195

Johnson, R. W. (2011). Phased retirement and workplace flexibility for older adults: Opportunities and challenges. *Annals of the American Academy of Political and Social Science, 638*(1), 68–85. doi: 10.1177/0002716211413542

Johnson, R. W., Mermin, G. B. T., & Resseger, M. (2011). Job demands and work ability at older ages. *Journal of Aging and Social Policy, 23*(2), 101–118. doi: 10.1080/08959420.2011.551465

Johnson, R. W., & Mommaerts, C. (2011). *Age differences in job loss, job search, and reemployment*. Washington, DC: The Urban Institute.

Judge, K. S., Yarry, S. J., Looman, W. J., & Bass, D. M. (2013). Improved strain and psychosocial outcomes for caregivers of individuals with dementia: Findings from project ANSWERS. *Gerontologist, 53,* 280–292. doi: 10.1093/geront/gns076

Juhn, C., & McCue, K. (2012). *Workplace characteristics and employment of older workers*. Paper presented at the 14th Annual Joint Conference of the Retirement Research Consortium, Washington, DC, August 2–3, 2012.

The Kaiser Commission on Medicaid and the Uninsured. (2013). Infographic: Medicaid spending & enrollment. Who is covered and what does the program spend on their care? Retrieved from http://kff.org/interactive/infographic-medicaid-spending-enrollment/

Kaiser Family Foundation. (2010). *Medicare. A primer*. Menlo Park, CA: The Henry J. Kaiser Family Foundation.

Kaufman, S. R. (2005). *And a time to die: How American hospitals shape the end of life*. New York, NY: Scribner.

Kaufman, S. R., Shim, J. K., & Russ, A. J. (2004). Revisiting the biomedicalization of aging: Clinical trends and ethical challenges. *The Gerontologist, 44*(6), 731–738. doi: 10.1093/geront/44.6.731

Kayser-Jones, J. (2002). The experience of dying: An ethnographic nursing home study. *The Gerontologist, 42*(SpecIssue3), 11–19. doi: 10.1093/geront/42.suppl_3.11

Kite, M. E., Stockdale, G. D., Whitley, B. E., Jr., & Johnson, B. T. (2005). Attitudes toward younger and older adults: An updated meta-analytic review. *Journal of Social Issues, 61*(2), 241–266. doi: 10.1111/j.1540-4560.2005.00404.x

Klein, D., Turvey, C., & Wallace, R. (2004). Elders who delay medication because of cost: Health insurance, demographic, health, and financial correlates. *Gerontologist, 44*(6), 779–787. doi: 10.1093/geront/44.6.779

Klonoff, E. A., & Landrine, H. (2000). Is skin color a marker for racial discrimination? Explaining the skin color-hypertension relationship. *Journal of Behavioral Medicine, 23*(4), 329–338. doi: 10.1023/a:1005580300128

Kozol, J. (2005). *The shame of the nation: The restoration of apartheid schooling in America*. New York, NY: Crown Trade Paperbacks/Crown Publishers.

Kunkel, S. R., Applebaum, R. A., & Nelson, I. M. (2003). For love and money: Paying family caregivers. *Generations, 27*(4), 74–80.

Lai, D. W. L., & Thomson, C. (2011). The impact of perceived adequacy of social support on caregiving burden of family caregivers. *Families in Society, 92*(1), 99–106. doi: 10.1606/1044-3894.4063

Langlois, J. A., Keyl, P. M., Guralnik, J. M., Foley, D. J., Marottoli, R. A., & Wallace, R. B. (1997). Characteristics of older pedestrians who have difficulty crossing the street. *American Journal of Public Health, 87*(3), 393–397. doi: 10.2105/Ajph.87.3.393

Lattanzi-Licht, M., & Connor, S. (1995). Care of the dying: The hospice approach. In H. Wass & R. A. Neimeyer (Eds.), *Dying. Facing the facts* (3rd ed., pp. 143–162). Washington, DC: Taylor & Francis.

Laumann, E. O., Leitsch, S. A., & Waite, L. J. (2008). Elder mistreatment in the United States: Prevalence estimates from a nationally representative study. *The Journals of Gerontology: Series B: Psychological Sciences and Social Sciences, 63B*(4), S248-S254. doi: 10.1093/geronb/63.4.S248

Leventhal, T., & Brooks-Gunn, J. (2000). The neighborhoods they live in: The effects of neighborhood residence on child and adolescent outcomes. *Psychological Bulletin, 126*(2), 309–337. doi: 10.1037/0033-2909.126.2.309

Lin, N. (1999). Social networks and status attainment. *Annual Review of Sociology, 25*, 467–487. doi: 10.1146/annurev.soc.25.1.467

Lind, M., Hill, S., Hiltonsmith, R., & Freedman, J. (2013). *Expanded Social Security. A plan to increase retirement security for all Americans.* Washington, DC: New America Foundation.

Luo, Y., & Waite, L. J. (2011). Mistreatment and psychological well-being among older adults: Exploring the role of psychosocial resources and deficits. *The Journals of Gerontology: Series B: Psychological Sciences and Social Sciences, 66B*(2), 217–229. doi: 10.1093/geronb/gbq096

Magnus, G. (2009). *The age of aging: How demographics are changing the global economy and our world.* Hoboken, NJ: Wiley.

Mallet, L., Spinewine, A., & Huang, A. (2007). The challenge of managing drug interactions in elderly people. *Lancet, 370*(9582), 185–191. doi: 10.1016/S0140-6736(07)61092-7

McNamee, M. J., & Edwards, S. D. (2006). Transhumanism, medical technology and slippery slopes. *Journal of Medical Ethics: Journal of the Institute of Medical Ethics, 32*(9), 513–518. doi: 10.1136/jme.2005.013789

Metzler, M. (2012). Introduction: Japan at an inflection point. *Asia Pacific Business Review, 18*(2), 135–147. doi: 10.1080/13602381.2011.561650

Miller, E. A. (2012). The Affordable Care Act and long-term care: Comprehensive reform or just tinkering around the edges? *Journal of Aging and Social Policy, 24*(2), 101–117. doi: 10.1080/08959420.2012.659912

Minkler, M. (1991). "Generational equity" and the new victim blaming. In M. Minkler & C. Estes (Eds.), *Critical perspectives on aging: The political and moral economy of growing old* (pp. 67–79). Amityville, NY: Baywood.

Mittelman, M. S., Roth, D. L., Haley, W. E., & Zarit, S. H. (2004). Effects of a caregiver intervention on negative caregiver appraisals of behavior problems in patients with Alzheimer's disease: Results of a randomized trial. *The Journals of Gerontology: Series B: Psychological Sciences and Social Sciences, 59B*(1), P27-P34. doi: 10.1093/geronb/59.1.P27

Mojtabai, R., & Olfson, M. (2003). Medication costs, adherence, and health outcomes among Medicare beneficiaries. *Health Affairs, 22*(4), 220–229. doi: 10.1377/hlthaff.22.4.220

Moody, H. R., & Sasser, J. R. (2012). *Aging. Concepts and controversies* (7th ed.). Thousand Oaks, CA: Sage.

Mort, J. R., & Aparasu, R. R. (2000). Prescribing potentially inappropriate psychotropic medications to the ambulatory elderly. *Archives of Internal Medicine, 160*(18), 2825–2831. doi: 10.1001/archinte.160.18.2825

Moses, S. A. (1990). Fallacy of impoverishment. *Gerontologist, 30*(1), 21–25. doi: 10.1093/geront/30.1.21

Mouallem, L. (2002). Oh no, grandma has a computer: How Internet fraud will take the place of telemarketing fraud targeting the elderly. *Santa Clara Law Review, 42*(2), 659–687.

Munnell, A., & Rutledge, M. (2013, March). The effects of the Great Recession on the retirement security of older workers. *National Poverty Center Working Paper Series, #13–03*. Retrieved from http://npc.umich.edu/publications/u/2013-03-npc-working-paper.pdf

Nerenberg, L. (2010). Elder abuse prevention: A review of the field. In J. C. Cavanaugh & C. K. Cavanaugh (Eds.), *Aging in America* (Vol. 3: Societal Issues, pp. 53–80). Santa Barbara, CA: Praeger.

Ogden, L. L., & Adams, K. (2009). Poorhouse to Warehouse: Institutional long-term care in the United States. *Publius, 39*(1), 138–163. doi: 10.1093/publius/pjn030

O'Rand, A. M., Binstock, R. H., & George, L. K. (2006). Stratification and the life course: Life course capital, life course risks, and social inequality. In R. H. Binstock, L. K. George, S. J. Cutler, J. Hendricks & J. H. Schulz (Eds.), *Handbook of aging and the social sciences* (6th ed., pp. 145–162). Amsterdam, The Netherlands: Elsevier.

O'Rand, A. M., Isaacs, K., & Roth, L. (2010). Age and inequality in global context. In D. Dannefer & C. Phillipson (Eds.), *The SAGE handbook of social gerontology* (pp. 127–136). Thousand Oaks, CA: Sage.

Ory, M., Hoffman, M. K., Hawkins, M., Sanner, B., & Mockenhaupt, R. (2003). Challenging aging stereotypes: Strategies for creating a more active society. *American Journal of Preventive Medicine, 25*(3,Suppl2), 164–171. doi: 10.1016/s0749-3797(03)00181-8

Palloni, A. (2006). Reproducing inequalities: Luck, wallets, and the enduring effects of childhood health. *Demography, 43*(4), 587–615. doi: 10.1353/dem.2006.0036

Peterson, P. G. (1996). *Will America grow up before it grows old? How the coming social security crisis threatens you, your family, and your country* (1st ed.). New York, NY: Random House.

Polivka, L. (2010). Neoliberalism and the new politics of aging and retirement security. In J. C. Cavanaugh & C. K. Cavanaugh (Eds.), *Aging in America* (Vol. 3: Societal Issues, pp. 160–202). Santa Barbara, CA: Praeger.

Post, L., Page, C., Conner, T., Prokhorov, A., Fang, Y., & Biroscak, B. J. (2010). Elder abuse in long-term care: Types, patterns, and risk factors. *Research on Aging, 32*(3), 323–348. doi: 10.1177/0164027509357705

Powell, J. (2010). The power of global aging. *Ageing International, 35,* 1–14. doi: 10.1007/s12126-010-9051-6

Pruchno, R., & Smyer, M. A. (Eds.). (2007). *Challenges of an aging society: Ethical dilemmas, political issues*. Baltimore, MD: Johns Hopkins University Press.

Rikard, R. V., & Rosenberg, E. (2007). Aging inmates: A convergence of trends in the American criminal justice system. *Journal of Correctional Health Care, 13*(3), 150–162. doi: 10.1177/1078345807303001

Ritter, K. P. (1995). Preparation for guardianship cases poses a constant challenge. *Journal of Long-Term Care Administration, 23*(3), 14–17.

Rosenberg, D. E., Huang, D. L., Simonovich, S. D., & Belza, B. (2013). Outdoor built environment barriers and facilitators to activity among midlife and older adults with mobility disabilities. *Gerontologist, 53*(2), 268–279. doi: 10.1093/geront/gns119

Sampson, R. J., Morenoff, J. D., & Gannon-Rowley, T. (2002). Assessing "neighborhood effects": Social processes and new directions in research. *Annual Review of Sociology, 28,* 443–478. doi: 10.2307/3069249

Schneider, E. L. (1993). Changing the debate about health care for the elderly. In G. R. Winslow & J. W. Walters (Eds.), *Facing limits. Ethics and health care for the elderly* (pp. 161–174). Boulder, CO: Westview Press.

Seidman, L. (2013). Medicare for all. An economist's case. *Challenge, 56*(1), 88–115. doi: 10.2753/0577-5132560105

Shugarman, L. R., Fries, B. E., Wolf, R. S., & Morris, J. N. (2003). Identifying older people at risk of abuse during routine screening practices. *Journal of the American Geriatrics Society, 51*(1), 24–31. doi: 10.1034/j.1601-5215.2002.51005.x

Shumway-Cook, A., Patla, A. E., Stewart, A., Ferrucci, L., Ciol, M. A., & Guralnik, J. M. (2002). Environmental demands associated with community mobility in older adults with and without mobility disabilities. *Physical Therapy, 82*(7), 670–681.

Simon-Rusinowitz, L., Mahoney, K. J., & Benjamin, A. E. (2001). Payments to families who provide care: An option that should be available. In M. B. Holstein & P. B. Mitzen (Eds.), *Springer series on ethics, law, and aging* (pp. 286–296). New York, NY: Springer Publishing Co.

Smirnova, M. H. (2012). A will to youth: The woman's anti-aging elixir. *Social Science & Medicine, 75*(7), 1236–1243. doi: 10.1016/j.socscimed.2012.02.061

Smith, S. P. (1991). Ending mandatory retirement in the arts and sciences. *American Economic Review, 81*(2), 106–110.

Smith, T. L., & Toseland, R. W. (2006). The effectiveness of a telephone support program for caregivers of frail older adults. *The Gerontologist, 46*(5), 620–629. doi: 10.1093/geront/46.5.620

Social Security Administration. (2012). *Income of the population 55 or older, 2010.* Washington, DC: Social Security Administration. Retrieved from http://www.ssa.gov/policy/docs/statcomps/income_pop55/2010/incpop10.pdf

Social Security Administration. (2013, May 3, 2013). Social Security. The official website of the U.S. Social Security Administration. Retrieved from http://www.ssa.gov/

Starfield, B. (2000). Is US health really the best in the world? *Jama-Journal of the American Medical Association, 284*(4), 483–485. doi: 10.1001/jama.284.4.483

State of Florida Correctional Medical Authority. (2010). *2009–2010 annual report and report on aging inmates.* Retrieved from http://edocs.dlis.state.fl.us/fldocs/dcor/CMA/annualreport09-10.pdf

Steinman, M. A., Landefeld, C. S., Rosenthal, G. E., Berthenthal, D., Sen, S., & Kaboli, P. J. (2006). Polypharmacy and prescribing quality in older people. *Journal of the American Geriatrics Society, 54*(10), 1516–1523. doi: 10.1111/j.1532-5415.2006.00889.x

Sullivan, A.D., Hedberg, K., & Fleming, D. W. (2000). Legalized physician-assisted suicide in Oregon—The second year. *The New England Journal of Medicine, 342*(8), 598–604. doi: 10.1056/NEJM200002243420822

Teno, J. M., Gozalo, P. L., Bynum, J. P. W., Leland, N. E., Miller, S. C., Morden, N. E., et al. (2013). Change in end-of-life care for Medicare beneficiaries: Site of death, place of care, and health care transitions in 2000, 2005, and 2009. *JAMA, 309*(5), 470–477. doi: 10.1001/jama.2012.207624

Thoits, P. A. (2011). Mechanisms linking social ties and support to physical and mental health. *Journal of Health and Social Behavior, 52*(2), 145–161. doi: 10.1177/00221 46510395592

Thompson, E. H., Futterman, A. M., Gallagher-Thompson, D., Rose, J. M., & Lovett, S. B. (1993). Social support and caregiving burden in family caregivers of frail elders. *Journal of Gerontology, 48*(5), S245-S254. doi: 10.1093/geronj/48.5.S245

Thurow, L. C. (1996). *The future of capitalism: How today's economic forces shape tomorrow's world* (1st ed.). New York, NY: W. Morrow.

Troxel, W. M., Matthews, K. A., Bromberger, J. T., & Sutton-Tyrrell, K. (2003). Chronic stress burden, discrimination, and subclinical carotid artery disease in African American and Caucasian women. *Health Psychology, 22*(3), 300–309. doi: 10.1037/0278-6133.22.3.300

Tucker, J. V., Reno, V. P., & Bethell, T. N. (2013). *Strengthening Social Security: What do Americans want?* Washington, DC: National Academy of Social Insurance.

Uhlenberg, P. (2013). Demography is not destiny: The challenges and opportunities of global population aging. *Generations, 37*(1), 12–18.

United Nations, Department of Economic and Social Affairs, Population Division. (2013). *World population prospects: The 2012 revision.* Retrieved from http://esa.un.org /unpd/wpp/index.htm

Van de Water, P. N., & Sherman, A. (2010). *Social security keeps 20 million Americans out of poverty: A state-by-state analysis.* Washington, DC: Center on Budget and Policy Priorities.

Victor, C. (2010). The demography of ageing. In D. Dannefer & C. Phillipson (Eds.), *The SAGE handbook of social gerontology* (pp. 61–74). Thousand Oaks, CA: Sage.

Vogel, J. (2002). Ageing and living conditions of the elderly: Sweden 1980–1998. *Social Indicators Research, 59*(1), 1–34. doi: 10.1023/a:1016082428082

Wahidin, A., & Aday, R. H. (2010). Later life and imprisonment. In D. Dannefer & C. Phillipson (Eds.), *The SAGE handbook of social gerontology* (pp. 587–596). Thousand Oaks, CA: Sage.

Warren, J. R., Hoonakker, P., Carayon, P., & Brand, J. (2004). Job characteristics as mediators in SES-health relationships. *Social Science & Medicine, 59*(7), 1367–1378. doi: 10.1016/j.socscimed.2004.01.035

Wenning, L., & Cruz, R. (2006). The ethics of artificial vision technology: An early step towards an ethics of cybernetic repair and augmentation. *Columbia University Journal of Bioethics, 1,* 59–64.

Wetle, T., & Besdine, R. W. (1990). Letting individuals decide. In P. Homer & M. Holstein (Eds.), *A good old age? The paradox of setting limits* (pp. 53–57). New York, NY: Simon & Schuster.

Wilber, K. H., & Reynolds, S. L. (1996). Introducing a framework for defining financial abuse of the elderly. *Journal of Elder Abuse and Neglect, 8*(2), 61–80. doi: 10.1300/J084v08n02_06

Williams, B. A., Sudore, R. L., Greifinger, R., & Morrison, R. S. (2011). Balancing punishment and compassion for seriously ill prisoners. *Annals of Internal Medicine, 155*(2), 122–126. doi: 10.7326/0003-4819-155-2-201107190-00348

Williams, D. R., & Neighbors, H. (2001). Racism, discrimination and hypertension: Evidence and needed research. *Ethnicity & Disease, 11*(4), 800–816.

Williamson, J. B., Watts-Roy, D. M., & Kingson, E. R. (1999). *The generational equity debate*. New York, NY: Columbia University Press.

Willson, A. E., Shuey, K. M., & Elder, G. H., Jr. (2007). Cumulative advantage processes as mechanisms of inequality in life course health. *American Journal of Sociology, 112*(6), 1886–1924. doi: 10.1086/512712

Winslow, G. R. (1993). Exceptions and the elderly. In G. R. Winslow & J. W. Walters (Eds.), *Facing limits. Ethics and health care for the elderly* (pp. 231–243). Boulder, CO: Westview Press.

Woodward, K. (2003). Against wisdom: The social politics of anger and aging. *Journal of Aging Studies, 17*(1), 55–67. doi: 10.1016/S0890-4065(02)00090-7

Zuvekas, S. H., & Taliaferro, G. S. (2003). Pathways to access: Health insurance, the health care delivery system, and racial/ethnic disparities, 1996–1999. *Health Affairs, 22*(2), 139–153. doi: 10.1377/hlthaff.22.2.139

Chapter 12

Social Justice and Poverty: Perspectives for Psychologists[1]

Laura Smith and Riddhi Sandil

Feminist, multicultural, and social justice critiques of traditional psychotherapy have long contended that conventional psychotherapeutic approaches are, at best, culture bound and, at worst, oppressive to people who are members of marginalized groups (Sue et al., 1998). Calls for a corresponding re-envisioning of professional mental health practice are not new in the field; in 1969, for example, former American Psychological Association (APA) president George Albee explicated emotional disturbance as the human consequences of an unjust, dehumanized society (Albee, 1969). Yet, four decades later, poverty and its survival still go missing from most considerations of mental health theory and application, with the result that interventions offered to poor clients may bear little relevance to their lives and experiences (Smith, 2005, 2008).

Counseling psychologists have consistently been among those at the forefront of efforts to advance social justice advocacy and multicultural competence within psychotherapeutic practice. Outlining the long-standing emphasis within counseling psychology on sociocultural factors in human development and well-being, Goodman et al. (2004) traced a thread that began with Frank Parson's vocational work in the early 1900s and extended through the development of the APA's *Guidelines on Multicultural Education, Training, Research, Practice, and Organizational*

Change for Psychologists (APA, 2002). Largely absent within this history, however, are integrative considerations of social class, classism, and poverty. Liu et al. (2004) revealed this gap in a content analysis of articles published in three counseling journals between the years 1981 and 2000: *Journal of Counseling Psychology*, *Journal of Counseling and Development*, and *Journal of Multicultural Counseling and Development*. They found that only 18% of the articles reviewed incorporated social class as a variable; even then, when social class was referenced, it was most often not a focus of the article but received mention in a methods section. Lott (2002) observed that classism is generally missing from psychological examinations even when multiculturalism is a central focus. Thus, although efforts have been made to include poverty and classism in the context of understanding human experience, these important constructs have been largely ignored in clinical and counseling psychological research and practice.

It should be noted that other fields of psychology, such as community and social psychology, have made significant contributions toward understanding the impact of poverty and social class oppression on mental health and well-being (e.g., Duncan & Brooks-Gunn, 1997; Marks, 2004). Although this research has helped enhance current awareness of poverty, it has also been criticized for being primarily Western in its perspective, for presenting narrow findings that are not generalizable on a global level, and for not providing suggestions for addressing inequities and injustices (Campbell & Murray, 2004; Murray & Campbell, 2003). Thus, it is imperative that attention be given not only to advance the understanding of poverty and its impact on psychological well-being, but also to suggest new directions for socially disadvantaged populations, many of whom may experience psychosocial distress (Campbell & Murray, 2004).

A SOCIAL JUSTICE FRAMEWORK FOR UNDERSTANDING POVERTY AND CLASSISM

Before outlining a social justice approach to an understanding of poverty and classism, it is important to address the language that is used to delineate social class membership in the United States. The language used to describe class groupings is notoriously wide-ranging (Baker, 1996). Descriptors include poor, low-income, disadvantaged, working-class, blue-collar, white-collar, wealthy, and upper-class; class indicators (the criteria used to differentiate class membership) are similarly multitudinous and include such considerations as income, attitudes and beliefs, education level, job prestige, power in the workplace, and differences between manual and physical labor.

What Is Social Class?

Each of these formulations captures some, but not all, of the truth about the lived experience of social class, and different formulations lend themselves more readily to different types of scholarly inquiry. Two authors who have offered basic typologies are Leondar-Wright (2005) and Zweig (2000). Their broad, conceptual formulations are similar to each other, and the following framework combines elements from their work regarding social class dynamics in the United States:

- *Poverty* includes predominantly working-class people who, because of unemployment, low-wage jobs, health problems, or other crises, are without enough income to support their basic needs.
- The *working* class includes people who have little power or authority in the workplace; little control over the availability or content of jobs; and little say in the decisions that affect their access to health care, education, and housing. They tend to have lower levels of income, net worth, and formal education than more powerful classes.
- The *middle* class includes professionals, managers, small-business owners, often college educated and salaried. Middle-class people have more autonomy and control in work settings than do working-class people, and more economic security; however, they rely on earnings from work to support themselves.
- The *owning* class includes people who own enough wealth that they need not work to support themselves; moreover, they are people who own and control the resources by which other people earn a living. As a result of their economic power, the owning class includes people who also have significant social, cultural, and political power relative to other classes.

Beyond the context of the United States, formulations of class membership vary so widely that they cannot be encompassed within a single chapter. Illustrative examples include Kharas's (2010) conception of the global middle class as including households with a daily per capita income of $10 to $100, and L. R. Bloom's (2009) delineation of global poverty as comprising the 1.4 billion people in the world who live at or below a poverty line of $1.25 a day. Fukuda-Parr (1999) cautioned that income should not be the sole determinant of poverty on a global scale, but rather that poverty is "best measured by indicators of the opportunities and choices that people have" (Fukuda-Parr, 1999, p. 100). To frame worldwide poverty within a multidimensional framework, the 1997 Human Development Report proposed the Human Poverty Index (HPI), a non-income based measure of poverty. This index measured four dimensions of deprivation: survival, knowledge, standard of living, and social participation. Although the HPI excludes contextual oppressions such as political persecution, safety, and marginalization due to minority status (e.g., gender, race), it allows researchers to gain a deeper understanding of poverty rather than just its economic implications. Similarly, the United Nations Conference on Trade and Development also suggested that the definition of global poverty be broadened to include "non-material deprivation" (UNCTAD, 2002a). These deprivations include limited access to education, health care, and an increased susceptibility to harm because of societal marginalization and disempowerment.

Applying a Social Justice Perspective to Social Class

For the purposes of this overview, the general typology for social class presented earlier lends itself well to a social justice framework. Social justice psychology itself has been explicated by a number of authors in recent years (e.g., Albee, 1969; Mays, 2000; Prilleltensky, 1994; Speight & Vera, 2004; Strickland, 2000). Most of these conceptualizations converge generally on a few central tenets. Goodman et al. (2004) explained that social justice psychology rejects the artificial separation of individual well-being from the sociocultural forces that can affect it critically, and comprises research and action designed to change societal values, structures, policies, and practices. For example, according to an ecological model of change presented by Prilleltensky and Nelson (2002), oppression, liberation, and well-being are connected to one another at multiple experiential levels, delineated as self, relationships with others, and society. Researchers have directed particular attention to the pathogenic impact of two forms of oppression, poverty and racism, upon individual and collective well-being. This body of work has revealed that oppression's destructive effects are mediated through such realities as environmental risk factors, physiological stress responses, psychosocial trauma, and community disintegration.

In their introductory chapter to the *Handbook for Social Justice in Counseling Psychology*, Fouad, Gerstein, and Toporek (2006) emphasized that social justice refers explicitly to the fair and equitable distributions of advantages and disadvantages within a society. In another chapter from this volume, Toporek and Williams (2006) referred back to the proceedings of the 2001 National Counseling Psychology Conference in adding that social justice implies the involvement of all individuals as co-participants in the decisions that affect their lives. These themes suggest a fundamental premise for a social justice approach to psychological practice. This premise begins with the acknowledgment that the current U.S. and global societal status quo is characterized by an inequitable distribution of power, resources, and access to same, within which psychology as a field and psychologists as individuals are inevitably located. Not only is one within this system, the system is within them: it is the medium in which current professional fields were conceived and from which their practices evolved. Importantly, this implies that doing nothing is not a neutral position. When psychologists, as practitioners, researchers, and educators, choose to avert their gaze and leave oppression unacknowledged, they implicitly support inequity by helping to obscure its existence.

Building on this premise, the application of a social justice framework to any professional endeavor begins with the identification of dominant-culture assumptions and actions that may be embedded within and perpetuated by a field's practices, even if unintentionally. Action toward the creation of new, socially just practices, policies, theories, and procedures can then be initiated and integrated within the field's activities and knowledge base. With regard to counseling and psychotherapy, this process leads to such considerations as the damaging impact of all forms of oppression on emotional and interpersonal well-being, the implications of relying on interventions that target the individual's "interior" while leaving sociocultural origins of distress unaddressed, and the possibility that conventional psychotherapeutic roles and practices reproduce power-over relationships in the lives of clients from marginalized groups.

Just as other aspects of sociocultural privilege are associated with characteristic forms of oppression, oppression expressed within the social class hierarchy is associated with *classism*, a form of structural oppression that intersects with the other, more familiar "-isms" (e.g., racism and sexism,). Again, within a social justice framework, the underlying supposition with regard to any form of oppression is that it is considered to exist in a real (as opposed to a relative) sense, and that these broad systems of power relations exist as a backdrop for discussions of the circumstances and well-being of members of dominant and subordinated groups. A social justice conceptualization of classism, therefore, corresponds to the third of three approaches to class-related inequalities as described by the APA Task Force on Socioeconomic Status (APA, 2006). These categories were identified as: (1) materialist approaches, or those that correlate differences in socioeconomic status (SES) with differential access to resources, goods, and services ("materials"); (2) gradient approaches, or those for which status is constructed as a continuum along which relative differences in class position may be considered; and (3) reproduction of power and privilege, or approaches that treat class inequity as a form of sociopolitical dominance by which some groups are systematically advantaged at the expense of others.

Psychologists have not extensively explored this third approach, although social psychologists have offered substantive treatments of class privilege (e.g., Lott & Bullock, 2007), as have community psychologists (e.g., Prilleltensky & Nelson, 2002), and feminist psychologists (e.g., Hill & Rothblum, 1996). A definition of classism that embodies this approach was offered by Bullock (1995), who defined classism as "the oppression of the poor through a network of everyday practices, attitudes, assumptions, behaviors, and institutional rules" (p. 119). Lott and Bullock (2007) further elaborated this definition to encompass institutional classism, through which social institutions function to perpetuate the deprivation and low status of poor people, and interpersonal classism, which is characterized by prejudice, stereotyping, and discrimination.

Seeing Classism in Everyday Life

If classism is conceptualized according to the definition presented earlier, then social class privilege can be understood as the advantageous net effect of all the everyday practices, attitudes, assumptions, behaviors, and institutional rules that operate to the benefit of people with higher class status. Social class privilege is made visible through such material advantages as increased educational opportunities and increased access to health care. Enhanced civic protection also accrues to those with social class privilege; for example, "dirty" industries and services such as waste dumps and bus depots are less likely to be located in neighborhoods where middle-class and wealthy people live (Bullard, 2005). In addition, cultural attitudes and images tend to reflect and perpetuate approval of people with privileged class status. Popular media demonstrate the widespread fascination with the lifestyles and habits of wealthy people (Lott & Bullock, 2007), whereas an analysis of televised representations of the poor indicated that, when they are seen at all, they are likely to be portrayed as dysfunctional, ignorant, unruly, promiscuous, drug users, or any combination of these (Bullock, Wyche, & Williams, 2001). Such considerations begin to sketch out the parameters of social class privilege—but they also underscore Lott and Bullock's (2007) call for more research attention to fundamental questions of class, power, and privilege.

Before psychologists can deepen their understanding of classism, they must develop their ability to see the operations of classism in everyday life. As is the case with other forms of oppression and privilege, some manifestations of classism are easily identifiable, whereas others are elusive and are perpetuated by well-intentioned people who are truly unaware of the classist implications of their thoughts or actions. As such, although it is important to learn about the circumstances of life in subordinated social classes, our learning should not end there. Understanding classism also means identifying the taken-for-granted social mechanisms that place obstacles in the paths of poor and working-class people as they simultaneously advantage members of the middle class and owning class—a subtle, often invisible bias that gives rise to the cliché "the rich get richer, and the poor get poorer." Examples of classism go beyond negative attitudes and beliefs regarding poor and working-class people to include tangible expressions of disadvantage such as lack of access to basic services and economic injustice.

Access to Basic Services

The provision of "essential human services, especially for those who are least able to help themselves," as the USDHHS (2007a) stated, is one of the foundational functions of the U.S. federal government. Yet, although they are often outside people's awareness, structural inequities operate so that the people most in need often receive the least adequate services. For example, the gap between the educational opportunities of children from poor families and their wealthier peers continues to widen (Fairchild, 1984; Fine, 1990; McGee, 2004). As documented by Kozol (2005), students in poor communities attend schools that have fewer computers, fewer library books, fewer classes, fewer extracurricular opportunities, and fewer teachers than wealthier students enjoy; their teachers are also more likely to be poorly paid and uncertified. Not surprisingly, academic attainment lags in such schools; the cumulative effect is summarized by the fact that the percentage of a school's children who are eligible for free lunch is inversely related to overall student performance (Day-Vines & Day-Hairston, 2005).

Along these lines, poor Americans have been largely left behind as medical innovations and expenditures have advanced health care here in the world's wealthiest country. Class, it was reported, is associated with everything from risk factors for chronic illnesses to quality of care, access to care, availability of social and financial support during illnesses, relationships with doctors, and overall stress level. And how do those at the bottom of American class structure fare? The medical and psychological risks associated with poverty are not particular to the United States, but the disparity between the health status of the rich and the poor in the United States is noteworthy: a recently released report on children's well-being by the United Nations Childrens's Fund (UNICEF, 2007) ranked the United States and Britain lowest overall among a list of 21 industrialized nations, with the United States occupying the lowest ranking with regard to child poverty and overall health and safety.

Belle, Doucet, Harris, Miller, and Tan (2000) affirmed that "poverty is associated with elevated rates of threatening and uncontrollable life events, noxious life conditions, marital dissolution, infant mortality, many diseases, violent crime, homicide, accidents, and deaths from all causes" (p. 1160). Psychologists are themselves part of this picture in that, despite decades of knowledge of the psychological damage exacted by poverty, psychological services remain embedded within the current configuration of the health care industry so that equitable access to them is precluded. Many psychologists choose to forego insurance reimbursement because of prodigious eligibility and claims-processing requirements and dwindling reimbursements, and even the lowest fee on most psychologists' sliding scale is out of the question for many poor families—assuming that a psychologist's office was even readily accessible by residents of poor communities.

Economic Injustice

Without people working in minimum-wage jobs to carry it along, everyday life in America would come to a standstill. Middle- and owning-class people rely regularly on these workers, who are all around them—working in child care and taking care of the elderly, cleaning offices, delivering food, washing dishes, and cutting grass. It seems safe to say that someone needs to do these things, yet the adults who perform these necessary jobs often cannot earn enough money to support themselves and their children. In the United States, the recent increase in the federal minimum wage was a welcome advance after years of stagnation, but at the rate of $7.25, it still lags behind estimates of what a living wage would be. A living wage is often considered to be the amount necessary to lift a family of four at least to the poverty line and no farther than 130% of the poverty line, 130% being the maximum that a family can earn and still be eligible for food stamps, and estimates for most locales begin at approximately $8.85 (Living Wage Resource Center, 2003).

The fact that an adult can work full time and yet live in poverty goes hand in hand with a report by the National Coalition for the Homeless (2005) that as many as 25% of people in U.S. homeless shelters have jobs—a statistic that makes clear the impact of this state of affairs on low-wage workers. Less obvious are the benefits and comforts that concurrently accrue to the middle and owning classes, who can afford to buy more products and services more cheaply when employers do not pay employees enough to live on. In a statement to Congress regarding the 1938 Fair Labor Standards Act, in which he advocated the establishment of a minimum wage, President Franklin D. Roosevelt had something to say about such acquisitions: "Goods produced under conditions which do not meet a rudimentary standard of decency should be regarded as contraband" (Grossman, 2006).

MENTAL HEALTH PRACTICE IN THE CONTEXT OF OPPRESSION

Having located poverty and social class within a social justice framework, how can one understand their implications for psychological practice? The emerging literature documenting the deleterious effects of oppression is logical and persuasive, and confirms the experiences of many clinicians who have worked in poor communities of people of color and who have seen the crushing influences that poverty and racism exact on the families who must survive them (Aponte, 1994; Dumont, 1996; Smith, 2005). Yet the literature can also leave therapists in a quandary: although they may accept the implications of a social justice perspective, and understand that theory and practice are limited in scope, the vast majority of them were trained according to conventional (and usually Western) psychotherapeutic models. The 50-minute individual talk therapy hour, derived from White middle-class culture (Javier & Herron, 2002), remains the primary tool in most therapists' toolboxes. Certainly, it can be (and must be) employed in the context of multicultural and social justice awareness, knowledge, and skills—but if therapists accept that oppression is the pathogen, can they offer anything *more* in the way of relevant, psychopolitically valid services for people impacted by oppression? And if so, what?

Participatory Action Frameworks

Participatory action approaches represent an opportunity for mental health professionals to address questions like these from a social and methodological stance that is less likely to reproduce dominant culture theories and practices. Most broadly, action research refers to "a cycle of inquiry involving *plan-act-observe-reflect*" (Herr & Anderson, 2005, p. 9); participatory action approaches build upon this orientation by incorporating the collaboration of local community members. These approaches have the potential to be psychopolitically valid by producing action and knowledge that contribute to social change: they offer researchers and community members the opportunity "to 'research back,' in the same tradition of 'writing back' or 'talking back' that characterizes much of the postcolonial or anticolonial literature" (Tuhiwai Smith, 1999, p. 7). Such fields as public health and education have established traditions of participatory action (e.g., Minkler & Wallerstein, 2003), yet these approaches are infrequently utilized across the mental health professions.

Participatory action research (PAR) is one of the best-known variants among action approaches, described by Kidd and Kral (2005) as "a process in which people (researchers and participants) develop goals and methods, participate in the gathering and analysis of data, and implement the results in a way that will raise critical consciousness and promote change in the lives of those involved—changes that are in the direction and control of the participating group or community" (p. 187). In PAR, therefore, the distinction between researcher and researched is challenged, so that participants are given the opportunity to be actively involved in identifying and addressing issues that affect them and their communities (Minkler & Wallerstein, 2003). Such approaches pose challenges for professional researchers. Kidd and Kral (2005) noted that participatory projects can be fraught with ambiguities that can tempt researchers to fall back on the comforts of a less egalitarian model in which they hold more power. As such, researchers must be prepared to engage in a personal struggle with their own deeply embedded beliefs about what constitutes knowledge. This idea of personal engagement contradicts the relatively neutral and distant posture to which mental health professionals are traditionally trained—a posture that ultimately separates them from those with whom they work through the establishment of a power dynamic.

The Positionality Continuum

The classic, fully elaborated form of PAR, which often requires years to develop, is, however, only one point on a spectrum of action research approaches that can incorporate community participation. Herr and Anderson (2005) offered a useful delineation of this spectrum based on their study of educators' initiatives to study their own practice. Based on this research, Herr and Anderson developed a "continuum of positionality" (p. 30) for action research that described six possible locations for practitioners and researchers with regard to the research setting itself. These positionalities are specified by the insider/outsider status of the researcher with regard to the organizational setting where the research takes place: insiders are researchers who are also practitioners within the setting, whereas outsiders are university or professional researchers who enter a particular setting to study it in collaboration with insiders and community members.

Herr and Anderson's continuum of positionalities cannot be thoroughly conveyed in the space of this chapter, but it begins with *insider* research, in which a practitioner studies his or her own practice in the tradition of narrative or case study research. Next is *insider in collaboration with other insiders*, where a team of insiders gathers to study an issue relevant to the setting's work, followed by *insiders in collaboration with outsiders*, in which such a team may invite outside researchers to participate or consult. Next on the continuum is the classic form of PAR, a *reciprocal collaboration* that is jointly initiated and implemented by true insider-outsider teams; *outsiders in collaboration with insiders* is, however, the more common version of PAR, wherein outsiders are the initiators of the project. The sixth category, *outsider studies insider*, approximates traditional university research but may contain participatory elements. Finally, each of these six positions intersects with a second research dimension called *mode of participation*, or the degree to which local people are involved in the research; possibilities range from token or symbolic community participation to full collective action.

The implications of such a framework for the evolution of socially just practice are momentous: it invites the possibility that some form of action research to transform practice in keeping with a social justice vision is within the reach of many practitioners working in community settings. PAR appears to offer more promise than many other approaches in this regard, yet it is important to point out that no approach, however promising, can be romanticized as an antidote to oppression in and of itself. Krumer-Nevo (2009), for example, cautioned against poverty-related projects that accomplish little more than to satisfy researchers' agendas, and recommended understanding "people in poverty as possessors of thoughts and ideas, not only as experiences" (p. 290). Similarly, Martinez-Salgado (2009) reflected on the impact of qualitative inquiry in Mexico City on researchers' professional identity. Martinez-Salgado described conducting a qualitative study on health risks with poor, urban families. Along the way, she and her research team struggled with emergent issues of uncertainty, rejection, confusion, misunderstanding, sadness and impotence, highlighting the value of honoring and reflecting on changes that occur within the researcher and the research team. Such examples provide important direction for researchers who wish to address poverty through the formation of participatory action research collaborations or other methodologies.

RELATED CHALLENGES EMERGING FROM A GLOBAL CONSIDERATION OF POVERTY

Consideration of the dynamics of poverty around the world raises still other issues for psychologists and others who wish to address it. Far from being an infrequent challenge to the world's peoples, poverty is a fact of life for many; the World Bank (2001) suggests that nearly half of the global population have a daily income of less than $2.50 a day, and that one in two children in the world live in poverty (Amoroso, 2007). A related phenomenon, sometimes called the *feminization of poverty*, refers to societal forces that make women and children most vulnerable to poverty, with women making up 70% of the world's poor while being relegated to the least desired and paid jobs. These inequities can be attributed generally to the fact that women are frequently excluded from participation in decisions that impact their lives, and excluded from choices and opportunities that are available to men (Fukuda-Parr, 1999. Other gender oppressive experiences—such as domestic violence, trauma, and patriarchy—further obstruct the ability of women around the world to climb out of economic oppression (Fishbach & Herbert, 1997).

The feminization of poverty is one example of how global poverty intersects meaningfully with gender, race, histories of colonization, and political instability to impact the well-being of marginalized groups. In order to gain a better understanding of poverty and dimensions of well-being, the World Health Organization (WHO) developed the Global Burden of Disease (GBD) index, a measure that provides information about mortality and loss of health due to diseases, injuries, and risk factors around the globe (World Health Organization [WHO], 2008). According to the 2008 WHO report, 13% of the GBD among the world's people corresponds to mental, neurological, and substance abuse disorders—higher than the rates of both cardiovascular disease and cancer. Within this group of disorders, depression, substance abuse, and suicide are leading contributors (Collins, Patel, & Joestl, 2011). Intersections with poverty can be seen via the contextual inequities that exist with regards to the GBD. For example, in low- and middle-income countries (LAMIC) and developing nations, there is frequently a lack of education regarding mental illness, psychiatric treatments are often unavailable, and practicing mental health professionals are relatively scarce. Furthermore, the psychological well-being of such nations is largely ignored in the psychological literature, with only 6% of the published research on mental health referring to populations from LAMIC (Saxena, Paraje, Shanan, Karam, & Sadana, 2006). So although mental health disorders (e.g., depression, schizophrenia, and alcohol use) comprise more than 11% of the GBD in LAMIC, there is little attention paid to addressing the mental health needs of these affected populations (Patel, 2007).

Mental health disorders in LAMIC also dovetail with other health concerns such as child nutrition, mortality, and suicide risk (Sachs & MacArthur, 2005). Patel (2007) suggested that mental health and poverty are a part of a detrimental circular process, with economic deprivation (resulting in lack of education, access to civic amenities, and debt) leading to mental health concerns, which in turn impacts the productivity of an individual and thereby increases the financial oppression experienced. Rapid societal changes in these countries also contribute to experiences of oppression and marginalization. For example, individuals who leave their homes in rural villages in search of better-paying jobs often report social isolation, insecurity, cultural alienation, and displacement, all of which are factors in the overall well-being of the individual (Rahim & Cederblad, 1989). Despite these linkages between poverty and mental health, there continues to be a lack of effective interventions for individuals living in LAMIC. Frequently, empirically validated interventions are developed in relatively affluent Western countries, and their generalizability and reliability in LAMIC are limited. Furthermore, these interventions are often not economically viable in countries where health care resources of every kind are already scarce (Patel, 2000, 2007). Other sociocultural factors such as globalization, stigma, and lack of awareness around mental illness, both within the general and health care provider population, also contribute to the existing disparities between needs and resources in LAMIC.

Economic trends themselves can also be understood to exacerbate these disparities. For example, economic globalization has been demonstrated to heighten poverty as opposed to increasing economic wealth (Diaz, Schnieder, & Mantal, 2012; Harrison & McMillan, 2007; Marsella, 2012). Free trade, which often saturates a LAMIC's market with cheaper, foreign alternatives, negatively impacts local small businesses, thereby reducing the income and wages of native populations. In turn, these events can contribute to psychological distress, depression, and other indicators of poor mental health (Corrigal, Plagerson, Lund, & Myers, 2008; Diaz et al., 2012; Weinreb et al., 2005). Globalization has also supported the continued Westernization of the mental health profession, whereby mental health care professionals often "import" Western ideologies and practices into LAMICs without considering the viability and applicability of these interventions to non-Western populations. Understandably, this practice often intensifies mistrust of mental health care professionals within LAMIC populations (Diaz et al., 2012). In order to meet the aforementioned challenges of mental health needs within LAMIC, researchers have suggested that culturally sensitive interventions must be developed to promote community health in minimally serviced areas that operate from a system of social inclusion and justice (Diaz et al., 2012; Patel et al., 2007; World Health Organization, 2007).

A number of recommendations regarding the development of culturally sensitive interventions in LAMIC have emerged. First, education regarding mental health symptoms and treatments (both for popular and for professional audiences) is essential (Patel, 2007). Many mental health disorders may go undiagnosed in LAMIC either due to somatic presentations by the client or short visit times, causing the mental health needs of marginalized individuals to potentially be overlooked. Accordingly, resources that facilitate awareness and education among primary care providers are vital; moreover, WHO (2007) recommends that traditional medical practitioners (TMP) should be included in education efforts in LAMIC. TMPs are well regarded in many cultures and often have a high level of influence in LAMIC. Thus, the training of TMPs, along with their inclusion in the treatment plan of patients in LAMIC, might be successful in aiding the effectiveness of psychological interventions (Patel, 2007).

Education, however, needs to extend beyond medical practitioners. Rahman, Mubbashar, Garter, and Goldberg (1998) developed a school-based intervention that sought to increase awareness of knowledge of mental illness with children between the ages of 12 and 16 years in rural Pakistan. A doctor, a psychologist, and a social worker from the Institute of Psychiatry in Rawalpindi incorporated such participatory educational methods as essay writings, poster creation, and student-led plays to highlight mental health symptoms that might be observed in the community. Parents and other community members were invited to participate in these activities. The researchers found that at the end of the four-month intervention, not only did the mental health awareness of the students increase but the mental health literacy of the local community also rose (Rahman et al., 1998).

CONCLUDING COMMENTS

As psychologists turn their attention toward the well-being of people living in poverty, their efforts should be informed by an understanding of classism as a parallel to other forms of oppression. In addition, poverty, as the lowest rung on the social class ladder, can be usefully conceptualized as the social location most affected by classism. PAR offers a comprehensive, revolutionary course of action for teams of researchers who wish to address these issues, and even psychologists who may be the only mental health professionals at their sites can study their own setting and practices, involving other members of the organization and the community to the extent possible. For psychologists of any specialty, advocacy on behalf of the poor must address mental health education and the eradication of stigma as well as world trends and events—such as economic globalization—that may be detrimental to the emotional well-being of vulnerable populations (Patel, 2007). The survival of individuals and communities living in poverty, the usefulness of mainstream psychological roles and approaches in this context, and the most effective methods of incorporating these and other aspects of social location into mental health practice are issues that invite the full attention of researchers as professional psychology develops a model of diversity that more fully incorporates dimensions of poverty and social class.

NOTE

1. Passages within this chapter have been adapted from the first author's previous work, and we gratefully acknowledge the permission granted for their use by the original publishers:

Published by the American Psychological Association:

Smith, L. (2005). Classism, psychotherapy, and the poor: Conspicuous by their absence. *American Psychologist*, 60(7), 687–696.

Smith, L. (2009). Enhancing training and practice in the context of poverty. *Training and Education in Professional Psychology, 3,* 84–93.

Smith, L., Chambers, D. A., & Bratini, L. (2009). When oppression is the pathogen: The participatory development of socially-just mental health practice. *American Journal of Orthopsychiatry, 79,* 159–168.

Published by Sage/Society:

Smith, L. (2008). Positioning classism within psychology's social justice agenda. *The Counseling Psychologist, 36,* 895–924.

REFERENCES

Albee, G. W. (1969). Who shall be served? *Professional Psychology, 1,* 4–7. doi: 10.1037/h0028786

American Psychological Association. (2002). *Guidelines on multicultural education, training, research, practice, and organizational change for psychologists.* Washington, DC: Author.

American Psychological Association. (2006). *Task Force on Socioeconomic Status (SES): Final report, August 2006.* Washington, DC: Author.

Amoroso, B. (2007). Globalization and poverty: Winners and losers. *Development, 50,* 12–19. doi: 10.1057/palgrave.development.1100374

Aponte, H. J. (1994). *Bread and spirit: Therapy with the new poor.* New York, NY: Norton.

Baker, N. L. (1996). Class as a construct in a "classless" society. In M. Hill & E. D. Rothblum (Eds.), *Classism and feminist therapy* (pp. 13–24). New York, NY: Harrington Park.

Belle, D., Doucet, J., Harris, J., Miller, J., & Tan, E. (2000). Who is rich? Who is happy? *American Psychologist, 55,* 1160–1161. doi: 10.1037//0003-066X.55.10.1160

Bloom, L. R. (2009). Global perspectives on poverty research for social justice. *International Journal of Qualitative Studies in Education, 22,* 253–261. doi: 10.1080/09518390902835447

Bullard, R. D. (2005). *The quest for environmental justice.* San Francisco, CA: Sierra Club.

Bullock, H. E. (1995). Class acts. In B. Lott & D. Maluso (Eds.), *The social psychology of interpersonal discrimination* (pp. 118–159). New York, NY: Guilford.

Bullock, H. E., Wyche, K. F., & Williams, W. R. (2001). Media images of the poor. *Journal of Social Issues, 57,* 229–246. doi: 10.1111/0022-4537.00210

Campbell, C., & Murray, M. (2004). Community health psychology: Promoting analysis and action for social change. *Journal of Health Psychology, 9,* 187–195. doi: 10.1177/1359105304040886

Collins, P. Y., Patel, V., & Joestl, S. S. (2011). Grand challenges in global mental health. *Nature, 475,* 27–30.

Corrigal, J., Plagerson, S., Lund, C., & Myers, J. (2008). Global trade and mental health. *Global Social Policy, 8,* 335–358. doi: 10.1177/1468018108095632

Day-Vines, N. L., & Day-Hairston, B. O. (2005). Culturally congruent strategies for addressing the behavioral needs of urban African American male adolescents. *Professional School Counseling, 8,* 236–243.

Diaz, J., Schneider, R., & Pwogwam Sante Mantal. (2012). Globalization as re-traumati zation: Rebuilding Haiti from the spirit up. *Journal of Social Issues, 68,* 493–513. doi: 10.1111/j.1540-4560.2012.01760.x

Dumont, M. P. (1996). *Treating the poor.* Belmont, MA: Dymphna Press.

Duncan, G. J., & Brooks-Gunn, J. (1997). Income effects across the life span: Integration and interpretation. In G. J. Duncan & J. Brooks-Gunn (Eds.), *Consequences of growing up poor* (pp. 596–610). New York, NY: Russell Sage Foundation.

Fairchild, H. (1984). School size, per-pupil expenditures, and academic achievement. *Review of Public Data Use, 12,* 221–229.

Fine, M. (1990). "The public" in public schools: The social construction/constriction of moral communities. *Journal of Social Issues, 46,* 107–119.

Fischback, R. L., & Herbert, B. (1997). Domestic violence and mental health: Correlates and conundrums within and across cultures. *Social Science and Medicine, 45,* 1161–1176.

Fouad, N. A., Gerstein, L. H., & Toporek, R. L. (2006). Social justice and counseling psychology in context. In R. L. Toporek, L. H. Gerstein, N. A. Fouad, G. Roysicar, & T. Israel, (Eds.), *The handbook for social justice in counseling psychology* (pp. 1–16). Thousand Oaks, CA: Sage.

Fukuda-Parr, S. (1999). What does feminization of poverty mean? It isn't just lack of income. *Feminist Economics, 5,* 99–103.

Goodman, L. A., Liang, B., Helms, J. E., Latta, R. E., Sparks, E., & Weintraub, S. (2004). Training counseling psychologists as social justice agents: Feminist and multicultural perspectives. *The Counseling Psychologist, 32,* 793–837. doi: 10.1177/0011000004268802

Grossman, J. (2006). *Fair labor standards act of 1938: Maximum struggle for a minimum wage.* Retrieved from http://www.dol.gov/oasam/programs/history/flsa1938.htm

Harrison, A., & McMillan, M. (2007). On the links between globalization and poverty. *Journal of Economic Inequality, 5,* 123–134.

Herr, K., & Anderson, G. L. (2005). *The action research dissertation.* Thousand Oaks, CA: Sage.

Hill, M., & Rothblum, E. D. (Eds.). (1996). *Classism and feminist therapy: Counting costs.* New York, NY: Harrington Park.

Javier, R. A., & Herron, W. G. (2002). Psychoanalysis and the disenfranchised: Countertransference issues. *Psychoanalytic Psychology, 19,* 149–166. doi: 10.1037//0736-9735.19.1.149

Kharas, H. (2010, January). *The emerging middle class in developing countries.* OECD Development Center: Working Paper Series, 285. Retrieved from http://unpan1.un.org/intradoc/groups/public/documents/UN-DPADM/UNPAN044413.pdf

Kidd, S. A., & Kral, M. J. (2005). Practicing participatory action research. *Journal of Counseling Psychology, 52,* 187–195. doi: 10.1037/0022-0167.52.2.187

Kozol, J. (2005). *The shame of the nation.* New York, NY: Crown.

Krumer-Nevo, M. (2009). From voice to knowledge: Participatory action research, inclusive debate and feminism. *International Journal of Qualitative Studies in Education, 22,* 279–295. doi: 10.1080/09518390902835462

Leondar-Wright, B. (2005). *Class matters.* Gabriola Island, CA: New Society.

Liu, W. M., Ali, S., Soleck, G., Hopps, J., Dunston, K., & Pickett, T. (2004). Using social class in counseling psychology research. *Journal of Counseling Psychology, 51,* 3–18. doi: 10.1037/0022-0167.51.1.3

Living Wage Resource Center. (2003). *Setting a living wage level.* Retrieved from http://www.livingwagecampaign.org/index.php?id=1954

Lott, B. (2002). Cognitive and behavioral distancing from the poor. *American Psychologist, 57,* 100–110. doi: 10.1037//0003-066X.57.2.100

Lott, B., & Bullock, H. E. (2007). *Psychology and economic injustice.* Washington, DC: American Psychological Association.

Lykes, M. B., & Coquillon, E. (2007). Participatory and action research and feminisms: Towards transformative praxis. In S. Hesse-Biber (Ed.), *Handbook of feminist research: Theory and praxis* (pp. 297–326). Thousand Oaks, CA: Sage.

Marks, D. (2004). Rights to health, freedom from illness: A life and death matter. In M. Murray (Ed.), *Critical health psychology* (pp. 61–82). London, UK: Palgrave.

Marsella, A. (2012). Psychology and globalization: Understanding a complex relationship. *Journal of Social Issues, 68,* 454–472. doi: 10.1111/j.1540-4560.2012.01758.x

Martinez-Salgado, C. (2009). Qualitative inquiry with women in poverty in Mexico City: Reflections on the emotional responses of a research team. *International Journal of Qualitative Studies in Education, 22,* 279–295. doi: 10.1080/09518390902835439

Mays, V. (2000). A social justice agenda. *American Psychologist, 55,* 326–327. doi: 10.1037//0003 066X.55.3.326

McGee, G. W. (2004). Closing the achievement gap: Lessons from Illinois' golden spike high-poverty high-performing schools. *Journal of Education for Students Placed at Risk, 9,* 97–125. doi: 10.1207/s15327671espr0902_2

Minkler, M., & Wallerstein, N. (Eds.) (2003). *Community-based participatory research for health.* San Francisco, CA: Jossey-Bass.

Murray, M., & Campbell, C. (2003). Living in a material world: Reflecting on some assumptions of health psychology. *Journal of Health Psychology, 8,* 231–236. doi: 10.1177/1359105303008002665

National Coalition for the Homeless. (2005). *Who is homeless? NCH Fact Sheet #3.* Retrieved from http://www.nationalhomeless.org/publications/facts/Whois.pdf

Patel, V. (2000). The need for treatment evidence for common mental disorders in developing countries. *Psychosocial Medicine, 30,* 743–746.

Patel, V. (2007). Mental health in low- and middle-income countries. *British Medical Bulletin, 81–82,* 81–96. doi: 10.1093/bmb/ldm010

Patel, V., Araya, R., Chatterjee, S., Chisholm, D., Cohen, A., De Silva, M, . . . van Ommeren, M. (2007). Treatment and prevention of mental disorders in low-income and middle-income countries. *Lancet, 15,* 991–1005. doi: 10.1016/S0140-6736(07)61240-9

Prilleltensky, I. (1994). *The morals and politics of psychology.* Albany, NY: SUNY Press.

Prilleltensky, I., & Nelson, G. (2002). *Doing psychology critically: Making a difference in diverse settings.* New York, NY: Macmillan.

Rahim, S. I., & Cederblad, M. (1989). Epidemiology of mental disorders in young adults of a newly urbanized area in Khartoum, Sudan. *British Journal of Psychiatry, 155,* 44–47. doi: 10.1192/bjp.155.1.44

Rahman, A., Mubbashar, M., Garter, R., & Goldberg, D. (1998). Randomized trial of impact of school mental health program in rural Rawalpindi, Pakistan. *Lancet, 352,* 1022–1025.

Sachs, J. D. & McArthur, J.W. (2005). *The millennium project: A plan for meeting the millennium development goals, Lancet,* 347–353.

Saxena, S., Paraje, G., Sharan, P., Karam, G., & Sadana, R. (2006). The 10/90 divide in mental health research: Trends over a 10-year period. *British Journal of Psychiatry, 188,* 81–82.

Smith, L. (2005). Psychotherapy, classism, and the poor: Conspicuous by their absence. *American Psychologist, 60,* 687–696. doi: 10.1037/0003-066X.60.7.687

Smith, L. (2008). Positioning classism within psychology's social justice agenda. *The Counseling Psychologist, 36,* 895–924. doi: 10.1177/0011000007309861

Speight, S. L., & Vera, E. M. (2004). A social justice agenda: Ready or not? *The Counseling Psychologist, 32,* 109–118. doi: 10.1177/0011000003260005

Strickland, B. R. (2000). Misassumptions, misadventures, and the misuse of psychology. *American Psychologist, 55,* 331–338. doi: 10.1037//0003-066X.55.3.331

Sue, D. W., Carter, R. T., Casas, J. M., Fouad, N. A., Ivey, A. E., Jensen, M., . . . Vazquez-Nutall, E. (1998). *Multicultural counseling competencies: Individual and organizational development.* Thousand Oaks, CA: Sage.

Toporek, R. L., & Williams, R. A. (2006). Ethics and professional issues related to the practice of social justice in counseling psychology. In R. L. Toporek, L. H. Gerstein, N. A. Fouad, G. Roysicar, & T. Israel (Eds.), *The handbook for social justice in counseling psychology* (pp. 17–34). Thousand Oaks, CA: Sage.

Tuhiwai Smith, L. (1999). *Decolonizing methodologies.* New York, NY: Zed Books.

UNCTAD (United Nations Conference on Trade and Development). (2002a). *The least developed countries report 2002: Escaping the poverty trap.* New York, NY and Geneva, CH: United Nations.

UNCTAD (United Nations Conference on Trade and Development). (2002b). Economic development in Africa: From adjustment to poverty reduction: What is new? New York, NY and Geneva, CH: United Nations.

United Nations Children's Fund. (2007). *Child poverty in perspective: An overview of child well-being in rich countries.* Retrieved from http://www.unicef-icdc.org/press-centre/presskit/reportcard7/rc7_eng.pdf

U.S. Department of Health and Human Services. (2007a). HHS: What we do. Retrieved from http://www.hhs.gov/about/whatwedo.html/

Weinreb, L., Wehler, C., Perloff, J., Scott, R., Hosmer, D., Sagor, L., & Gundersen, C. (2005). Hunger: Its impact on children's health and mental health. *Pediatrics, 4,* 1–9. doi: 10.1542/peds.110.4.e41

World Bank. (2001). *World Development Report 2000/2001: Attacking poverty.* New York, NY: Oxford University Press.

World Health Organization. (2007). *Integrating mental health services into primary health care.* Geneva, CH: World Health Organization. Retrieved from http://www.who.int/mental_health/policy/services/3_MHintoPHC_Infosheet.pdf.

World Health Organization. (2008). The global burden of disease: 2004 Update.

Zweig, M. (2000). *The working class majority.* Ithaca, NY: Cornell University Press.

Chapter 13

Criminal Justice and Its Many Injustices: Focus on Prison Psychology within the United States[1]

Kathryn M. Whiteley, Tina Bloom, and Harris L. Friedman

Social justice ideally entails maintaining basic rights and liberties of human beings, while ensuring all are treated with dignity and respect (D. Miller, 1999; Walzer, 1983), and this applies especially to prisoners who are placed in almost total dependency on those who care for them. The criminal justice system is a major social institution that supposedly furthers ideals of social justice, such as protecting the public (including those accused of crimes, but who might be innocent), rehabilitating those who are legal transgressors so they can return to a productive social life, and maintaining social order (i.e., redirecting the emotional motives of victimized individuals to being under the more rational purview of the state). The bulwark of criminal justice in the United States is embedded within rule of law, but laws are constructed by fallible humans who have varying and often competing interests, and hence laws may not always be just.

One way to address the relative degree of justice or injustice of any law is by taking a conflict perspective, such as by examining who benefits and who suffers from the law. This introduces the notion of power, as the vested interests of those holding greater power will tend to benefit, whereas laws tend to function to the detriment of those with lesser power. Through such mechanisms, privileging inures to some groups as well as to some individuals. When criminal laws become profoundly unjust, based on a variety of ways that might be used to ascertain injustice, then the very term, *criminal justice*, becomes an oxymoron, as incongruous as analogous oxymoronic terms, such as *large shrimp*. Our chapter focuses on the relationship between psychology and social justice in U.S. prisons, and represents a sampling of issues prevalent in the larger area of criminal justice, which in turn is just a sample of how the even larger legal system in general operates. Therefore, consider from a justice perspective the following representative scenarios of people serving time in U.S. prisons.

In a state where medical marijuana is not legalized, a frail elderly woman with glaucoma is sent to prison for possessing a small amount she herself grew and used to treat her own medical condition. An 18-year-old man, who impregnated his then 15-year-old girlfriend when he was 17 (note: it was not considered a crime then, as they were both minors), is sent to prison as a sexual predator once he turned 18 and continued their relationship, while his girlfriend and their newborn await being reunited with him to form a family unit after he completes his sentence. An African American man continues to serve time in prison for rape, based on a White person's eye-witness testimony of dubious validity and despite that there is new DNA evidence exonerating him, because the new evidence is ruled inadmissible in court. A homeless mentally ill man is given a life sentence for shoplifting junk food of trivial value from a convenience store, because he is a multiple offender caught in mandatory sentencing laws. A demented elderly man is kept in a squalid prison isolation cell serving a life sentence, despite that he is now both mentally and physically incapacitated, and that he poses little possible further threat to society. Lastly, a political prisoner has been tortured in a U.S. prison on territory outside of the United States and has spent over 11 years incarcerated without being formally charged with a crime; even if somehow found innocent, the speculation is that he can never be released because it is thought that he now is so filled with hate that he would only seek revenge.

Contrast these unfortunate scenarios, all based on true cases, with wealthy people convicted of so-called white-collar crime, such as robbing the financial hopes and dreams of thousands, but who regularly receive only probation or, at worst, are sentenced to countryclub-style prisons built for the elite. These contrasting scenarios represent some of the types of injustices perpetrated regularly within the U.S. criminal justice system.

This is not to state that the criminal justice system in the United States lacks all virtue, or that prisons are totally bad institutions. People accused of crimes within the United States are guaranteed legal representation, trial by a jury of their peers, and many other rights that are denied in some other countries. However, the brutal reality is that these rights are often more aspirational than actual. For example, legal representation may be woefully inadequate for the U.S. low socioeconomic population who often rely on overworked public defenders, and jury trials are routinely circumvented, even for the innocent, in the United States by strong prosecutorial pressure to accept plea deals to avoid the chances of conviction under a climate of harsh mandatory punishment. In this regard, the United States can be seen as simultaneously having one of the best and worst criminal justice systems, and the same conclusion is warranted for its prisons.

THE PREVALENCE OF PRISON INJUSTICES

As an example of a severe problem within one U.S. prison system, over 3,000 prisoners held by the California Department of Correction and Rehabilitation remain in indefinite solitary confinement, despite court orders mandating their release from such isolation (Curtin, 2013). This isolation could qualify as torture under international law and could lead to serious psychological harm, as these prisoners are individually confined for approximately 22 hours each day within small window-less rooms, behind doors that block fresh air circulation and most light, and they are denied opportunities to attend group activities (but can leave their cells daily for brief individual exercise periods). Many of these inmates have been in isolation for over a decade, and Amnesty International claims conditions are actually deteriorating rather than improving for them. Contrast this with many Western European prison systems, which appear not only more humane in numerous ways, but also are more efficient in reducing recidivism through providing ample educational and rehabilitative services (e.g., Kenis, Kruyen, Baaijens, & Barneveld, 2010; Mauer, 2003).

It is recognized that the United States has the highest rate of criminal incarceration in the world (Langan & Levin, 2004), and has many forms of abuse, from prison rape to gang violence, in the confines of its prisons. In fact, the United States remains one of the few modern industrialized countries to retain the death penalty, which is condemned by many throughout the world as a cruel and unusual punishment (e.g., Bessler, 2012). These, and similar problems, have recently become exacerbated by *law-and-order* rhetoric, which plays upon the U.S. public's understandable desire for security, but also is part of a larger cultural war between opposing political leanings. However, there is more to the story than simple splits based on political ideology. For example, private correctional companies actively lobby for creating harsh sentencing laws, which favor their economic interests as they profit from the mass incarceration within the United States (Jones & Mauer, 2013). In some states, young Black males, who are more likely to serve time in prison than go to college, are disenfranchised as felons, diluting their future political influence as a minority voting class that tends to vote in the liberal direction, thus benefitting politicians who tend to support laws oppressing this group (Pager, 2009).

This tough on crime legacy, especially with its emphasis on strict mandatory prison sentences for relatively minor offenses, usually committed by members of oppressed groups, such as related to the so-called crack/powder racial disparity (Kurtzleben, 2010), has been at least one cause of the dramatic increases in the numbers incarcerated. For example, toughening guidelines for sentencing has led to the number of offenders serving life sentences without parole in the United States to jump 22% between the years of 2003 and 2008 (Nellis, 2010). This sadly also includes many adolescents and even children convicted as adults despite their youth and sentenced to life in prison. Of course, these youths' minds have not yet fully developed and adolescents are more subject to peer influences than their adult counterparts. Although psychologists and mental health experts were instrumental in a recent U.S. Supreme Court ruling reversing the procedure that juveniles could be tried as adults in capital murder, which had applied to over 2,500 prisoners who committed murder prior to the age of 18, life sentences are still common for this group (Mears, 2012). The glaring disparities between who gets prosecuted for various crimes suggests a flawed criminal justice system far from being just, as in terms of free from discriminatory biases. Particularly glaring injustices include offenses going unpunished by rich bankers and corporate chief executives who steal openly and with impunity, whereas the prison door is slammed shut for minor offenses committed by the poor and marginalized.

Perhaps on the surface, it seems that underlying these trends is a dual process driven by increasing fear (e.g., mistrust of policing to adequately protect against crime, which spurs mandatory sentencing laws) and pessimism as to whether personal reformation may be possible (especially when applied to minority groups). In an editorial in *The Economist* (2011), a former California legislator and convicted felon addressed the fact that, in the recent two decades, crime rates fell but incarceration rates continued to rise, and stated: "[W]e build jails for people we're afraid of, and fill them with people we are mad at" (n.p.). To place this into historical context, in the mid-1970s, the United States incarcerated only 110 per 100,000 people, whereas by the late 1990s, the rate had risen to nearly 700 per 100,000 (Pratt, 2011). Although the United States has the highest per capita rate of incarceration among the Westernized world, many alternatives to incarceration appear to offer superior benefits. For example, two international studies suggest that probation is better than incarceration in relation to recidivism. The Scottish Centre for Crime and Justice Research (Armstrong & McNeill, 2012) published a comparative study of six jurisdictions to include Scotland, England and Wales, Northern Ireland, Ireland, Norway, and New Zealand. Across the period of 2001 to 2004, it found that people released from prison, compared to those who received a lesser sentence of probation, had significantly higher recidivism. Similarly, an Irish study conducted by the Probation Service and the Central Statistics Office (2012) followed individuals sentenced to probation and community service in 2007. This research looked at 3,576 offenders for two years and found that 63% had no convictions over the next two years. Re-offending rates in general in Ireland range up to 50%, therefore a key conclusion is that re-offending treatment programs based in the community are more effective than prison sentences at reducing recidivism. Consequently, the

U.S. strategy to incarcerate more individuals, while less frequently offering probation as an alternative, appears counterproductive. This illustrates some of the deep systemic problems in the U.S. prison system related to social justice.

Perhaps the worst injustice in U.S. prisons has to do with demographics, especially the disproportionate number of minorities and poor who are imprisoned. This largely has related to systemic injustices, such as selective prosecution and varying opportunities for being caught for widespread practices that are criminalized, such as smoking marijuana (e.g., those using this substance in the privacy of their homes within wealthy gated communities are much less likely to be arrested than those engaging openly on the street within poor neighborhoods). Aldarondo (2007) described social justice as seeking to decrease suffering and promote human values of equality and justice, but this ideal is often far from the reality in U.S. prisons. Instead, the criminal justice system in the United States too often worsens, rather than rectifies, injustices by unnecessarily ruining lives, and not just of those incarcerated but also their families, who are often thrown into dire poverty that appears incompatible with any reasonable notion of social justice (Robinson, 2010). Our chapter examines some of these disturbing trends from a psychological vantage with the hope that deeper understanding might sway outcomes toward more meaningful social justice in this setting.

THE ROLE OF MENTAL HEALTH IN U.S. PRISONS

Mental health issues are a central part of the work performed by most professional psychologists, and psychologists play many roles in prisons attending to the mental health needs of inmates. In addition, it is worth emphasizing that prisons now serve as the warehouse for many of society's rejected. For example, Berzins and Trestman (2004) noted that, due to widespread deinstitutionalization that closed many mental hospitals, there are three times as many men and women with mental illness in U.S. jails and prisons than in any of the remaining mental hospitals.

Serious Mental Illnesses

With the closure of these many mental hospitals and the drastic cuts in funding to community mental health centers, prisons in the United States have become the *de facto* dumping ground for many mentally ill people. The largest psychiatric facility in the United States is known as the Twin Towers, a wing of a Los Angeles County Jail as, on any given day, there can be up to 1,400 inmates housed with a diagnosable mental illness (Montagne, 2008). The U.S. Department of Justice Statistics (2006) reported 700,000 U.S. prison and jail inmates had signs of mental illness, many of whom suffered from serious mental illnesses (SMI).

Offenders with SMI are caught in a revolving door as a result of limited mental health interventions available within prisons, as well as limited community supports upon release (Lamb & Weinberger, 2001; Lovell, Gagliardi, & Peterson, 2002). Subsequently, cycles of decompensation and escalation of behaviors result in successive arrests and incarcerations. The injustice of limited and inadequate mental health intervention in U.S. prisons is shown in many studies, such as that by Cloyes, Wong, Latimer, and Abarca (2010), who reported that people with SMI in Utah were re-incarcerated on average at 385 days from release, as compared to those without SMI who were re-incarcerated on average at 743 days.

Discrimination against offenders with SMI has also been identified in relation to parole decisions, the conditional release of prisoners which operates within 30 U.S. states (Matejkowski, Caplan, & Cullen, 2010). A key consideration to parole is whether the individual is capable of remaining crime free in the community. A host of factors are assessed, among which mental status rises to prominence. In their examination of mental health and recidivism, Carroll, Weiner, Coates, Galegher, and Alibrio (1982) found that people with SMI tended to fare worse on overall risk assessments for parole. Herein lies another example of a criminal justice system that penalizes inmates with SMI for problems that the system does not adequately address.

One mechanism to understand how this might operate is through a signal detection perspective (Swets, 1961), which can be utilized to clarify a common trap into which psychologists often place inmates when considering the inmates' diagnoses and prognoses (e.g., their potential dangerousness). Assessors, often psychologists, are asked to opine about whether danger is present (justifying keeping the inmate imprisoned) or absent (justifying parole or otherwise releasing the inmate). Given this binary choice, psychologists can never with 100% assuredness know whether an inmate is truly dangerous or not, but the penalty to an examining psychologist from releasing a dangerous person whose future actions could demonstrate the psychologist's error is grave. In contrast, the false alarm of keeping an inmate who is not dangerous incarcerated has little consequence as, by remaining incarcerated, inmates will never show the assessor to be wrong. This signal detection bias undeniably slants toward concluding that danger is present, inadvertently keeping nondangerous inmates incarcerated unfairly. However, the societal cost of these false alarms is not often considered by the decision makers.

In 2010, the financial cost of incarceration across 40 states was estimated to be over $39 billion, or between $31,300 and $60,000 per inmate (Hendrichson & Delaney, 2012), and no doubt the cost of keeping SMI inmates would be toward the high end if they were to receive adequate treatment. In addition to the financial costs of keeping individuals incarcerated, other related social costs are immense. For example, incarceration greatly decreases inmates' future ability to secure gainful employment, and it drains local economies of able-bodied employees (Western, Kling, & Weiman, 2001). The effect of incarceration on an inmate's families is also profound, such as poorer health in family members and poorer performance of inmates' children in school, as well as increases in their behavior problems (Hagan, 2010).

Sex Offenders

To illustrate the dynamics of keeping some people who are not deemed very dangerous incarcerated, there is one subgroup of offenders of whom society is especially afraid and mad, namely sex offenders. Sex offending encompasses a myriad of offenses, and these can be as trivial as indecent exposure for public urination, a crime that is much more likely to occur in minority neighborhoods with less access to public restroom facilities. Psychologists play a pivotal role in the initial assessment, treatment, and later assessment of risk for re-offending for this group. The Association for the Treatment of Sexual Abusers (ATSA, 2010) reported that, although certain subtypes of sex offenders (e.g., pedophiles who molest boys and rapists of adult women) present a great risk for recidivism, overall sex offence recidivism rates are much lower than for many other crimes, namely between 5 and 20%. In a report for the Bureau of Justice based on 1994 statistics from 15 states regarding 9,691 released sex offenders, Langan, Schmitt, and Durose (2004) presented data indicating that 339 sex offenders committed a new sex crime over the three-year follow-up period, yielding a recidivism rate of only 3.5% for subsequent sex offending. When nonsex crimes were included for sex offenders' re-arrest rate (e.g., parole violations, such as missing an appointment with a parole officer), it jumped to 43%, but was still much lower than the re-arrest rate for nonsex offenders, who were at 68%.

Despite the very low sex-offense recidivism rate for most sex offenders, they tend to face harsh penalties that do not likely protect society or reduce the likelihood of their future offending, but instead reflect societal fear and anger (Agudo, 2008). Because some sex offenders commit crimes considered particularly heinous and often against society's most vulnerable, their civil liberties can even be stripped from them, such as through a lifetime of involuntary civil incarceration after serving their legal sentence. There is a balancing act needed between protecting society from its most despised members' potentially dangerous behaviors, while simultaneously remaining aware of their human rights and the actual likelihood of danger. The statistics suggest that although the current harsh laws may help society feel protected, the manner in which sex offenders are incarcerated provides little actual protection (Agudo, 2008). Specifically, in almost half of molestation cases involving a victim who was under 18 years, 46% of the time the molester was a relative (Langan et al., 2004). The ATSA (2010) noted that the myth of "stranger danger" is largely unfounded, and that sexually abused children are molested most often by family, friends, or acquaintances (93%). This is confirmed in Langan et al.'s (2004) data, in which only 6.7% of the cases in which the victim was under 18 years were committed by a stranger; in contrast, when the victim was older than 18 years, strangers were perpetrators less than half (34%) of the time.

Another common myth about the sex offender is that treatment does not work. This was based on early studies that have been essentially debunked, whereas more recent investigations report efficacy from a variety of approaches (ATSA,

2010). The ATSA claims there is now increased ability to predict sexual dangerousness, and risk assessments can, with some accuracy, identify those offenders who pose the greatest threat to public safety, so that limited resources can be used most effectively when high-risk offenders are intensively managed, with low-risk offenders less intensively handled. When low-risk offenders are targeted merely because they are labeled as a sex offender, however, not only are limited resources strained, but the low-risk offenders are destabilized, resulting in the unintended consequence of increasing their likelihood to reoffend. The ATSA concluded that "about one-third to one-half of adult sex offenders subjected to community notification experience unintended consequences such as job loss, housing instability, threats or harassment, vigilantism, or property damage. About 19% of adult sex offenders report that these negative consequences have affected other members of their households. Notification may actually undermine public safety by exacerbating factors (e.g., unemployment, instability) correlated with criminal recidivism" (p. 3–4).

The ATSA (2010) warned that offense-based classification systems, such as the Adam Walsh Act (in which sex offenders are categorized by the severity of their conviction) may inflate the risk of some offenders while erroneously deflating the risk of other offenders (e.g., those who accept plea bargaining for lesser crimes). The ATSA noted that such offense-based categorization is unverified, and suggested that actuarial models that have been assessed for predictive validity may be more accurate in appropriate risk management. The ATSA further stated that, without community education and involvement, public notification (i.e., making public aware of the location of released sex offenders) is less likely to be helpful in the management of sex offenders. Additionally, because victims are so often family members, victim advocacy groups admonish that such notification systems lead to inadvertent identification of victims and a tendency for victims to not report sexual abuse by family members. The ATSA summarized that "prevention of sexual violence requires a well-planned, comprehensive, inter-disciplinary response. Prevention efforts must begin with developing clear goals and objectives, implementing strategies based on empirical research, and collecting and analyzing data on an ongoing basis. Lawmakers and citizens should advocate for research-based social policies that both protect communities and also support the rehabilitation of perpetrators to effectuate long-term community safety" (pp. 3–4).

The plight of convicted sex offenders who have committed relatively trivial crimes is one example of a special population impacted by unjust laws. The rights and liberties of those convicted of sex offending are at risk, and they often require specialized treatment units and protection from other inmates. Upon release, they are required to openly register as sex offenders and become a public spectacle. Communities have even rallied to forbid sex offenders access to housing. It appears that sex offenders, more than any other group, have attained what social psychologist Lewin (1948) would classify as "out-group hostility."

Elderly

Another special population of inmates is the incarcerated elderly, and giving life sentences without parole to children who grow old in prison is one especially egregious example of a practice counterproductive to social justice. Toch (2010) concluded that the best established statistical fact regarding criminal recidivism is that reoffending decreases with age. In support of this assertion, Laub and Sampson (2003) declare that criminality peaks in adolescence and early adulthood, and decreases thereafter with age. Research by Mauer, King, and Young (2004) found that released lifers were one third less likely to reoffend within a three-year period than all other prisoners released. In an analysis of 285 lifers in one U.S. state, most of whom were incarcerated for violent offending and were released between the years of 1933 and 2005, only seven were re-incarcerated, which reinforces the conclusion that, with aging, reoffending decreases (Advisory Committee on Geriatric and Seriously Ill Inmates, 2005). Within this group there were 100 inmates aged 50 and older and, within this subset, only one person was sent back to prison. Furthermore, Bedau (1982) reported in another study that less than 1% of released murderers were returned to prison for committing another murder.

Social justice within the context of aging inmates is a double-edged sword. Lengthy incarcerations of the elderly do not lower crime rates, and are very expensive. With the rapidly growing number of aging prisoners comes a need for more health care and other geriatric services. Chiu (2010) estimated that the number of inmates 55 and older housed in U.S. federal and state prisons increased by nearly 77% from 1999 to 2007, accompanied by an estimate that elderly inmates may cost two to three times the annual rate for incarceration of a younger prisoner. Clearly the graying of the prison population in the United States poses challenges from a social justice perspective.

A related topic not often addressed is, what are the leading causes of death within a prison? In 2001, a total of 3,008 inmates died within U.S. prisons as a result of prison violence, with only 2% of the prison deaths caused by another person (Pastore & Maguire, 2003). Although suicide among inmates is significantly higher compared to their peers in the general population, Pastore and Maguire (2003) concluded that for 2001, 75% of inmate deaths were related to natural causes other than AIDS, largely categorized as chronic illness and old age, suggesting that, for many inmates, their end of sentence is their dying.

If this group of aging prisoners is costing significantly more and are at far less risk of reoffending, why are they not being released? One simple explanation is that most aging prisoners are serving time for violent offenses toward which the public is mad. For example, Price (2006) found that 60% of North Carolina's inmates 50 years of age and older were convicted of violent crimes, which included violent sex offenses. In an effort to reduce prison populations and in recognition that many offenders no longer posed a risk for violence, 15 states and the District of Columbia established paths for older inmates to receive geriatric releases (Chiu,

2010). The same study found that complex procedures and lengthy response times discouraged inmates from pursuing such releases, and many of those who did pursue them simply died before their request was granted.

Furthermore, Wright and Bronstein (2007) discussed the introduction of hospice programming into prisons. In a balanced overview of the organizational challenges to introducing this intense level of programming to a highly structured setting, these researchers also gathered the perceptions of prison staff involved at all levels with implementing hospices. It should be noted that many staff were receptive to hospice. However, most disheartening was the presence of staff whose belief was that inmates were not deserving of compassionate care (e.g., nursing staff who resented the time it took to oversee hospice volunteers). Perhaps not surprising, Wright and Bronstein disclosed that newer, less experienced wardens especially struggled to embrace an appreciation of such programs. Perhaps these types of perceptions require change prior to any meaningful implementation of approaches to the care of inmates who are terminally ill.

Many public officials remain reluctant to release elderly prisoners despite the overwhelming evidence that they reoffend at lower rates than young, repeat offenders. A classic example of this deeply entrenched attitude was heard in the remarks of the then California governor Arnold Schwarzenegger in addressing a compassionate release request (Gottschalk, 2011). The offender was Susan Atkins, an accomplice of Charles Manson in the infamous Tate-La Bianca murders. Ms. Atkins had been a role-model prisoner for 40 years, and was paralyzed and dying of a cancerous brain tumor. The governor was quoted in a 2008 CNN interview stating, "I don't believe in compassionate release. I think they have to stay in; they have to serve their time. Those kinds of crime are just so unbelievable that I'm not for compassionate release" (cited in Gottschalk, p. 126). In contrast, throughout the 19th century and much of the early 20th century, presidents and governors were moved to issue clemency regularly, but that was a different era.

This stance parallels the increase in being tough on crime and advocating strict sentencing guidelines. This shift prompted the American Bar Association Justice Kennedy Commission (American Bar Association, 2004) to analyze the state of pardons. They concluded that "pardon power" is rarely employed in contemporary times. This commission recommended that state and the federal governments revitalize pardons across numerous scenarios, including age, disability, exigent family matters, and unusual suffering—and in accordance with changing laws. However, in this era of toughness on crime, politicians worry that a release leading to a serious reoffending will lead to community outrage, and to their own political demise (related to the signal detecting bias previously mentioned).

White-Collar Criminals

Crimes of a violent nature garner the most attention, outrage, fear, and mount the greatest challenge to the principles of social justice. As a nation, the United

States fears violence and wrestles with the capacity for a violent offender to change, whereas so-called white-collar crime (WCC) seemingly is held to a lesser standard. Although not an especially large population of inmates, we think it important to cover those whose public perception is captured well in the title of an article by Perri (2011), "White Collar Criminals: The Kinder, Gentler Offender." Apart from a few highly publicized cases, such as the well-documented Bernard Madoff scandal, less is read and heard about WCC than street crime. This fact is realized in a landmark paper by Wilson (2011), who commented about violent and property crimes being at an all-time low but still highly visible in public fora, although conspicuously absent is any discussion of WCC. In comparing street crime to WCC, Friedrichs (2007) argued that the financial costs of WCC far exceeds those of street crime, as does the chances of a U.S. resident being a victim of WCC.

When speaking in terms of social justice, it is necessary to think of financial, as well as other, costs. Writing in relation to the social impact of WCC, Ford (2007) suggested this crime not only serves to undermine the economy but also widens the gap between poverty and wealth. The extent of the financial costs of WCC is enormous, and arguably robs monies that could be used for the greater good. In research seeking to assess damage from the lack of financial disclosure and fraudulent disclosure to U.S. corporations, COSO (2010) found the staggering loss among 347 public corporations at over $120 billion between the years of 1998 and 2007.

This gravitation toward addressing crimes of violence, while seemingly ignoring WCC, has for decades been widely cited in criminology and criminal justice literature. Cullen, Link, and Polazi (1982) and Croall (2007) argued how this double standard has infiltrated the courts and academics. Perhaps the sting of this double standard is most felt when referring to WCC as *victimless* crimes, which is clearly false. This designation arises primarily from what Gustafson (2007) and Perri (2011) believed is the premise that no one feels the injury uniquely and that, as it is widely dispersed, it is seen as a rather painless injury, in contrast to the horrors of crimes of personal violence. However, Price and Norris (2009) wrote that WCC victims may have as many emotional consequences and experience as severe a blow to their quality of life as those victimized from street crime. By classifying WCC as victimless crime, Croall pointed out that its victims are often not included in victimology literature, further promulgating WCC as nonviolent offending.

A term that seeks to debunk the victimless crime myth is the labeling of a WCC perpetrator as a social predator. A typical profile of white-collar criminals identified by Dorminey, Fleming, Kranacher, and Riley is "middle aged and well educated, good citizens and hard workers, and a first time offender" (cited in Perri, 2011, p. 219). Further, their criminal acts are often portrayed as well outside of their usual character, and rationalized as due to their having yielded to overwhelming pressures, quite different from the tendency to blame other criminal perpetrators for their personal faults or even for being evil. It is understood that fraud can be deemed as accidental, but this raises the question of the identity of those who operate with intent and premeditation as social predators. In writing on how white-collar criminals seek to neutralize their criminality, Hare (1993, p. 122) quoted a convicted white collar criminal as that offender addressed his sentencing judge, "I have been sitting in jail for two months now and have experienced living in a cell with a poor ignorant illegal alien, a career criminal, a drug user and smuggler, and a killer. I can tell you without hesitation that I am not at all similar. I don't look the same, talk the same, act the same, or feel the same." This statement fits squarely within the frame of Perri's article in which he argued that the white-collar criminal is unfairly viewed differently from other criminals. They are seen as not violent and relatively harmless, and often sympathetically judged as victims themselves.

In an analysis of law enforcement's perceptions of WCC, Brody and Kiehl (2010) concluded that law enforcement has largely embraced this kinder and gentler view of WCC criminals and approaches them accordingly. It is no coincidence that these criminals tend to not be from oppressed and marginalized groups, and have privilege in many other domains of life. For the sake of completeness of coverage, however, it should be recognized that there exists a subgroup of white-collar criminals who do resort to violence. The act of violence is most often murder that seeks to prevent their fraud from being fully exposed; in fact, this event occurs with enough frequency that it has come to be recognized with its own term, "fraud-detection homicide" (Perri, 2011).

Psychology's relative ignoring of WCC, as compared to other crime, parallels the way society grants privilege to this type of criminal. One pioneering criminologist addressing WCC was Sutherland (1940) who, according to Friedrich (2007), argued that WCC could not be understood at the individual level; although it has been addressed increasingly by sociologists and criminologists, it largely remains absent from the psychological literature (Briggs & Sarre, 2010). According to Ramamoorti (2008), this lacuna of missing literature particularly needs more psychological examination of WCC in terms of how psychological factors might underlie that criminal behavior (e.g., such as how WCC is motived; Alalehto, 2003).

In addressing traits of white-collar criminals, Carozza (2008) identified several attitudes and behaviors that defy a kind and gentle offender portrayal. These include a sense of entitlement, skill at deceit, cheating, and manipulation, an inability to engage in empathy, and the belief that others are simply resources to be exploited. As mentioned earlier, the most prominent recent WCC is arguably Bernard Madoff's case; the sentencing judge in his case countered the victimless crime argument by stating, "the message must be sent that this kind of manipulation of the system is not just a bloodless crime that takes place on paper, but one instead that takes a staggering toll" (as cited in Perri, 2011). Perri concluded that more empirical research with white-collar criminals is warranted. Perri also quoted Hare, one of most widely known psychological scholars of psychopathy, who stated that "if he [Hare] was not studying psychopaths in prison, he would be studying them at the New York Stock Exchange" (as cited in Perri, p. 236). Unfortunately, psychopathic traits among those in power are often considered to be admirable, rather than despicable (Millon, Grossman, Millon, Meagher, & Ramnath, 2004).

THE PSYCHOLOGICAL ASSESSMENT AND TREATMENT OF CRIMINALS

There are many theoretical approaches, most stemming from the field of sociology, for explaining deviancy, including criminal behavior as one type of deviancy. Among these are general strain (Agnew, 1992), pathways to crime (Chesney-Lind, 1989), social structure and anomie (Merton, 1938), and Lemert's (1972) primary and secondary deviance theories, all emphasizing the need to examine where society failed to help an individual achieve goals in a more acceptable way. These sociological approaches take into consideration not just individual behavior, but the larger social context of the individual. However, most psychological theories of criminal behavior tend to emphasize the individual as an isolated being, rather than as embedded in a social context, and resultingly focus on issues emphasizing individual responsibility. Such an example is Samenow's (1984) widely used approach to criminal thinking, which disputes that society has any shared responsibility for criminal behavior by placing the blame squarely on the individual.

Different approaches to psychology describe varying etiologies of criminal behaviors, and thus, emphasize diverse strategies for prevention and treatment, including approaches from personality, cognitive-behavioral, psychoanalytic, humanistic-existential, and social learning theories. Together they all, except perhaps the social learning approach, tend to focus on the individual, and in that sense have a commonality of blaming the individual rather than looking at the social structures that afford or deny opportunities related to criminal deviancy.

Personality

Psychology has leaned heavily upon blaming faulty personality traits and other individual properties of offenders for their deviancy. This focus upon either psychopathology or being bad (or even evil) is depicted in diagnostic criteria that have guided psychology's predominant approach to deviance. For adolescents, the diagnosis of conduct disorder and for adults, antisocial personality disorder (ASPD) have been keys to understanding criminality (see *Diagnostic and Statistical Manual of Mental Disorders*, *DSM-IV-TR*, 2000), and place culpability on the individual and tend to ignore or minimize sociocultural and physical circumstances. ASPD is defined by a constellation of intrusive behaviors that violate the rights of others, such as nonconformity, callousness, deceitfulness, irresponsibility, recklessness, impulsivity, and aggressiveness.

Utilization of exclusively behavioral criteria for this diagnosis may enhance diagnostic reliability, but may yield a collection of people with vastly diverse personality traits (Millon, 1981). Additionally, individuals with personality characteristics representative of this so-called disorder may manage to keep their behavior contained, and thus, remain excluded from the diagnosis (Hare, Hart, & Harpur, 1991). Although the *DSM-IV-TR* notes, "Antisocial Personality Disorder appears to be associated with low socioeconomic status and urban settings," and cautions that such behaviors may be "part of a protective survival strategy" and that "it is helpful for the clinician to consider the social and economic context in which the behaviors occur" (APA, 2000, p. 703–704), in actuality assessment using the *DSM-IV-TR* does not usually take that advice into account. Instead, there is rampant blame inherent in individualizing this diagnosis as a personality flaw, and one which is associated with a poor prognosis for change—and often accompanied by tacit moral condemnation from those giving the label. When a personality approach to criminality is maintained, those given the ASPD label tend to be dismissed as extremely difficult, even impossible, to change, which is often then used in a process of circular reasoning to justify incarceration without hope of redemption.

A term associated with ASPD is *psychopathy* (e.g., see Hare's, 1991, Psychopathic Checklist-Revised; PCL-R). The terms *psychopath* and *ASPD* are often used interchangeably in criminal and broader forensic settings, but they have key differences. ASPD is defined by a constellation of antisocial behaviors, whereas psychopathy is defined as something even worse: a constellation of antisocial behaviors in addition to a set of personality factors that are described as aggressive narcissism, which according to Hare includes grandiosity, superficial charm, a complete lack of empathy and remorse, and failure to take responsibility for actions. Psychopaths can also be seen as an extreme subset of ASPD, and Ogloff (2006) claims that 50 to 80% of prisoners fall under the rubric of ASPD, whereas only 15% fit that of psychopath. However, in current popular usage, the term psychopath conjures up the scariest profile, such as violent serial killers, which further justifies the attitude of being tough on crime for those given this personality label that goes beyond mere ASPD.

Skeem, Monahan, and Mulvey (2002) reviewed myths perpetuated about the untreatableness of psychopaths. One common myth is that treatment causes psychopaths, seen as sneaky and intelligent deviants, to become more likely to recidivate, and even more likely to recidivate violently because treatment only teaches them what normal people expect, so they become better at playing manipulative games. Then, these so-called depraved individuals can tailor their charming, manipulative presentations in an even more convincing fashion. This conclusion appears primarily based on one key study that examined the use of radical techniques on coerced participants of a therapeutic community housed within a maximum security prison, where results were unsuccessful (Rice, Harris, & Cormier, 1992). In this paper, it was acknowledged by Rice and colleagues that the bizarre methods used in this investigation were not appropriate for the treatment of psychopaths, or perhaps any other disorder. These so-called radical practices included nude encounter groups, administration of LSD, and dispensation of meals via feeding tubes strung through the walls. Yet the stereotype persists of the untreatable psychopath, justifying the belief that such people cannot change and deserve to be incarcerated forever.

However, there are some hopeful trends when examining criminals from a personality vantage. There is some recognition of a confounding problem with most research on treatment of psychopaths, as identified by Skeem et al. (2003, p. 583) as the "dose-response effect." Due to psychopaths being prematurely terminated from treatment more often than nonpsychopaths, with this termination sometimes due to their own quitting and other times because of their removal from treatment due to noncompliance, they are less likely to get adequate treatment. Skeem and colleagues (2002) concluded that psychopaths responded favorably to appropriate treatment, when given, and that intensive treatment was more helpful, described in terms of such broad categories as "medication, verbal therapy only, combination of medication and verbal therapy, drug and alcohol treatment, group therapy only, or other therapy" (p. 587).

Some treatments have been shown especially effective with those seen as having so-called criminal personality disorders, such as Dialectical Behavior Therapy (DBT; see Linehan, 1987), which combines psychoanalytic and cognitive-behavioral approaches in order to target personality disorder. DBT has been found to decrease negative moods and interpersonal conflicts in a forensic unit comprising individuals diagnosed with ASPD (McCann, Ball, & Ivanoff, 2000), as compliance with treatment was higher and staff burnout was lower than when using other methods. This clearly shows that, as distasteful as some may find criminals diagnosed with ASPD and even labeled as psychopaths, change is possible.

In a different approach to treating personality disorder in those identified as psychopaths, Newman (1998) emphasized that these individuals have a specific information processing deficit that is akin to a learning disability. Wallace, Vitale, and Newman (1999) found that once psychopaths engaged in reward-based behavior, they had difficulty attending to cues that would modulate their goal-directed responses. Psychopaths' early attention bottleneck are thought to prevent them from noticing some stimuli, such as fearful facial expressions, that nonpsychopaths would detect and then accordingly adjust their goal-directed behaviors. Baskin-Sommers, Wolf, Buckholtz, Warren, and Newman (2012) found that computerized training, similar to the playing of video games, can teach psychopaths to attend to peripheral stimuli, instead of being brutally focused on their goals. For decades, such computer-assisted cognitive rehabilitation has been successful in other populations, such as those suffering from brain injury (Bracy, 1983), and offers promise for treating these supposedly untreatable people.

In another approach, Kiehl (2006) identified psychopaths as having paralimbic dysfunction, which is often due to brain injuries similar to many of whom Bracy's (1983) colleagues found so amenable to cognitive rehabilitation. In support of Kiehl's (2006) neurobiological approach to identifying psychopaths, Fallon (2010) found consistent biological abnormalities utilizing brain imaging techniques in identified psychopaths. His team linked these brain abnormalities to genetic correlates and, to his surprise, he also found the same abnormal brain functioning and genetic markers in himself and some of his family members, suggesting that biology in this case is not necessarily destiny. After this revealing finding, he concluded that environment is extraordinarily important in shaping a person's genetic propensities, a finding in itself highly supportive of the need to bring social justice perspectives to this population, rather than just discarding them through incarceration. It is ironic that the inmate population, often overly representative of marginalized groups (Alexander, 2012), might need to be trained to be less goal-directed for this theoretical vantage, as being goal-oriented is a quality that is often considered advantageous in an individualistic society. Millon et al. (2004) noted that some of the most admired qualities in U.S. culture are traits of the antisocial personality: adventuresomeness, willingness to do things their own way regardless of social pressure, limit-stretching, pushing forward out of sheer will, and using clever maneuvers and aggressive postures to overturn obstacles. In addition, in some professional settings, this personality style is highly desired and effective. No matter which treatment modality one prefers, such as personality-targeted DBT or neurobiologically based cognitive rehabilitation, to withhold treatment from 15% of the prison population due to their label as psychopaths is not only socially unjust, it is costly, amounting to $460 billion per year or 10 times the cost of treating depression (Price, 2002).

Other Psychological Approaches

In addition to the predominant personality approach that tends to focus on the so-called individual shortcomings of incarcerated individuals, there are many other psychological approaches that are applicable. These may overlap with personality approaches, and with each other, but add to the overall picture of how criminals can be viewed.

Cognitive-Behavioral

Ellis (Ellis & Dryden, 1997) and Beck (Beck & Weishaar, 2000) are cofounders of classic cognitive-behavioral (CBT) approaches. Ellis deemed some thoughts to be irrational, and then focused on disputing their veracity, whereas Beck described disruptive thoughts, primarily about self and world as being distorted. Gonzalez-Prendes (2012) argued that CBT is congruent with a social justice perspective because it is a strength-based approach that encourages self-respect. He stated that CBT seeks out clients' input and thus empowers them throughout the psychotherapeutic process, but he was concerned about CBT being primarily Eurocentric in nature, such that less culturally competent CBT practitioners might pathologize cultural differences, something problematic in prison settings where many inmates are from marginalized cultures (Alexander, 2012).

Holmes (2002) was not convinced that CBT can be effective in culturally diverse populations, leaving possible problems in applying it within prisons. In corrections, thinking errors and cognitive distortions related to violence and other criminal behaviors are often targeted by CBT (e.g., Barriga, Hawkins, & Camelia, 2008), and several prepackaged brand-name programs such as *Thinking for a Change* (Bush, Glick, & Taymans, 1997), *Reasoning and Rehabilitation* (Ross, Fabiano, & Ewles, 1988), and *Aggression Replacement Therapy* (Goldstein, Glick, Gibbs, 1998) are frequently used and generally considered effective interventions (Clark, 2010). However, R. Miller (2013) proposed that labeling thoughts behind heinous actions as irrational or distorted, as is done in CBT, sanitizes these actions in a way that diminishes their gravity. He described CBT's attempt to claim morally neutral status by using words such as "inappropriate, dysfunctional, destructive, violent, antisocial, or predatory" (p. 221), instead of directly speaking of "evil," to be a minimization of the malevolent actions. Alternatively, pathologizing as a sickness different patterns of thought that may be adaptive in difficult environments, such as in low socioeconomic ghettos and barrios, can be seen as a further example of psychological blaming, whereas reducing criminals to being evil denies them even more of their dignity.

There is now a third wave of CBT approaches that draws heavily from spiritual and contemplative traditions, and these begin to address Miller's (2013) concerns regarding the sanitization of heinous actions. In their embrace and acceptance of suffering, instead of labeling and disputing the thoughts surrounding the suffering, they overlap with the humanistic-existential approaches in psychology (Prasko, Mainerova, Jelenova, Kamaradova, & Sigmundova, 2012). Third wave traditions include Acceptance and Commitment Therapy (ACT, Hays, 2005), Mindfulness-Based Stress Reduction (Kabat-Zinn, 2003), Mindfulness-Based Cognitive Therapy (Segal,Williams, & Teasdale, 2002), and DBT (Linehan, 1993), all of which are percolating into prison work. A review by Chiesa and Malinowski (2011) meticulously outlined the commonalities and differences among these third wave approaches, and Fuchs, Lee, Roemer, and Orsillo (2013) found that mindfulness- and acceptance-based treatments relieved the suffering of clients from nondominant cultures and marginalized backgrounds, as well as those more culturally mainstream. They speculated that, due to the non-European underpinnings of these approaches, perhaps these treatments might be more congruent with culturally responsive therapy. As applied to prisons, Howells, Tennant, Day, and Elmer (2010) found that offenders in forensic mental health and criminal justice services benefited from mindfulness-based techniques, and these reduced risk of recidivism, alleviated distress, and facilitated coping. Howells (2010) reviewed third wave approaches aimed directly at forensic populations and stated that the Good Lives Model (Ward & Stewart, 2003) and the What Works Model (Hollin & Palmer, 2006) are highly effective, structured approaches. These approaches attempt to build on the strengths of the offenders in order to construct a positive identity, instead of focusing solely on eliminating problems and abnormalities.

Humanistic-Existential

In the Rogerian tradition, Bohart (2013) maintained that every human, despite any former "evil" behaviors, is worthy of respect as a person, and is capable of positive change. Schneider (2013) similarly argued that the humanistic-existential principles emphasizing finding meaning is important, which is in line with Lifton's (1969) conclusion that, when overcome by meaninglessness, men are more likely to murder. Frankl (1963) believed criminality and meaning in life are inversely related, something others have found useful in working with prisoners (Shrum, 2004). Knoll (2009), who primarily interviewed inmates with life sentences, noted that individuals who had no hope for parole became less behaviorally problematic and less suicidal when they discovered meaning and purposefulness, as compared to lifers who reported no purpose or meaning in their lives. When discussing inmates who were able to be paroled, Knoll (2009) reported that incarceration can place behavioral problems in a veritable deep freeze during the prison sentence, but these problems often reappear after release; therefore Knoll argued that an existential approach might be helpful in reducing recidivism rates outside of prisons.

Psychoanalytic

Meloy and Shiva (2007) described a psychoanalytic view of the psychopath that includes a lack of attachment, low arousal and anxiety, grandiose self with omnipotent fantasies, primitive internalization of objects (resulting in enhancement of self and devaluation of other), a failure to internalize values, a range and depth of emotions similar to that of a toddler, and lack of struggle with ego-dystonic aggression resulting in immediate violent acting out or cold, carefully planned, predatory aggression. When discussing the psychopath's limited internalization of objects, they noted the predator-prey dynamic in the counter-transference responses of adult psychopaths. The emphasis on individual blame inherent in this approach is obvious, and the lack of an evidence base for applying this approach within corrections, as well as the inordinate time required for treatment using these methods, puts psychoanalysis on the retreat in prisons. However, hybrids drawing from this tradition, such as DBT that combines CBT with psychoanalytic approaches, have been found successful in treating narcissistic personality (Marra, 2005), which is often associated with the psychopathy (Hare, 1991).

Social Learning Theories

Social justice requires treating inmates with dignity and respect, so pathologizing individuals or, worse, labeling them as evil is contrary to its tenets. Social learning theory advances the idea that culturally transmitted beliefs can lead to devaluation of certain groups, which in turn makes them susceptible to exploitation. Such imbalanced power relationship can lead to deviancy, wherein those without power act out against those with power through means deemed illegitimate (e.g., criminal). For example, when easily delineated factions possessing strong group identities compete for scarce resources, bitterness, hostility, and even violence may ensue between the rivaling groups (Sherif & Sherif, 1956).

Similarly, when one group is given social power over another via societally prescribed roles, such as being assigned the roles of guard and prisoner, the presiding group's oppression can lead to learned helplessness and depression in the oppressed group, as well as zealous, even sadistic, behaviors in the empowered group (Haney, Banks, & Zimbardo, 1973). Displaying aggressive behavior, even when a role model verbally discourages such behavior, can lead to emulation of the undesirable behavior by observers (Bandura, 1971). Thus, social learning theory provides a strong psychological basis not only for understanding criminals but also for providing milieus more conducive to positive outcomes. Although it is less tied just to the individual level of analysis than other psychological approaches reviewed in this chapter, nevertheless its emphasis is on learning that occurs within the individual, although also within a social context.

Biological

The use of psychopharmacological agents has become the mainstay of social control of the SMI within prisons, as well as first-line treatment for other inmates voicing a variety of complaints, often for social gains (e.g., to get out of a difficult situation by claiming a psychological problem). This bias toward using medications is based on underlying assumptions about the biological nature of humans, including criminals. It is also less expensive to medicate rather than to work psychologically with the incarcerated population. Nevertheless, this biological reductionism is not unique to prisons in the United States, but reflects larger societal trends in which use of medications for psychological problems has become commonplace. Clearly there are effective alternatives to medication in treating even inmates with SMI, such as Mosher's (1991) interpersonal treatment of schizophrenia, which was found to be as effective as psychopharmacological agents in several studies. Many scholars (e.g., Leitner, 2013), have argued that mental health professionals should pursue alternatives to biological treatment, but when the profession of psychology has not successfully advocated for the unincarcerated in this venue, it is not to be expected that it could do so for the incarcerated. This is clearly a social justice issue, as so many prisoners are languishing under the effects of powerful, and often iatrogenic, psychotropic medications that make them easier to be docilely warehoused, which is perhaps the most extreme form of dehumanization.

Psychological Dilemmas

Psychologists working in U.S. prisons face many social justice dilemmas. One of the most daunting is that they are often called upon to make decisions that place them in ethical binds. Consider what happens when one is asked to rehabilitate mentally ill inmates who cannot be executed due to being legally insane, knowing that, if they are successfully treated to achieve sanity, then these inmates will face the ultimate penalty. Or one might consider the dual role of being a psychotherapist to inmates, yet being expected under various forms of pressure, such as duty-to-warn provisions in prisons that circumvent usual professional confidentiality, to snitch on inmates in ways that could result in their severe punishment. One particularly vexing issue is the rampant increase of privatization in health care to inmates, in which the profit motive erodes the availability of many needed psychological, and even basic medical, services to inmates. Governments often outsource these services specifically so they can avoid direct liability for denying them, but allow private companies to bid low, saving the governments' money, while the governments know fully that any cost savings comes out of services to inmates, a vulnerable population due to being incarcerated and having no health care alternatives.

With such a large percentage of the U.S. prison population suffering from mental health disorders, mental health and related professionals are confronted with alarmingly high caseloads of inmates with a wide range of mental illnesses. Inmates often express frustration with limited services for their mental health needs, and typically there exists a bureaucratic maze to negotiate in order to receive any mental health interventions, while inmates often wait lengthy periods to receive the help they require. Many inmates will simply forgo requesting help in light of these hurdles.

This also applies to health care in general within prisons, as depicted in *A Woman Doing Life: Notes from a Prison for Women* (George, 2009). This story chronicles female inmates' ongoing struggles to obtain their basic health care needs, such as gynecological and dental care, and convincingly argues that many women simply stop seeking routine care given the challenges in receiving what most citizens simply take for granted; and clearly this also applies to male inmates. What are psychologists to do in such circumstances? Are they expected to be complicit with such government-corporate alliances by knowingly performing in settings where substandard levels of psychological service are being provided to the most needy individuals, or to leave for ethical reasons, which would be an action that would only further deny such services to this vulnerable population? Perhaps the extreme of this type of dilemma involves those who worked in U.S. military prisons outside of the United States where torture was accepted policy, and who participated in delivering torture under orders, as well as under the weak justification that their presence as psychologists mitigated some of the harm from torture. These are just some of the many dilemmas faced by psychologists working with incarcerated populations.

In addition, prison staff suicide rates in the United States are higher than inmate suicide rates (Waugh, 2000), which evidence some of the toxic carry-over in working in these types of settings. Stack and Tsoudis (1997) found that correctional officers had a 39% higher rate of suicide than did other professions. Spinaris

(2006) noted that inmates come and go, whereas staff spend a lifetime behind bars in highly stressful, and often thankless, positions. She articulately described the no-win situation staff can often experience by coining the term "corrections fatigue" to describe what can be seen as endemic of posttraumatic stress disorder within prison staff members. Prison staff are also often portrayed in the media as being corrupt and even more evil than the inmates they manage, and staff often function under a climate of continuous surveillance and suspicion in which investigations abound. Compounding the stress of being constantly watched and suspected of misdeeds, inmates pose very real physical dangers to staff and can be litigious, as frivolous grievances and lawsuits are common. When this happens, paperwork proliferates and staff time becomes allocated to administrative and legal self-defense. Due to constant budget cuts, workload is often unmanageable, compromising quality and leading to even the most diligent staff often becoming disgruntled. These conditions tend to demoralize prison staff, including psychologists, and also tend to increase the likelihood of them unfairly treating inmates.

More broadly, the effects of the many social injustices related to incarceration hurt and impact others within our society way beyond the prison walls. To know that innocent people are incarcerated due to prosecutorial malfeasance, that rape and other horrendous abuses are not uncommon within prisons, and that going to prison tends not to rehabilitate people but, rather, to only make them more likely to recidivate as criminals (facts that are widely acknowledged), and to be unable to change these sordid facts dehumanizes everyone concerned. It is no wonder that much animosity becomes deflected onto all who are incarcerated, as it is a way to avoid a sense of complicity with injustice.

CONCLUSION

This chapter examined social justice issues related to criminal justice with a focus on U.S. prisons. Worldwide, many prison systems are much worse, as well as many are much better, but we have focused on the United States merely because we are more familiar with these prisons. The statistics in the United States are overwhelming, as they depict a nation that has captured the reputation as the country that incarcerates far more of its citizens than any of its closest rivals, which is an incarceration rate that continues to climb while the overall crime rate has fallen. With more adults entering prison, more children are left without the presence of parents, and there are many ripples of social injustice from this penal system. In one of the most often cited analyses of the effectiveness of prisons in curtailing recidivism, Langan and Levin (2002) found that, within three months, 30% of United States released inmates had been rearrested and, within three years, the rate jumped to 67.5%. An interesting question is raised by Cullen, Johnson, and Nagin (2011), that is, if two-thirds of hospital patients left with their ailments not cured and only to be soon readmitted for the same problem, what would be the societal response?

How does any measure of social justice gauge such practices as found in some Texas prisons where inmates are awakened at 3:30 a.m, not paid for their labor, and limited to one five-minute phone call every 90 days based upon good behavior (Wacquant, 2009). The use of indefinite solitary confinement in near soundproof rooms void of most light and mental stimulation has become common practice within the growing number of super-max prisons, since they were first introduced in 1984 (Cullen et al., 2011). Enforced shaved heads and no facial hair, along with no clothing from the outside world, are also common practices and serve a dehumanizing purpose. Social justice as it relates to prisons is eloquently and profoundly espoused by Johnson (2002), "[P]risons pose difficult tests of our values because the conditions of our prisons are a measure of our capacity to recognize and respect the humanity of offenders, people we fear and hate" (p. 12).

Recognizing the limits of what we have discussed, as this is a huge topic whose surface has only been selectively skimmed, we nevertheless hope our chapter has raised awareness of social injustice as it relates to criminal offenders from a psychological perspective within U.S. prisons. The charge of bringing social justice to those incarcerated is daunting, but there do exist numerous entry points. The renewed interest in social justice among psychologists is encouraging, and can play a significant future role in addressing these issues. Further, through research, education, and practice, as well as professional advocacy, psychology can impact the criminal justice system and ensure social justice has a seat at the bargaining table. A word of caution is in order, however, as in the perception of Arrigo (1998) that the criminal justice system resists change due to its many vested interests and, consequently, the challenge becomes all the greater. Last, we turn to the origin of the word *penitentiary*, which relates to a place where people can repent, or turn away from their previous misdeeds to live a renewed life of virtue. One goal of social justice in prisons is to evolve institutions that can better, rather than simply contain or even worsen, the lives of those who are incarcerated, and the many lives interconnected with them.

NOTE

1. None of the statements, representations, or viewpoints contained herein has been sanctioned, approved, or endorsed by the Commonwealth of Pennsylvania or the Pennsylvania Department of Corrections. Nothing contained herein should be deemed to represent the official views of the Commonwealth or the Department.

REFERENCES

Advisory Committee on Geriatric and Seriously Ill Inmates (2005). *Report of the Joint State Government Commission*. Harrisburg, PA: General Assembly of the Commonwealth of Pennsylvania. Retrieved from http://jsg.legis.state.pa.us/publications.cfm?JSPU_PUBLN_ID=40

Agnew, R. (1992). Foundation for a general strain theory of crime and delinquency. *Criminology, 5,* 373–387.
Agudo, S. (2008). Irregular passion: The unconstitutionality and inefficacy of the sex offender residency laws. *Northwestern University Law Review, 102*(1), 308–342.
Alalehto, T. (2003). Economic crime: Does personality matter? *International Journal of Offender Therapy and Comparative Criminology, 47*(3), 335–355.
Aldarondo, E. (2007). Rekindling the reformist spirit in the mental health professions. In E. Aldarondo (Ed.), *Advancing social justice through clinical practice* (pp. 3–17). Mahwah, NJ: Erlbaum.
Alexander, M. (2012). *The new Jim Crow: Mass incarceration in the age of colorblindness.* New York, NY: The New Press.
American Bar Association (Justice Kennedy Commission). (2004). *Reports with recommendations to the ABA House of Delegates.* Washington, DC: Author. Retrieved from http://www.abanow.org/wordpress/wp-content/files_flutter/1267822633_20_1_1_7_Upload_File.pdf
American Psychiatric Association. (2000). *Diagnostic and statistical manual of mental disorders* (4th ed.). Arlington, VA: American Psychiatric Association.
Armstrong, S., & McNeill, F. (2012). *Reducing reoffending: Review of selected countries. Final report for audit Scotland. Report No. 4.* Glasgow, Scotland: The Scottish Centre for Crime and Justice Research.
Arrigo, B. (1998). Justice with prejudice. *Justice Quarterly, 15,* 199–205.
Association for the Treatment of Sexual Abusers (ATSA, 2010). *The registration and community notification of adult sexual offenders.* Beaverton, OR: Author. Retrieved from http://www.atsa.com/registration-and-community-notification-adult-sexual-offenders
Bandura, A. (1971). *Social learning theory.* Morristown, NJ: General Learning.
Barriga, A. Q., Hawkins, M. A., & Carmelia, C. R. (2008). Specificity of cognitive distortions to antisocial behaviors. *Criminal Behavior and Mental Health 18*(2), 104–116.
Baskin-Sommers, A., Wolf, R., Buckholtz, J., Warren, C., & Newman, J. (2012). Exaggerated attention blink response in prisoners while externalizing. *Journal of Research in Personality, 46,* 688–693.
Beck, A. T., & Weishaar, M. E. (2000). In R. J. Corsini & D. Wedding (Eds.). *Current psychotherapies* (6th ed., pp. 241–272). Itasca, IL: F.E. Peacock.
Bedau, H. A. (1982). Prisoners' rights. *Criminal Justice Ethics, 1*(1), 26–41.
Berzins, L. G., & Trestman, R. L. (2004). The development and implementation of Dialectical Behavioral Therapy in forensic settings. *International Journal of Forensic Mental Health, 3*(1), 93–103.
Bessler, J. (2012). *Cruel and unusual: The American death penalty and the founders' Eighth Amendment.* Boston, MA: Northeastern University Press.
Bohart, A. C. (2013). Darth Vader, Carl Rogers, and self-organizing wisdom. In A. C. Bohart, B. S. Held, E. Mendelowitz, & K. J. Schneider (Eds.), *Humanity's dark side: Evil, destructive experience and psychotherapy* (pp. 141–156.). Washington, DC: APA.
Bracy O. L. (1983). Computer based cognitive rehabilitation. *Cognitive Rehabilitation, 1*(1), 7–8.
Briggs, S., & Sarre, R. (2010). *Using personality profiling to identify potential fraudsters.* San Francisco, CA: American Accounting Association Annual Meeting. Retrieved from http://aaahq.org/AM2013/abstract.cfm?submissionID=1451

Brody, R. G., & Kiehl, K. A. (2010). From white-collar crime to red-collar crime. *Journal of Financial Crime, 17*(3), 351–364.

Bureau of Justice Statistics. (2006). *Mental health problems of prison and jail inmates* (NCJ 213600). Washington, DC: U.S. Department of Justice.

Bush, J., Glick, B., & Taymans, J. (1997). *Thinking for a change: Integrated cognitive behavior change program.* Washington, DC: The National Institute of Corrections.

Carozza, D. (2008, July-August). These men know "snakes in suits." *Fraud Magazine, 22*(4), 36–43.

Carroll, J. S., Weiner, R., Coates, D., Galegher, J., & Alibrio, J. (1982). Evaluation, diagnosis, and prediction in parole decision making. *Law and Society Review, 17,* 199–228.

Chesney-Lind, M. (1989). Girls, crime and woman's place: Toward a feminist model of female delinquency. *Crime and Delinquency, 35,* 5–29.

Chiesa, A., & Malinowski, P. (2011). Mindfulness-based approaches: Are they the same? *Journal of Clinical Psychology, 67*(4), 404–424.

Chiu, T. (2010, April). *It's about time: Aging prisoners, increasing costs, and geriatric release.* New York, NY: Vera Institute of Justice, Center on Sentencing and Corrections.

Clark, P. (2010). Preventing future crime with cognitive behavioral therapy. *National Institute of Justice Journal, 265,* n.p. Retrieved from http://www.nij.gov/journals/265/therapy.htm#note4

Cloyes, K. G., Wong, B., Latimer, S., & Abarca, J. (2010). Time to prison return for offenders with serious mental illness released from prison: A survival analysis. *Criminal Justice and Behavior, 37*(2), 175–187.

COSO. (2010). *Fraudulent financial reporting: 1998–2007.* Ewing, NJ: Author. Retrieved from http://www.coso.org/FraudReport.htm

Croall, H. (2007). Victims of white collar crime and corporate crime. In P. Davies, P. Francis, & C. Greer (Eds.), *Victims, Crime and Society* (pp. 78–108). London, UK: Sage. Retrieved from http://www.uk.sagpub.com/stout/croall_white_collar20%-%20vics_crim_soc.pdf.

Cullen, F. T., Johnson, C. L., & Nagin, D. S. (2011). Prisons do not reduce recidivism: The high cost of ignoring science. *The Prison Journal, 91*(3), 48S–65S.

Cullen, F. T., Link, B. G., & Polazi, C. W. (1982). The seriousness of crime revisited: Have attitudes towards white collar crimes changed? *Criminology, 20,* 83–102.

Curtin, A. (2013). Prisoners in California's solitary confinement units to start hunger strikes. *Nation of Change, July 6,* n.p. Retrieved from http://www.nationofchange.org/

Dorminey, J. W., Fleming, A. S., Kranacher, M., & Riley, R. A. (2010). Beyond the fraud triangle: Enhancing deterrence of economic crimes. *The CPA Journal, July,* 17–23.

Economist (2011). Conservatives and criminal justice: Right and proper (with a record of being tough on crime, the political right can afford to start being clever about it), *Author, May 26,* n.p. Retrieved from http://www.economist.com/node/18744617a

Ellis, A., & Dryden, W. (1997). *The practice of rational-emotive therapy* (Rev. ed.). New York, NY: Springer.

Fallon, J. (2010). *A neuroscientist uncovers a dark secret.* Washington, DC: NPR Special Series: Inside the Criminal Mind. Retrieved from http://www.npr.org/templates/story/story.php?storyId=127888976

Ford, M. A. (2007). White-collar crime, social harm, and punishment: A critique and modification of the sixth circuit's ruling in United States v. Davis. *St. Johns Law Review, 83,* 383–399.

Frankl, V. (1963). *Man's search for meaning*. Boston, MA: Beacon.

Friedrichs, D. O. (2007). *Trusted criminals: White collar crime in contemporary society* (3rd ed.). Belmont, CA: Thomson Wadsworth.

Fuchs, C., Lee, J. K., Roemer, E., & Orsillo, S. M., (2013). Using mindfulness- and acceptance-based treatments with clients from nondominant and/or marginalized backgrounds: Clinical considerations, meta-analysis findings, and introduction to the special series: Clinical considerations in using acceptance based- and mindfulness-based treatments with diverse populations. *Cognitive and Behavioral Practice, 20*(1), 1–12.

George, E. (2009). *A woman doing life: Notes from a prison for women*. New York, NY: Oxford University Press.

Goldstein, A. P., Glick, B., & Gibbs, J. C. (1998). *Aggression replacement training: A comprehensive intervention for aggressive youth*. Champaign, IL: Research Press.

Gonzalez-Prendes, A. A. (2012). Cognitive behavioral therapy and social work values: A critical analysis. *Journal of Social Work and Ethics, 9*(2), 21–33.

Gottschalk, M. (2011). Extraordinary sentences and the proposed police surge. *Criminology & Public Policy, 10*(1), 123–136.

Gustafson, J. L. (2007). Cracking down on white collar crime: Analysis of the recent trend of severe sentences for corporate officers. *Suffolk University Law Review, XL*(3), 865–701.

Hagan, J. (2010). Social costs of incarceration. *Researching the Law, 21* (3), n.p. Retrieved from http://www.americanbarfoundation.org/uploads/cms/documents/abf_rl_summer_2010.pdf

Haney, C., Banks, C., & Zimbardo, P. (1973). Interpersonal dynamics in a simulated prison. *International Journal of Criminology and Penology, 1*, 69–97.

Hare, R. (1993). *Without conscience*. New York, NY: Guilford.

Hare, R. D., Hart, S. D., & Harpur, T. J. (1991). Psychopathy and the DSM-V criteria for antisocial personality disorder. *Journal of Abnormal Psychology, 100*, 391–398.

Hays, C. (2005). *Get out of your mind and into your life: The new Acceptance Commitment Therapy*. Oakland, CA: New Harbinger.

Hendrichson, C., & Delaney, R. (2012). *The price of prisons: What incarceration costs taxpayers*. New York, NY: Vera Institute of Justice. Retrieved from http://www.vera.org/pubs/price-prisons-what-incarceration-costs-taxpayers

Hollin, C. R., & Palmer, E. J. (2006). (Eds.). *Offending behaviour programmes: Development, application, and controversies*. Chichester, UK: Wiley.

Holmes, J. (2002). All you need is cognitive behaviour therapy. *British Journal of Medicine, 324* (7332), 288–294.

Howells, K. (2010). The "third wave" of cognitive-behavioral therapy and forensic practice. *Criminal Behaviour and Mental Health, 20*, 251–256.

Howells, K., Tennant, A., Day, A., & Elmer, R. (2010). Mindfulness in forensic mental health: Does it have a role? *Mindfulness, 1*, 4–9.

Johnson, R. (2002). *Hard time: Understanding and reforming the prison*. Belmont, CA: Wadsworth.

Jones, S., & Mauer, M. (2013). *Race to incarcerate*. New York, NY: New Press.

Kabat-Zinn, J. (2003). Mindfulness-based interventions in context: Past, present, and future. *Clinical Psychology, Science and Practice, 10*, 144–156.

Kenis, P., Kruyen, P. M., Baaijens, J., & Barneveld, P. (2010). The prison of the future? An evaluation of an innovative prison design in the Netherlands. *Prison Journal, 90*(3), 313–330. doi: 10.1177/0032885510373506

Kiehl, K. A., (2006). A cognitive neuroscience perspective on psychopathy: Evidence for paralimbic system dysfunction. *Psychiatry Research, 142* (2–3), 107–128.

Knoll, J. L., (2009). Discussing the meaning of life with a lifer. *Psychiatric Times, 26*(9), n.p. Retrieved from http://www.psychiatrictimes.com/news/content/article/10168/1442823#

Kurtzleben, D. (2010). Data show racial disparity in crack sentencing. *US News, August 3*, n.p. Retrieved from http://www.usnews.com/news/articles/2010/08/03/data-show-racial-disparity-in-crack-sentencing.

Lamb, H., & Weinberger, L. (2001). Persons with severe mental illness in jails and prisons: A review. *Psychiatric Services, 49,* 483–492.

Langan, P. A., & Levin, D. (2002). Bureau of Justice special report: Recidivism of prisoners released in 1994. *Bureau of Justice Statistics.* Washington, DC: U.S. Department of Justice. Retrieved from www.ojp.usdoj.gov/bjs/

Langan, P., A., Schmitt, E. L., & Durose, M. R. (2004). Recidivism of sex offenders released from prison in 1994. *Bureau of Justice Statistics.* Washington, DC: U.S. Department of Justice. Retrieved from www.ojp.usdoj.gov/bjs/

Laub, J. H., & Sampson, R. J. (2003). *Shared beginnings, divergent lives: Delinquent boys to age 70.* Cambridge, MA: Harvard University Press.

Leitner, L. M., (2013). Evil: An experiential constructivist understanding. In A. C. Bohart, B. S. Held, E. Mendelowitz, & K. J. Schneider (Eds). *Humanity's dark side: Evil, destructive experience and psychotherapy* (pp. 119–140). Washington, DC: American Psychological Association.

Lemert, E. M. (1972). *Human deviance, social problems, and social control* (2nd ed.). Englewood Cliffs, NJ: Prentice-Hall.

Lewin, K. (1948). *Resolving social conflicts.* New York, NY: Harper.

Lifton, R. J. (1969). *History and human survival.* New York, NY: Random House.

Linehan, M. M. (1987). Dialectical Behavior Therapy for treatment of borderline personality disorder: *Theory and method. Bulletin of the Menninger Clinic, 51*(3), 261–276.

Linehan, M. M. (1993). *Cognitive behavioral treatment of borderline personality disorder.* New York, NY: Guilford Press.

Lovell, D., Gagliardi, G., & Peterson, P. (2002). Recidivism and use of services among persons with mental illness after release from prison. *Psychiatric Services, 53,* 1290–1296.

Marra, T. (2005). *Dialectical Behavior Therapy in private practice: A practical & comprehensive guide.* Oakland, CA: New Harbinger Publications, Inc.

Matejkowski, J., Caplan, J. M., & Cullen, S. W. (2010). The impact of severe mental illness on parole decisions. Social integration within a prison setting. *Criminal Justice and Behavior 37*(9), 1005–1029.

Mauer, M. (2003). *Comparative international rates of incarceration: An examination of causes and trends*: U.S. Commission on Civil Rights. Washington, DC: The Sentencing Project.

Mauer, M., King, R. S., & Young, M. C. (2004). The meaning of "life": Long prison sentences in context. Washington, DC: The Sentencing Project. Retrieved from www.sentencingproject.org

McCann, R. A., Ball, E. M., & Ivanoff, A. (2000). DBT with an inpatient forensic population: The CMHIP forensic model. *Cognitive and Behavioral Practice, 7*(4), 447–456.

Mears, B. (2012). Justices rule for underage killers sentenced to life without parole. *CNN Justice, June 25*, n.p. Retrieved from http://www.cnn.com/2012/06/25/justice/scotus-juvenile-life-sentences

Meloy, J. R., & Shiva, A. (2007). A psychoanalytic view of the psychopath. In A. Felthous & H. Sass (Eds.), *The International Handbook of Psychopathic Disorders* (pp. 335–346). New York, NY: Wiley.

Merton, R. (1938). Social structure and anomie. *American Sociological Review, 3,* 672–682.

Miller, D. (1999). *Principles of social justice.* Cambridge, MA: Harvard University Press.

Miller, R. (2013). Deny no evil, ignore no evil, reframe no evil: Psychology's moral agenda. In A. C. Bohart, B. S. Held, E. Mendelowitz, & K. J. Schneider (Eds.), *Humanity's dark side: Evil, destructive experience and psychotherapy* (pp. 141–156.). Washington, DC: American Psychological Association.

Millon, T. (1981). *Disorders of personality: DSM-III: Axis II.* New York, NY: Wiley.

Millon, T., Grossman, S., Millon, C., Meagher, S., & Ramnath, R. (2004). *Personality disorders in modern life* (2nd ed.). Hoboken, NJ: Wiley.

Montagne, R. (2008). Inside the nation's largest mental institution. *National Public Radio, August 14,* n.p. Retrieved from http://www.npr.org/templates/story/story.php?storyId=93581736

Mosher, L. R. (1991). Soteria: A therapeutic community for psychotic patients. *International Journal of Therapeutic Communities, 12*(1), 53–67.

Nellis, A. (2010). Throwing away the key: The expansion of life without parole sentences in the United States. *Federal Sentencing Reporter, 23*(1), 27–32.

Newman, J. P. (1998). Psychopathic behavior: An information processing perspective. In D. J. Cooke, R. D. Hare, & A. Forth (Eds.), *Psychopathy: Theory, research and implications for society* (pp. 81–104). Alphen aan den Rijn, The Netherlands: Kluwer Academic.

Ogloff, J. R., (2006). Psychopathy/antisocial personality disorder conundrum. *Australian and New Zealand Journal of Psychiatry, 40,* 519–528.

Pager, D. (2009). *Marked: Race, crime, and finding work in an era of mass incarceration.* Chicago, IL: University of Chicago Press.

Pastore, A. L., & Maguire, K. (Eds.). (2003). *Sourcebook of criminal justice statistics.* Washington, DC: U.S. Department of Justice, Bureau of Justice Statistics. Retrieved from http://www.albany.edu/sourcebook/

Perri, F. S. (2011). White-collar criminals: The "kinder, gentler" offender? *Journal of Investigative Psychology and Offender Profiling, 8,* 217–241.

Prasko, J., Mainerova, B., Jelenova, D., Kamaradova, D., & Sigmundova, Z. (2012). Existential perspectives and cognitive behavioral therapy. *Activitas Nervosa Superior Rediviva, 54*(1) 3–14.

Pratt, J. (2011). The international diffusion of punitive penalty: Or, penal exceptionalism in the United States? *Australian & New Zealand Journal of Criminology, 44*(1), 116–128.

Price, C. A. (2006). *Aging inmate population.* Raleigh, NC: North Carolina Department of Corrections, Division of Prisons.

Price, J. (2012). [Mis]guided light. *On Wisconsin, 113*(3), 22–29.

Price, M., & Norris, D. M. (2009). White collar crime: Corporate and securities and commodities fraud. *The Journal of the American Academy of Psychiatry and the Law, 37*(4), 538–544.

The Probation Service. (2012). *Probation Service Recidivism Study 2007–2011, Report No. 2.* Dublin, Ireland: Author. Retrieved from www.probation.ie

Ramamoorti, S. (2008,). The psychology and sociology of fraud: Integrating the behavioral sciences component into fraud and forensic accounting curricula, *Issues in Accounting Education, November,* 351–363.

Rice, M. E., Harris, G. T., & Cormier, C. A. (1992). An evaluation of a maximum security therapeutic community for psychopaths and other mentally disordered offenders. *Law and Human Behavior, 16*(4), 399–412.

Robinson, M. (2010). Assessing criminal justice practice using social justice theory. *Social Justice Research, 23,* 77–97.

Ross, R. R., Fabiano, E. A., & Ewles, C. D. (1988). Reasoning and rehabilitation. *International Journal of Offender Therapy and Comparative Criminology, 32*(1), 29–35.

Samenow, S. (1984). *Inside the criminal mind.* New York, NY: Times Books.

Schneider, K. J. (2013). Radical openness to radical mystery: Rollo May and the awe-based way. In A. C. Bohart, B. S. Held, E. Mendelowitz, & K. J. Schneider (Eds.), *Humanity's dark side: Evil, destructive experience and psychotherapy* (pp. 19–33). Washington, DC: American Psychological Association.

Segal, Z. J., Williams, M. G., & Teasdale, J. D. (2002). *Mindfulness-based cognitive therapy for depression: A new approach to preventing relapses.* New York, NY: Guilford Press.

Sherif, M., & Sherif, C. W. (1956). *An outline of social psychology* (2nd ed.). New York, NY: Harper & Row.

Shrum, H. (2004). No longer theory: Practices that work. *Journal of Correctional Education, 55*(3), 225–235.

Skeem, J. L., Monahan, J. & Mulvey, E. P. (2002). Psychopathy, treatment involvement, and subsequent violence among civil psychiatric patients. *Law and Human Behavior, 26*(6), 577–603.

Spinaris, C. (2006). Factors that contribute to correctional fatigue. *Archives of Suicide Research, 3*(3), 183–186.

Stack, S. J., & Tsoudis, O. (1997). Suicide risk among correctional officers: A logistical regression analysis. *Archives of Suicide Research, 3*(3), 183–186.

Sutherland, E. H. (1940). The white collar criminal. *American Sociological Review, 5,* 1–12.

Swets, J. A. (1961). Is there a sensory threshold? *Science, 134,* 168–177.

Toch, H. (2010). I am not now who I used to be then: Risk assessment and the maturation of long-term prison inmates. *The Prison Journal, 90*(1), 4–11.

Wacquant, L. (2009). *Prisons of poverty: Expanded edition.* Minneapolis, MN: University of Minnesota.

Wallace, J. F., Vitale, J. E., & Newman, J. P. (1999). Response modulation deficits: Implications for the diagnosis and treatment of psychopathy. *Journal of Cognitive Psychotherapy, 13*(1), 55–70.

Walzer, M. (1983). *Spheres of justice.* New York, NY: Basic Books.

Ward, T., & Steward, C. A. (2003). The treatment of sex offenders: Risk management and Good Lives. *Professional Psychology: Research and Practice, 34,* 353–360.

Waugh, P. (August 30, 2000). Jail union seeks to cut high staff suicide rate. *The Independent.* Retrieved from http://www.independent.co.uk/news/this britain/jail union seeks action to cut high staff suicide rate 710823.html

Western, B., Kling, J. R., Weiman, D. F. (2001). Labor market consequences of incarceration. *Princeton Labor Relations Section,* n.p. Retrieved from http://dataspace.princeton.edu/jspui/bitstream/88435/dsp01kw52j807k/1/450.pdf

Wilson, J. Q. (2011). Hard times, fewer crimes. *Wall Street Journal, May 28–29,* C1.

Wright, K. N., & Bronstein, L. (2007). An organizational analysis of prison hospice. *The Prison Journal, 87*(4), 391–407.

Index

Abeles, R. P., 104
Accompaniment, 120, 122
Adams, J. S., 12
Adam Walsh Act, 248
Adorno, Theodor, 87
AFN. *See* Assembly of First Nations
African Americans, 116; government criticisms by, 100–101; miseducation of, 98–99, 104, 107; psychology of nigrescence and, 103; on racial colorblindness, 101
African Commission on Human and Peoples' Rights, 161
African Spring movement, 108–9
Afuape, T., 123
Aglioti, S. M., 44
Ahmadinejad, Mahmoud, 155
AIM. *See* American Indian Movement
Albee, George W., 39–40, 223
Alcantara, C., 136
Alcatraz Island occupation, 146
Alcoholism, 138
Aldarondo, E., 245
Alderson, J., 158
Alfred, Taiaike, 143–44
Algeria, 99
Alibrio, J., 246
Allocation, 4–5, 13
Alterglobalization, 45
Altschiller, D., 161
American Anthropological Association, 164
American Bar Association Justice Kennedy Commission, 250
American Community Survey, 164–65
American Indian Movement (AIM), 146
American Indian/Native Alaskan, 135, 148; boarding school era and, 137; demographics of, 136; discrimination, micro-aggression, racism and, 140–41; federal governmental policies and, 136–38, 149nn1–2; healing practices of, 141–43; health and mental disparities within, 138–39; historical resistance stories of, 145–47; reclaiming and reconstructing histories of, 144–45; storytelling and, 141–44; trauma response of, 139–40
Americanization, 107–8
American Psychiatric Association, 164

American Psychological Association (APA), 59, 141, 166, 169–70; Guidelines on Multicultural Education, Training, Research, Practice, and Organizational Change for Psychologists, 223–24; Resolution on Marriage Equality for Same-Sex Couples, 164; Resolution on Poverty and Socioeconomic Status, 40; Resolution on Sexual Orientation Parents, and Children, 164–65; Statement on Reforming the Juvenile Justice System, 40; Task Force on Socioeconomic Status, 227
American Sociological Association, 164
Americans with Disabilities Act, 180
The American Dream, 107–8
Anderson, G. I., 231–32
Antisocial personality disorder (ASPD), 253–54
Anzeldua, Gloria, 121
APA. *See* American Psychological Association
Aporia, 45
Arab movement, 108–9
Aristotle, 4–5, 11, 21nn9–10, 22n12, 68
Arrigo, B. A., 37
Asians, 101, 105
ASPD. *See* Antisocial personality disorder
Assembly of First Nations (AFN), 146–47
Association for the Treatment of Sexual Abusers (ATSA), 247–48
Atkins, Susan, 250
ATSA. *See* Association for the Treatment of Sexual Abusers
Avenanti, A., 44
Ayala, J., 121

Ban Ki-moon, 170
"Base and Superstructure in Marxist Cultural Theory," 86
Baskin-Sommers, A., 255
Batson, C. D., 44
Beard, J., 40
Beck, A. T., 256
Bedau, H. A., 249
Behavior, 80; criminal, 37; just, 18, 21n10; sexual, 159. *See also* Classic cognitive-behavioral approach
Bell, L. A., 144–45, 148
Belle, D., 229
Bemak, F. P., 54, 58–59
Bentham, Jeremy, 7
Berscheid, E., 12
Bertram, C., 123
Berzins, L. G., 245
BIA. *See* Bureau of Indian Affairs, U.S.
Bies, R. J., 17, 35
BigFoot, Delores S., 142
Billies, M., 122
Blacks, 99, 103–4, 243–44. *See also* African Americans
Blau, P. M., 12
Bling: A Planet Rock (Cepeda and Bozotti), 43
Blood Struggles (Wilkinson), 146
Bloom, L. R., 225
Bohart, A. C., 258
Bonilla-Silva, E., 104
Bourdieu, P., 70
Bourgeois revolutions, 80
Bozotti, F., 43
Bracy, O. L., 255
Brasfield, C. R., 137
Brave Heart, Maria Y. H., 139
Brazaitis, S., 46
Brockner, J., 16
Brody, R. G., 252
Bronfenbrenner, U., 121, 186
Bronstein, L., 2
Brown, L. S., 56
Brown, R., 106, 109
Brown v. the Board of Education, 41

Brydon-Miller, M., 119
Buckholtz, J., 255
Bulhan, H., 116
Bullock, H. E., 227–28
Buranajakoenkij, D. N., 129
Bureau of Indian Affairs, U.S. (BIA), 137, 146
Bureau of Justice, U.S., 247
Burke, Edmund, 10–11, 14
Burman, E., 65
Burton, M., 120
Bush, George W., 101
Bush, J., 257
Butler, G., 158

California, 166, 243
Canada, 137, 146–47, 164
Canadian Psychological Association, 164
Capeheart, L., 38
Capitalism, 6; alternatives to, 81; governments and, 81; ideology and, 94n3; individualism and, 57; labor and, 81; multinational corporations and, 81–82; universal commodification by, 83
Caregivers, 206
Carozza, D., 252
Carroll, J. S., 246
Carter, R. T., 40
Cattaneou, L. B., 44
CBT. *See* Classic cognitive-behavioral approach
Central and Eastern Europe (CEE), 178, 181–85
Cepeda, R., 43
Certificate in Lesbian and Queer Culture, 124
Chapman, A. R., 44
Chauca-Sabroso, R. L., 120
Chaudry, L., 123
Cheung, M. H., 105
Chiesa, A., 257
Children, 183, 194, 197, 229, 244; in Latin American, 120; youth LGBTQI and, 164–65
China. *See* People's Republic of China
Chiu, T., 249
Christensen, M., 137
Chung, R. C.-Y., 54, 58–59
Classic cognitive-behavioral approach (CBT), 256–57
Classism: conceptualization of, 227; in everyday life, 227–30; framework for understanding, 224–30
Cliché, 86
Coates, D., 246
CoBRAS. *See* Color-Blind Racial Attitudes Scale
Colonialism, 81, 109n1; domination and, 99; of lifeworld, 82; racism and, 99
Color-Blind Racial Attitudes Scale (CoBRAS), 101
The Communist Manifesto (Marx), 6
Compromise formation, 82–88, 94n1
Conflict resolution, 34–35
Conscientization, 118–19, 126
Consciousness, 121, 126
Consciousness-raising, 55–56
Conservatism, 58; justice and, 14–15; liberalism, socialism and, 10–11, 21n7
Coquillon, E., 119
Corntassel, Jeff, 144
COSO, 251
Council of Europe, 161
Counseling, 51, 57, 224, 226; practice of, 54–56, 60–61; professional hubris within, 57–60; theories, 53
Criminal: assessment and treatment of, 253–56; behavior, 37; justice system, 241–43; white-collar, 250–53
Critique of the Gotha Program (Marx), 6
Croall, H., 251

Crosby, A., 121
Cross, W. E., Jr., 103–4
Cullen, F. T., 37, 251, 261

Daly, K., 37
Danziger, K., 68
Day, A., 257
Death: penalty, 37, 243; in prison, 249; women and, 73
Decety, J., 44
Decision-making: equality, inequality and, 9–10; the original position of, 8; principles, 8–10; process and procedural justice, 34–35; third-party, 15–16; under veil of ignorance, 8
Decolonization, 88, 94
Decolonizing Methodology (Smith, Linda T.), 143
Demuth, S., 37
Denham, A. R., 147
Department of Justice Statistics, U.S., 245
Deprivation, 108; non-material, 225–26; social comparison and, 106
Deracialization, 103
Derrida, J., 45
Descartes, R., 71
Desymbolization, 82–88
Deutsch, M., 6, 46
DeVinney, L. C., 106
Diagnostic and Statistical Manual of Mental Disorders (*DSM*), 59, 167–68, 254
Dialogue: attempts at, 91–93; connotation of, 91; role of, 79–80, 94
Diamond trade, 43–44
Dion, K. L., 106
Disability, 188; activists, 185–87; in CEE, 181–85; civil rights and, 180–81; human rights and, 179–80; recognition of, 177–78; rights, 178–79
Distribution, 6, 15, 34
Distributive justice, 8; characterization of, 21n2; comparative allotment in, 21n3; focus of, 34; history of concept and, 4–5, 21n3; socialism and, 5–7, 21n4
District of Columbia, 249
Domination, 98–99
Dorminey, J. W., 251
Doucet, J., 229
Douglass, Frederick, 97
Drug abuse, 138
DSM. See Diagnostic and Statistical Manual of Mental Disorders
Dube-Simard, L., 104
Duran, Eduardo, 141
Durose, M. R., 247
Dworkin, R., 21n6

Economy, 80, 86
Education, 234; of LGBTQI, 165–66; people with disabilities and, 180
Egalitarians, 21n8
Elderly: abuse and neglect of, 206–9; challenges with, 210–13; effects of, 191–93; generational equity of, 194–202; long-term care for, 205–6; mental and physical health of, 202–5; population of world's, 193–94; in prisons, 209–10, 249–50; psychological costs of, 201–2; retirement of, 200–201
Ellis, A., 256
Elmer, R., 257
El Salvador, 122
Emotions, 37, 42–43
Empathy, 43–44
Employee Benefit Research Institute, 198
Empowerment, 44
Engels, Friedrich, 6, 21n4, 98–99
Entrepreneurship, 44
Environment, 81, 87–88

Equality, 9–10; concept of, 15; just apportionment and, 5; liberty and, 74; principles of need and, 13–14, 21nn8–9; of ratios, 11–12; understandings of, 41–42
Equity: allocation of resources and, 4–5, 13; concerns of groups, 109; establishment or restoration of, 12–13; generational, 194–202; intergenerational, 195–96; intragenerational, 196–98; perceptions of, 13; theory, 11–13
Ethics, 72–73
Europe, 80–81, 161, 167–68. *See also* Central and Eastern Europe
European Parliament, 161
European Union Agency for Fundamental Rights, 167–68
Evans-Campbell, T., 139
Ewes, C. D., 257

Fabiano, E. A., 257
Fair Labor Standards Act, 230
Fallon, J., 255–56
False consciousness, 18, 22n12, 55, 79; globalization and, 106–9; group/personal identity, identification and, 102; individual/national/political ideology and, 104–5; injustice and, 97–98; justice and, 98; as psychological construct, 99–100; social comparison and, 105–6; social identity awareness models and, 102–4; system justification theory and, 100–101
Fanon, Franz, 75, 99, 109n1, 117
Feinberg, J., 8
Feminism, 232–33; cycles, 125; liberation psychology and, 118, 120–23; women and, 103
Feminism & Psychology, 116, 121–22
Feminist psychology: approach, 115–16, 129–30; key concepts in, 118; liberation and oppression cycles in, 125; participants' voices in, 118, 124–29; structural analysis in, 125
Feuerbach, Ludwig, 65
Fieland, K. C., 138
15 movement, 92
Fine, M., 119
Fixico, Donald, 138
Fleming, A. S., 251
Fonagy, P., 94n2
Forgiveness, 36
Fouad, N. A., 226
France, 99
Frankena, W. K., 8, 17–18, 21n3
Frankfurt, H., 21n8
Frankfurt School, 82–83
Frankl, V., 258
Free trade, 234
Free Trade agreement, 147
Freidrichs, D. O., 251
Freire, P., 117–19, 143
Frohlich, N., 10
Fromm, Erich, 87
Fry, W. R., 16
Fryer, John E., 167
Fuchs, C., 257
Fuentas-Polar, S., 120
Fukuda-Parr, S., 225
Fukuyama, F., 93

Galegher, J., 246
Galtung, J., 75
Garter, R., 234
Gates, G., 158
Gathering of Native Americans (GONA), 143
Gay British Crime Survey, 160
Gays, 103, 115, 160, 169
GBD. *See* Global Burden of Disease
GBV. *See* Gender-based violence
Gender: identity, 156–57; third, 157
Gender-based violence (GBV), 122

Gender Identity disorder (GID), 167
George, E., 259
Gergen, K. J., 68
Gerontology, 191–93. *See also* Elderly
Gerstein, L. H., 226
GID. *See* Gender Identity disorder
Gilligan, C., 35–36
Gilmour, J. A., 158
Glick, B., 257
Global Burden of Disease (GBD), 233
Globalization: characteristics of, 38–39; communications and, 44–45; false consciousness and, 106–9. *See also* Alterglobalization
Goldberg, D., 234
GONA. *See* Gathering of Native Americans
Gone, Joseph P., 136, 148
Gonzalez-Prendes, A. A., 256
Good Lives Model, 257
Goodman, L. A., 40, 52–53, 123, 223, 226
Gough, B., 158
Gould, C. C., 37–38
Government, 36, 81, 136–38, 149nn1–2; criticisms by African Americans, 100–101; Latinos' trust of, 101
Graham, J., 11
Gramsci, Antonio, 98
Great recession, 200
Greenberg, J., 13
Grief, 139
Groups: equity concerns of, 109; higher-status, 98; low-status, 100–101, 105; oppressed, 116; personal identity, identification, and false consciousness of, 102; subordinate, 98; U.S. social, 103
Guatemala, 119–20
Guilt feelings, 42–43
Guimond, S., 104
Gustafson, J. L., 251
Habermas, Jürgen, 82, 90
Hacking, I., 68
Hafer, C. L., 99
Haidt, J., 11
Haines, E. L., 100
Halliburton, C., 41
Handbook for Social Justice in Counseling, 226
Happiness, 7–8, 15
Hardin, C. D., 105
Hare, R., 252, 254
Harris, J., 229
Hatfield, E., 12
Hayek, F. A., 21n7
Healing: circles, 36–37; forgiveness and, 36; justice and, 36; recovery process, 120; through storytelling, 141–43
Healthy Lesbian, Gay, and Bisexual Students Project, 165–66
Hegel, G., 66
Heinz dilemma, 35–36
Henry, P. J., 105
Hermaphrodite, 157
Hermeneutic deficit, 73
Hermeneutic surplus, 73
Hernández, E., 120
Herr, K., 231–32
Higgitt, A., 94n2
Hillier, L., 160, 165
Hiltonsmith, R., 201
Hinduism, 72–73
Hispanics, 105
Hoffman, F. L., 124
Holmes, J., 257
Holzkamp, K., 71
Homans, G. C., 12
Homosexuality, 157, 167
Howells, K., 257
Hoxie, F., 146
HPI. *See* Human Poverty Index
Human capability, 38
Human development, 37–38

Human Development Report, 225
Human nature, 66
Human Poverty Index (HPI), 225
Human reasoning, 8
Human rights: approaches to, 38; of people with disabilities, 179–80. *See also* United Nations
Humans: nature of, 66–68; treatment of, 68
Hunter, J., 160
Huntington, A., 158

IAT. *See* Implicit Association Test
Identity, 102. *See also* Social identity
Ideology, 94; capitalism and, 94n3; compromise formation and, 82–88; concept of, 79–80, 94n3; desymbolization and, 82–88; false consciousness and individual/national/political, 104–5; resymbolization and, 88–90; social justice, 51–52
Idle No More movement, 147
Ikenberry, G. J., 107
ILGA. *See* International Lesbian, Gay, Bisexual, Trans, and Intersex Association
Implicit Association Test (IAT), 44
Incarceration, 246
Individualism, 138; capitalism and, 57; deficit model of, 36; society and, 67–68; understanding of, 41–42, 80
Individuals with Disabilities Education Act, 180
Industrialization, 80–81
Inequality: concept of, 68–69; decision making and, 9–10; economic, 6, 15; resources and, 40–41; societal, 39–40
Inequity, 13
Informal justice. *See* Interactional justice
Injustice: criminal justice and, 241–43; economic, 229–30; experiences with, 35; false consciousness and, 97–98; prison, 243–45
Interactional justice, 17; characterization of, 21n2; interpretation of, 35–36
Inter-American Commission on Human Rights, 161
International Lesbian, Gay, Bisexual, Trans, and Intersex Association (ILGA), 159
Interpretations, 73–74
Intersex, 157
Ireland, 244
Iyer, A., 42

Japan, 81
Johnson, C. L., 261
Johnson, J., 122
Johnson, R., 262
Johnson, Scott, 61
Jost, John T., 15, 34–35, 41, 100–101
Journal of Counseling and Development, 224
Journal of Counseling Psychology, 224
Journal of Multicultural Counseling and Development, 224
Jurisprudence, concept of, 6
Justice, 8; appraisals, 16–17; conceptions of, 6–7, 17–18; conservatism and, 14–15; disagreements regarding, 18; false consciousness and, 98; healing and, 36; liberalism and, 14–15; morality and, 21n11; motivation for, 18–19, 22n12; multidimensional approach to, 13; relationships and, 35–36; theories of, 18–19; triple burden and, 37. *See also specific areas of justice*

Kant, Immanuel, 6, 8, 68
Karuza, J., 16
Kawakami, K., 106

Kay, A. C., 34–35, 41
Kharas, H., 225
Kidd, S. A., 119, 231
Kiehl, K. A., 252, 255
Kinder, D., 98
King, R. S., 249
Kjaerum, M., 169
Knapp, Curtis, 155
Knoll, J. L., 258
Knowledge, 69–72
Kohlberg, L., 8
Kozol, J., 228
Kral, M. J., 119, 231
Kranacher, M., 251
Krumer-Nevo, M., 232
Kupchan, C. A., 107

Labor, 81, 198–200
LAMIC. *See* Low- and middle-income countries
Lamm, C., 44
Langan, P. A., 247, 261
Latin American: children in, 120; liberation psychology, 118–20
Latinos, 160; as defendants, 37; low-income, 100; on racial colorblindness, 101; trust of government by, 101
Laub, J. H., 249
Leach, C. W., 42
Lee, J. K., 257
Lemert, E. M., 253
Leondar-Wright, B., 225
Lerner, M. J., 6, 13, 14
Lesbian, gay, bisexual, transgendered, queer, or intersex (LGBTQI), 170; children and youth, 164–65; discrimination and violence against, 156–57, 160–63; education of, 165–66; employment and housing of, 168–69; family and relationships of, 163–65; health care of, 166–68; social justice issues of, 160–69; status of, 158–60
Lesbian, gay bisexual transgendered (LGBT), 122, 127–28
Lesbians, 103, 115, 122
Leventhal, G. S., 16
Levin, D., 261
Lévinas, E., 71
Lewin, Kurt, 17, 20
LGBT. *See* Lesbian, gay bisexual transgendered
LGBTQI. *See* Lesbian, gay, bisexual, transgendered, queer, or intersex
Liberalism: conservatism and, 10–11, 21n7; deontological approach to, 8–10, 21n6; happiness and, 15; justice and, 14–15; -progressive tradition, 7–10, 21nn5–6; utilitarianism and, 7–8, 21n5
Liberation psychology: activism, intervention and, 117; approach, 115–17, 129–30; feminism and, 118, 120–23; Latin American, 118–20; liberation and oppression cycles in, 125; modules, 125, 127; oppression and, 117, 125; participants' voices in, 118, 124–29; structural analysis in, 125
Libertarians, 21n7
Life expectancy, 193–94
Lifeworld: of colonialism, 82; of people, 141
Lind, E. A., 16, 17
Link, B. G., 251
Linton, S., 185
Liu, W. M., 224
Looping effect, 68
Lorasdagi, B. K., 123
Lorenzer, A., 84, 86
Los Angeles County Jail, 245
Lott, B., 227–28
Low- and middle-income countries (LAMIC), 233–34
Lukács, G., 82–83
Lykes, M. B., 119, 122

MacCartney, D., 42
MacKenzie, D., 158
Madoff, Bernie, 251
Madrigal, L. J., 121
Maguire, K., 249
Malinowski, P., 257
Manifest destiny, 137, 149n2
Manson, Charles, 250
Manson, S., 137
The Man Made of Words (Momaday), 142
Marcus, E. C., 46
Mardi Gras Made in China (Redmon, Smith, D., Smith, D., and Sabin), 43
Marketplace, global, 39
Marriage, same-sex, 164
Martín, Baró, 67, 117–19
Martin, J., 68
Martinez-Salgado, C., 232
Marx, Karl, 5–7, 65–66, 71, 98–99
Marxism: principles of allocation and, 4–5, 13; theories of, 86; during 20th century, 92–94
Maton, K., 65, 76
Mauer, M., 249
Maximin principle, 8
MDRI. *See* Mental Disability Rights International
Medicaid, 211
Medicare, 195–96, 203, 206, 211
Mellers, B. A., 10, 15
Meloy, J. R., 258
Memmi, A., 117
Memory, historical, 123–24
Men, 198–200
Mental Disability Advocacy Centre, 184
Mental Disability Rights International (MDRI), 183
Mental health: disorders, 233–34; oppression and, 230–32; positionality continuum and, 231–32; poverty and, 230–32; in prisons, 245–53
Merit, 14, 41–42
Mexico, 147
Middle class, 225
Middle East, 107
Milavanovic, D., 38
Mill, John Stuart, 7–8, 19
Miller, D. T., 7, 10, 14, 18, 22n11, 42
Miller, J., 229
Miller, R., 257
Millon, T., 256
Minkler, M., 196
Minorities, 116, 202–3
The Mirage of Social Justice (Hayek), 21n7
The Miseducation of the Negro (Woodson), 98–99
Miseducation: of African Americans, 98–99, 104, 107; degrees of, 99
Mitchell, G., 10, 15
Moag, J. S., 17
Moghaddam, F. M., 107–8
Momaday, Scott, 142
Monahan, J., 254–55
Montero, M., 117, 119
Moral exclusion, 42
Morality, 59–60; intuitions and, 11; justice and, 21n11; nature of, 49; understandings of, 41–42
Moran, G., 94n2
Mosher, L. R., 259
Mount Rushmore, 140
Mubbashar, M., 234
Mulvey, E. P, 254–55
Murders, 161
Murungi, K., 122
Muslim women, 123

Nagin, D. S., 261
Napier, J. L., 15
National Academy of Social Insurance, 196

National Coalition for the Homeless, 230
National Counseling Psychology Conference (2001), 53–54, 226
National Indian Child Welfare Association, 143
National Transgender Discrimination Survey, 161, 162
NCS. *See* Nice Counselor Syndrome
Nelson, G., 226
Neville, H. A., 40
Newman, J. P., 255
NGOs. *See* Nongovernmental organizations
Nice Counselor Syndrome (NCS), 58–59
Nicomachean Ethics (Aristotle), 4–5
Nobus, D., 71
Nongovernmental organizations (NGOs), 183–84
Noori, N., 107
Norris, D. M., 251
Norsworthy, K. L., 129
North Carolina, 249
Nozick, R., 21n7
Nussbaum, M. C., 38

Object relations theory: characterization of, 84, 94n1; stereotyped, 84–85, 94n2
Occupy movement, 91–93
Ogloff, J. R., 254
Olson, J. M., 99
"Open Letter to the DSM," 59
Opotow, J., 46
Oppenheimer, J. A., 10
Oppression, 54, 58, 123; liberation psychology and, 117, 125; as limit situations, 118; mental health and, 230–32; success of, 97–98
Ordóñez, L. D., 10, 15
Organization for Security and Cooperation in Europe (OSCE), 161
Orsillo, S. M., 257
OSCE. *See* Organization for Security and Cooperation in Europe
Other: commitment of, 71; consideration of, 71; idealization of, 74; interpretation of, 73–74; reflection on, 70–71
Owning class, 225

Panama, 120
PAR. *See* Participatory action research
Parents, 89, 94n2
Pareto, Vilfredo, 21n7
Parfit, D., 14
Parker, I., 66, 70
Parsons, Frank, 223
Participation, 119, 232
Participatory action frameworks, 230–31
Participatory action research (PAR), 119, 120–21, 231–32
Pastore, A. L., 249
Patel, V., 233–34
Penitentiary, 262
Pennsylvania, Commonwealth of, 262n1
Pennsylvania Department of Corrections, 262n1
Pensions, 200
People, 146–47, 179–80; lifeworld of, 141; virtues of, 119
People's Republic of China (PRC), 81
Perceptions, 42
Perkins, K., 104
Perri, F. S., 251, 252
Piaget, J., 8
Pieterse, A. L., 40
Pine Ridge Indian Reservation, 146
PIP. *See* Positive Indian Parenting
Polazi, C. W., 251
Political mobilization, 90–94
Politics, 60

Positive Indian Parenting (PIP), 143
Potok, M., 160
Poverty, 40, 165; feminization of, 232–33; framework for understanding, 224–30; global considerations regarding, 232–35; mental health and, 230–32; rates, 194, 197–98; understanding, 38
Power, 44; equalizing, 53; knowledge, money and, 70; of situation, 60
PRC. *See* People's Republic of China
Price, C. A., 249
Price, M., 251
Prilleltensky, I., 46, 74, 226
Prilleltensky, O., 46
Prison, 98, 259; elderly in, 209–10, 249–50; injustices, 243–45; mental health in, 245–53; psychology, 241–43; solitary confinement in, 243
Prison Notebooks (Gramsci), 98
Probation Service and Central Services Office, 244
Procedural justice: aspects of, 34–35; characterization of, 21n2; decision control and, 16; decision-making process and, 34–35; perceptions of, 16–17; pioneers of, 15–17; process control and, 16
Proportionality principles, 5
Psychoanalysis, 84, 94n1
Psychoanalytic view, 258
Psychologists, 71; as activists, 185–87; duties of, 51
Psychology, 61; critics of, 115–16; dilemmas in, 259–61; history of, 3–20; of nigrescence, 103; professional hubris within, 57–60; social justice and, 39–41, 51–52, 55–56; subdisciplines of, 40; transformative potential of, 56
Psychopathy, 254, 258
Pugh, R., 122
Queer, 158
Quinn, M., 71

Rabenstein, K. L., 119
Racial colorblindness: African Americans on, 101; Asians on, 101; assessment scale for, 101–2; concept of, 101; Latinos on, 101
Racism, 37; American Indian/Native Alaskan and, 140–41; assessment of, 44; colonialism and, 99; critiques of, 115
Rahman, A., 234
Ramamoorti, S., 252
Rape: as hate crime, 161; women and, 122
Rawls, J., 8–9, 19, 21n6
Reasoning and Rehabilitation (Ross, Fabiano, and Ewes), 257
Redmon, D., 43
Reflexivity, 76; epistemological, 69–72; ethical, 72–75; importance of, 65; narcissistic, 65–66; ontological, 66
Relational justice, 35–36
Relative deprivation theory, 108
Relocation Act of 1956, 137
Republicans, 58
Residential school syndrome, 137
Resources, 40–41; distribution of, 34; equity and allocation of, 4–5, 13
Restorative justice, 36–37
Resymbolization, 94; decolonization and, 88; ideology and, 88–90
Retirement, 198; of elderly, 200–201; income, 201
Retirement Confidence Survey, 198
Retributive justice, 37
Rice, M. E., 254
Richardson, F. C., 72
Rifkin, J., 43
Riley, R. A., 251
Robinson, F., 38–39

Roemer, E., 257
Ross, R. R., 257
Rostogi, S., 123

Sabin, A., 43
Samenow, S., 253
Sampson, E. E., 20
Sampson, R. J., 249
Sandel, M. J., 7
Sati ritual, 72–73
Saul, A., 105
Schmitt, E. L., 247
Schneider, K. J., 258
Scholte, J. A., 106
Schwarzenneger, Arnold, 250
Schwinger, T., 6–7
Scientific Enlightenment, 11
Scott, L., 39
Scottish Centre for Crime and Justice Research, 244
Sears, D. O., 98
Self-hatred, 104
Sen, Amartya, 38, 178
Serious mental illness (SMI), 245–46, 259
SES. *See* Socioeconomic status
Sex, 159, 164; characterization of, 156; offenders, 247–48; third, 157
Sexual assaults, 123, 138–39
Sexual orientation, 156–57, 167–68
Shalhoub-Kevorkian, N., 123
Shapiro, I., 11
Shermis, S. S., 52–53
Shiva, A., 258
Shiva, V., 108
Shrader McMillan, A., 120
Sign (Zeiche), 86
Silko, Leslie Marmon, 142
Simoni, J. M., 138
Sirigu, A., 44
Skeem, J. L., 254–55
Slife, B. D., 72
SMI. *See* Serious mental illness
Smith, Laura, 51–52
Smith, Linda T., 143
Smith, R., 75–76
Smith, D., 43
Snider, N., 42
Social class: characterization of, 224–26; perspective on, 226–27
Social comparison: deprivation and, 106; false consciousness and, 105–6; theory, 108
Social identity: awareness models and false consciousness, 102–4; stage-models of, 103–4; theory, 105, 108–9
Social interactions, 17
Socialism: conservatism and, 10–11, 21n7; distributive justice and, 5–7, 21n4; state, 93; tradition of, 5–7
Socialization, theory of, 87
Social justice: characterization of, 21n2, 33–34, 53–54; concepts of, 10, 21n7, 33–34, 68–69; dimensions of, 34–37; emotions and, 42–43; empathy and, 43–44; empowerment and, 44; false consciousness and, 18, 22n12; global, 38–39; history of, 3–20; human development and, 37–38; ideology, 51–52; information in, 44–45; integration of, 33–34; issues of LGBTQI, 160–69; moral exclusion and, 42; objective and subjective, 17–20, 21n10; orientation, 52–53; psychology and, 39–41, 51–52, 55–56; relationships and, 45–46; as social construction, 41–42; study of, 18; theory development of, 3–4, 21n2, 52–54; truncated subjectivism in, 20; work, 6, 73–74
Social Justice and Ethics Social Group, 53–54
Social learning theories, 258–59
Social movements, 102–4

Social psychological theories: development of, 52–54; equity theory as, 11–13; principles of equality and need as, 13–14, 21nn8–9
Social Security, 195–96, 210–11
Social structure, 34
Social systems, 3–4
Society: individualism and, 67–68; just, 39–40; open, 108; understanding, 66
Society for Humanistic Psychology, 59
Socioeconomic status (SES), 40, 196–97, 227
South African Government of Reconciliation, 36
Southern Poverty Law Center, 165
Soviet Union, 81
Spain, 92
Spartacus, 75
Speight, S. L., 54, 56
Spinaris, C., 260–61
Spivak, G. C., 73
Sprecher, S., 12
Stake, J. E., 124
Star, S. A., 106
State of Florida Correctional Medical Authority, 209
Steele, H., 94n2
Steele, M., 94n2
Stereotype: distrust of, 90; internalization of African Americans, 104; object relations theory and, 84–85, 94n2; one-sided, 84
Stoner, M., 158
Storytelling: approaches, 143–44; healing through, 141–43
Storytelling for Social Justice: Connecting Narratives and the Arts in Antiracist Teaching (Bell), 144
Stouffer, S. A., 106
Suchman, E. A., 106
Sue, D. W., 140
Sugarman, J., 68
Suicides, 73, 139, 161, 260–61
Survivance, 149n3
Symbols, 84
System justification theory, 105; false consciousness and, 100–101; low-status groups and, 100–101

Tan, E., 229
Taymans, J., 257
Teaching Tolerance Project, 165
Tejeda, W. V., 121
Tennant, A., 257
Terrorism, 94
Tetlock, P. E., 10, 15
Thibaut, J., 15–16, 34–35
Thinking for a Change (Bush, Glick, and Taymans), 257
Thompson, C. E., 52–53
TMP. *See* Traditional medical practitioners
Toch, H., 249
Todd, N. R., 40
Toporek, R. L., 226
Torre, M. E., 121
Toynbee, A. J., 3–4, 17
Traditional medical practitioners (TMP), 234
Transgender National Discrimination Survey, 169
Transhumanism, 212–13
Trauma: historical, 139–40; response of American Indian/Native Alaskan, 139–40
Trestman, R. L., 245
Tropp, R. L., 106
Tyler, T. R., 17

UCD. *See* University College Dublin
United Nations (U.N.), 183, 225–26; Childrens' Fund, 229; Committee against Torture, 162; Convention on the Rights of Persons with Disabilities, 180; Declaration of

Indigenous Rights of Indigenous People, 146–47; General Assembly, 180; International Covenant on Civil and Political Rights, 159; International Covenant on Economic, Social and Cultural Rights, 159, 166; International Rights of the Child, 41; Millennium Development Goals, 33–34; organizations within, 169–70; Special Rapporteur, 159, 161; Universal Declaration of Human Rights, 33–34, 38, 41, 159
United States (U.S.), 203, 211, 228, 243–45, 261–62; Constitution, 146; governmental policies of, 136–38, 149nn1–2; immigration, 43; social groups in, 103; Supreme Court, 164
University College Dublin (UCD), 124
Unnever, J. D., 37
U.S. *See* United States
Utilitarianism: act and rule, 21n5; theory of, 7–8, 21n5

Values: imposition of, 56–57, 107; promotion of, 54; of Whites, 99
Vasquez, M., 54
Vasquez, M. J. T., 40
Vera, E. M., 54, 56
Vico, G., 66
Victim Offender Mediation (VOM), 36
Victim Offender Reconciliation Program (VORP), 36
Violence, 122; domestic, 138; epistemological, 73–74; of hip-hop lyrics, 43–44; issue of, 74–75; against LGBTQI, 156–57, 160–63; sexual assaults as, 123, 138–39; women and, 123
Voice: dissenting, 58; effect, 16
VOM. *See* Victim Offender Mediation
VORP. *See* Victim Offender Reconciliation Program

Walker, L., 15–16, 34–35
Walster, E. G., 12
Walster, G. W., 12
Walters, K. L., 138
Walters, Karina, 140
Warren, C., 255
Wealth: distribution of, 15; white-collar crimes and, 242
Weiner, R., 246
Weisenfeld, B., 16
Welfare Warriors Research Collaborative, 122
Westernization, 106–8, 234
Weyman, N., 158
What Works Model, 257
White, A., 123
White-collar: crimes and wealth, 242; criminals, 250–53
Whites, 99
WHO. *See* World Health Organization
Wilkinson, Charles, 146
Wilkinson, S., 116
Williams, C. R., 37
Williams, R. M., 106
Williams, Raymond, 86–87
Wilson, J. O., 251
Wolf, R., 255
A Woman Doing Life: Notes from a Prison for Women (George), 259
Women, 124, 163, 198–200, 202, 206, 232–33; death and, 73; discrimination and oppression of, 123; feminism and, 103; migrant, 123; Muslim, 123; rape and, 122; sexual assaults of, 123; violence and, 123
Women's Studies Outreach Programme, 124
Woodson, Carter, G., 97, 98–100, 103
Woolf, L. M., 42
Worker: conditions, 85–86; older, 198–200; relations, 85

Working class, 225
Workplace: discriminations, 168–69; organization of, 85
World Bank, 232
World Health Organization (WHO), 167, 177–78, 233
World-system context, 80–82
Wright, C. S., 106
Wright, K. N., 2

Yoder, K., 140
Young, M. C., 249
Yunus, Mohammad, 44

Zagefka, H., 106, 109
Zapatista movement, 147
Zeiche. *See* Sign
Žižek, S., 67
Zweig, M., 225

About the Editors and Contributors

ABOUT THE EDITORS

JEANNETTE DIAZ, PhD is an assistant professor of psychology at the University of West Georgia. Dr. Diaz's scholarship focuses on globalization, social justice, and community-based approaches to mental health with an emphasis on critical and humanistic approaches to praxis. She is involved as a community psychologist both in her local community, where she is engaged in asset-based approaches to community development, and in Haiti where she is assisting in the establishment of a community-based mental health program.

ZENO FRANCO, PhD, is assistant professor of community engagement at the Medical College of Wisconsin (MCW) in the Department of Family and Community Medicine's Center for Healthy Communities and Research. He is also faculty in MCW's NIH-supported Clinical and Translational Science Institute Community Engagement group. His research focuses on improving mental health and community resilience outcomes in collaboration with veteran, Hispanic, and African American–serving organizations in the city of Milwaukee. Dr. Franco's recent publications include "Heroism: A Conceptual Analysis and Differentiation between Heroic Action and Altruism"—in *Review of General Psychology*; "The Dirty Dozen: Twelve Key Failures of the Hurricane Katrina Response & How Psychology Can Help"—in *American Psychologist*; and "Community Engagement for Translational Disaster Research: Fostering Public, Private & Responder Group Partnerships"—in the *Proceedings of the Ninth International Conference on Information Systems for Crisis Response and Management.*

HARRIS L. FRIEDMAN, PhD, is a Florida-licensed psychologist specializing in clinical psychology and organizational development/consulting. He recently retired as research professor of psychology at University of Florida, where he remains on the courtesy faculty, and he is also professor emeritus at Saybrook University. He has over 200 professional publications, mainly in the areas of clinical and organizational psychology, as well as research methodology, and he has special interest in transpersonal psychology. He is a fellow of the American Psychological

Association, and serves as senior editor of the *International Journal of Transpersonal Studies* and associate editor of *The Humanistic Psychologist*.

CHAD V. JOHNSON, PhD, is an associate professor of human relations, clinical assistant professor of psychiatry, and a project director in the Center of Applied Research for Nonprofit Organizations at the University of Oklahoma. His scholarship and clinical interests include spirituality and psychology, social justice, group psychotherapy, and humanistic/existential/transpersonal studies. He has conducted community-based participatory research projects with several organizations and community groups, such as Indian Health Care Resource Center of Tulsa, Oklahomans for Equality, the Oklahoma Center for Community and Justice, the YWCA, and the Johns Hope Franklin Center for Reconciliation. His scholarship and clinical work include social justice (e.g., LGBTQ rights, race relations), spirituality, and group psychotherapy. He serves on the editorial boards for *The Journal of Counseling Psychology* and *The International Journal for Transpersonal Psychology*. He is also a licensed psychologist and has a private psychotherapy practice in Tulsa, Oklahoma. Dr. Johnson holds a doctorate in counseling psychology from Pennsylvania State University.

BONNIE K. NASTASI, PhD, is an associate professor in the Department of Psychology at Tulane University. Dr. Nastasi's research focuses on the use of mixed methods designs to develop and evaluate culturally appropriate assessment and intervention approaches for promoting mental health and reducing health risks, such as sexually transmitted infections (STIs) and HIV, both within the United States and internationally. She has worked in Sri Lanka since 1995 on the development of school-based programs to promote psychological well-being and is currently directing a multicountry study of psychological well-being of children and adolescents with research partners in 12 countries. She has worked in India since 2001 as one of the principal investigators of an interdisciplinary public health research program to prevent STIs among married men and women living in the slums of Mumbai. She is active in promotion of child rights and social justice within the profession of school psychology, and is an associate of the International Institute of Child Rights & Development (IICRD), Centre for Global Studies, University of Victoria, British Columbia. She directed the development of a curriculum for training school psychologists internationally on child rights, *School Psychologist as Advocate for Child Rights*, a joint effort of International School Psychology Association, IICRD, and Tulane University's School Psychology Program. Her published works include the book, *School-Based Mental Health Services: Creating Comprehensive and Culturally Specific Programs*, published by the American Psychological Association in 2004. Dr. Nastasi is immediate past-president for Division 16 (School Psychology) of the American Psychological Association. She holds a doctorate in school psychology and early childhood education from Kent State University.

ABOUT THE CONTRIBUTORS

MONIKA ARDELT, PhD, is associate professor of sociology and a founding faculty member and member of the Advisory Committee of the Center for Spirituality and Health at the University of Florida. She is also a 1999 Brookdale National Fellow, a 2005 Positive Psychology Templeton Senior Fellow, and a fellow of the Gerontological Society of America. Her research focuses on successful human development across the life course with particular emphasis on the relations between wisdom, spirituality, aging well, and dying well.

TINA BLOOM, PhD, NCC, LPC, works as a psychological service specialist for the Pennsylvania Department of Corrections. Her doctorate is in clinical psychology from Walden University. Additionally, she has an MS in general psychology from University of Wisconsin, Madison, and an MS in physical education (exercise physiology) from Penn State, University Park. Her interests include attachment issues related to criminal behavior and emotional communication within and between species. In a previous career, she was a police and sport dog trainer.

WILLIAM E. CROSS JR., PhD, coordinates the higher education program within the College of Education, University of Denver. He holds professor emeritus status with the Social-Personality Program, The Graduate Center—CUNY.

NICOLAS CULP is a graduate student in clinical psychology at the Minnesota School of Professional Psychology.

WILLIAM R. EARNEST, PhD, works as a licensed psychologist in private practice in Tallahassee, Florida. He earned his doctorate in psychology at the University of Michigan in Ann Arbor. His website, addressing the use of psychoanalytic social psychology in critical social practice, is www.ideologystop.net.

MARY A. FUKUYAMA, PhD, is a licensed psychologist and clinical professor at the University of Florida Counseling & Wellness Center, where she has worked for the past 30 years counseling students, supervising interns, teaching, and writing on multicultural topics. She is a graduate in counseling psychology from Washington State University. Her current interests include spirituality and counseling, and international initiatives such as promoting study abroad programs. She is a fellow in Division 17 (Counseling Psychology) of the American Psychological Association.

ZHIPENG GAO is a PhD candidate at York University, Toronto, Canada, specialized in the theory and history of psychology with a social justice orientation. His major area of research focuses on epistemological and methodological issues in psychology; specifically, it addresses impacts of culture and power on researcher's interpretation, explanation, and ethics through dialogue, reflexivity, and discourse analysis. His secondary research area focuses on the history and theory of Chinese psychology.

DANIEL HOLLAND, PhD, MPH, is principal and director of the Neurobehavior Center of Minnesota and a core faculty member in the Clinical Psychology Program at Fielding Graduate University. His research has focused on disability issues across time and cultures. He has been a two-time Fulbright recipient, a fellow of the Solomon Asch Center for the Study of Ethnopolitical Conflict, a research scholar at the Woodrow Wilson International Center, a Mary E. Switzer Distinguished Fellow in Rehabilitation Research, and a Contemplative Practice Fellow with the American Council of Learned Societies. He is a graduate of Oberlin College and received his PhD in clinical psychology from Southern Illinois University.

DEIDRA HOLLAND, MSOT, EdD, is a pediatric occupational therapist in the public schools of St Paul, Minnesota. Her research, advocacy, and clinical work have focused on models for fostering optimal learning opportunities for students with disabilities in public school settings. She has a BA from the University of Washington, a master's in occupational therapy from Western Michigan University, and a doctorate in education from the University of Arkansas.

JOHN T. JOST (PhD, Yale University, 1995) is professor of psychology and politics at New York University and co-director of the Center for Social and Political Behavior. He has published over 120 journal articles and book chapters and four co-edited book volumes, including *Social and Psychological Bases of Ideology and System Justification* (Oxford, 2009). For this work, he has received the Gordon Allport Intergroup Relations Prize, Erik Erikson Award for Early Career Research Achievement in Political Psychology, International Society for Self and Identity Early Career Award, Society for Personality and Social Psychology Theoretical Innovation Prize, Society of Experimental Social Psychology Career Trajectory Award, and the Morton Deutsch Award for Distinguished Scholarly and Practical Contributions to Social Justice.

AARON C. KAY (PhD, Stanford University, 2005) is an associate professor of management and an associate professor of psychology and neuroscience at Duke University. He has published over 50 peer-reviewed articles on topics relevant to social justice. For this work, he has won early career awards from the American Psychological Society, the International Society of Justice Research, and the Society of Personality and Social Psychology.

TERESA D. LAFROMBOISE, PhD, is a professor of developmental and psychological sciences in the Graduate School of Education at Stanford University. She is a contributor to a number of American Indian mental health initiatives and author of prevention interventions for American Indian/Alaska Native youth resilience. Her scholarship and clinical work include suicide prevention, social emotional development, bicultural competence, and school-based mental health. She teaches courses in cultural psychology, racial and ethnic identity development, and psychology and American Indian/Alaska Native mental health. LaFromboise holds a doctoral degree in counseling psychology from the University of Oklahoma.

DANIELLE MACCARTNEY, PhD, is an associate professor of sociology, an International Human Rights Fellow, and the chair of the Women and Gender Studies program at Webster University in Saint Louis, Missouri. She conducts research on the effects of local, national, and international policies on women and sexual minorities and holds a doctorate in sociology from the University of California, Irvine.

GERALDINE MOANE, PhD, is a senior lecturer and director of the Higher Diploma in Psychology in the School of Psychology, and is also a teaching associate with the School of Social Justice at University College Dublin. She is a writer and activist for women and for LGBT rights. She holds PhD in psychology from the University of California at Berkeley.

VIRGIL MOOREHEAD, PsyD candidate, is a predoctoral clinical psychologist intern at the University of Michigan, and an enrolled member of Big Lagoon Rancheria. His scholarship and clinical work include social justice issues related to Native Americans. Mr. Moorehead holds a master's degree in marriage and family therapy from Sacramento State University and another master's degree in clinical psychology from the Wright Institute in Berkeley, California.

KRYSTAL M. PERKINS, PhD, is an assistant professor of psychology at the University of West Georgia. Her scholarship documents and explores how "devalued" members of society form, manage, and negotiate their identity in relation to other groups—dominant, Americans, immigrants, or politically subordinated—and the conditions under which critical or false consciousness can be documented. Perkins holds a doctorate in social/personality psychology from the City University of New York.

JONATHAN D. RASKIN, PhD, is a professor of psychology and counseling at the State University of New York at New Paltz. He is a licensed psychologist and fellow of the American Psychological Association. Dr. Raskin's scholarship focuses on constructivist counseling and psychotherapy, as well as on articulating and clarifying constructivist theories and their central role in human meaning-making. He holds a doctorate in counseling psychology from the University of Florida.

RIDDHI SANDIL, PhD, is a lecturer and Ed.M. program coordinator in the Department of Counseling and Clinical Psychology at Teachers College, Columbia University. She received her PhD in counseling psychology from University of

Iowa and is a licensed psychologist. Dr. Sandil was formerly the practicum coordinator and staff psychologist at the University of Utah Counseling Center and visiting assistant professor in the Department of Educational Psychology at the University of Utah. Her scholarly interests include counseling expectations of racial and ethnic minorities (in particular South Asian Women and South Asian sexual minorities), complex trauma and its impact on women's well-being and minority stress.

RAHA SHEIVARI is a second year MA student at York University (Keele campus), Toronto, Canada, specialized in the history and theory of psychology. Her research is focused on the impact of systemic economic inequalities on mental health. She investigates the adverse effects of socioeconomic injustice on psychosocial well-being.

TOD S. SLOAN, PhD, is professor in counseling psychology in the Lewis and Clark Graduate School of Education and Counseling. He earned his doctorate in psychology at the University of Michigan in Ann Arbor. He is the author of *Damaged Life: The Crisis of the Modern Psyche* (1996).

LAURA SMITH received her PhD in counseling psychology from Virginia Commonwealth University. Now an associate professor in the Department of Counseling and Clinical Psychology at Teachers College, Columbia University, Dr. Smith has previously worked in a variety of applied settings in New York City. She was formerly the director of Training of the APA-accredited predoctoral internship program at Pace University, the founding director of the Rosemary Furman Counseling Center at Barnard College, and the Director of Psychological Services at the West Farms Center, where she provided services, training, and programming within a multifaceted community-based organization in the Bronx. Dr. Smith's research interests include social class and poverty, the influence of classism on psychological theory and practice, the development of socially just practice models for psychologists at the community level, and participatory action research (PAR) in schools and communities.

LAURA STURM is a graduate student in clinical psychology at the Minnesota School of Professional Psychology.

THOMAS TEO, PhD, is professor in the History and Theory of Psychology Program at York University (Toronto), editor of *The Journal of Theoretical and Philosophical Psychology* and of *The Encyclopedia of Critical Psychology*. He has been analyzing the historical and theoretical foundations of the social sciences, the human sciences, and psychology, and he has been discussing the ontological, epistemological, and ethical-political challenges to these fields from a critical-psychological perspective.

KATHRYN M. WHITELEY, PhD, is an assistant professor in the Department of Sociology, Anthropology, and Criminal Justice at Messiah College of Pennsylvania. Her doctorate is from the Queensland University of Technology, Department of Law, School of Justice in Brisbane Queensland, Australia, and her scholarship focus is criminology, especially gender and crimes, such as violent crimes committed by women. She is a Pennsylvania Prison Society Official Visitor, specifically visiting women serving long sentences, such as those sentenced as juveniles to life without parole.

LINDA M. WOOLF, PhD, is a professor of psychology and international human rights at Webster University in Saint Louis, Missouri. She has researched and written extensively on topics such as human rights (LGBTI and women's rights), the Holocaust, genocide, hate groups, terrorism, torture, and peace psychology. Dr. Woolf is past-president of the Society for the Study of Peace, Conflict, and Violence (Peace Psychology—Division 48 of the American Psychological Association).